Statistical Symbol	Meaning
s^2	sample variance
z	z-score
ρ	Spearman rank-difference correlation coefficient (Greek letter rho)
r	Pearson product-moment correlation coefficient
r^2	coefficient of determination
H_0	null hypothesis
H_1	alternative hypothesis
df	degrees of freedom
n	number of scores in a group
k	number of independent groups
grand ΣX	sum of all scores in all groups
grand ΣX^2	sum of the square of all scores in all groups
SS_T	total sum of squares
SS_W	sum of squares within groups
SS_B	sum of squares between groups
MS_W	mean square for the sum of squares within groups
MS_B	mean square for the sum of squares between groups
F distribution	table value required to reject null hypothesis
$N - k$	degrees of freedom within groups
$k - 1$	degrees of freedom between groups

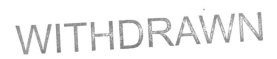

Measurement by the Physical Educator

Why and How

Fourth Edition

David K. Miller

University of North Carolina at Wilmington

Boston   Burr Ridge, IL   Dubuque, IA   Madison, WI   New York   San Francisco   St. Louis
Bangkok   Bogotá   Caracas   Kuala Lumpur   Lisbon   London   Madrid   Mexico City
Milan   Montreal   New Delhi   Santiago   Seoul   Singapore   Sydney   Taipei   Toronto

McGraw-Hill Higher Education

A Division of The McGraw-Hill Companies

MEASUREMENT BY THE PHYSICAL EDUCATOR: WHY AND HOW
FOURTH EDITION

Published by McGraw-Hill, a business unit of The McGraw-Hill Companies, Inc., 1221 Avenue of the Americas, New York, NY 10020. Copyright © 2002, 1998, 1994, 1988 by The McGraw-Hill Companies, Inc. No part of this publication may be reproduced or distributed in any form or by any means, or stored in a database or retrieval system, without the prior written consent of The McGraw-Hill Companies, Inc., including, but not limited to, in any network or other electronic storage or transmission, or broadcast for distance learning.

Some ancillaries, including electronic and print components, may not be available to customers outside the United States.

This book is printed on acid-free paper.

3 4 5 6 7 8 9 0 QPF/QPF 0 9 8 7 6 5 4 3 2

ISBN 0–07–232909–2

Vice president and editor-in-chief: *Thalia Dorwick*
Executive editor: *Vicki Malinee*
Developmental editor: *Lynda Huenefeld*
Senior marketing manager: *Pamela S. Cooper*
Project manager: *Mary E. Powers*
Production supervisor: *Sherry L. Kane*
Coordinator of freelance design: *Michelle D. Whitaker*
Cover/interior designer: *Rokusek Design*
Supplement producer: *Jodi K. Banowetz*
Media technology producer: *Judi David*
Compositor: *ElectraGraphics, Inc.*
Typeface: *10/12 Times Roman*
Printer: *Quebecor World Fairfield, PA*

Library of Congress Cataloging-in-Publication Data

Miller, David K. (David Keith)
    Measurement by the physical educator: why and how / David K. Miller.—4th ed.
      p. cm.
    Includes bibliographical references (p.) and index.
    ISBN 0–07–232909–2
    1. Physical fitness—Testing. 2. Physical fitness—Testing—Statistics. I. Title.

GV436 .M54 2002
613.7—dc21
                                       2001032711
                                               CIP

www.mhhe.com

To the students who have taught and continue to teach me so much.

CONTENTS

vi   Contents

PREFACE

Purpose and Content

Students in measurement and evaluation classes often are bombarded with an abundance of information. Regrettably, some students complete the class with a little knowledge in many areas but no confidence or skills to perform the procedures and techniques presented in the class. As professionals in school or nonschool settings, these same students often do not measure and assess knowledge, physical performance, and affective behavior in the proper way.

The purpose of this text is to help the physical education, exercise science, or kinesiology major develop the necessary confidence and skills to conduct measurement techniques properly and effectively. However, more than just measurement techniques are presented. Emphasis is placed upon the reasons for the measurement and how the results of the measurement should be used. These inclusions should help the student develop an appreciation of the need for measurement in a variety of settings. In addition, every effort has been made to present all the material in an uncomplicated way, and only practical measurement techniques are included.

Upon successful completion of the chapter objectives, the user of this text should be able to

1. Use and interpret fundamental statistical techniques;
2. Select appropriate knowledge and psychomotor tests;
3. Construct good psychomotor tests;
4. Construct good objective and subjective knowledge tests;
5. Objectively assess and grade students who participate in a physical education class;
6. Administer psychomotor and sports skills tests, interpret the results, and prescribe activities for the development of psychomotor and sports skills;
7. Administer body structure and composition tests, interpret the results, and prescribe scientifically sound methods for attainment of a healthy percent body fat;
8. Administer posture and body mechanics tests, interpret the results, and prescribe activities for the development of proper posture and body mechanics;
9. Administer psychomotor tests to special populations, interpret the results, and prescribe activities for the development of psychomotor skills; and
10. Administer affective behavior tests and interpret the results.

Audience

Until the 1980s, most undergraduate physical education majors planned to teach in grades K through 12. Today many majors in physical education, exercise science, kinesiology, and other similar subject areas anticipate a career in the nonschool environment. This book is designed for use by majors preparing for either environment—

school or nonschool. With the exception of grading skills, all of the competencies presented in this book will be expected of the physical educator in a variety of settings.

Organization

The text is organized so that the student will develop fundamental statistics skills early in the course (chapters 1–3). These skills are to be demonstrated throughout the text. Chapter 4, "What Is a Good Test," describes the criteria of a good test. Since these criteria and related terms are used throughout the text, it is recommended that this chapter be covered before the chapters that follow. Chapter 5, "Construction of Knowledge Tests," and chapter 6, "Assessing and Grading the Students," may be covered in the sequence presented or later in the course. It is recommended that chapter 7, "Construction and Administration of Psychomotor Tests," be presented before any discussion of psychomotor testing. The components of health-related fitness, skill-related fitness, and good posture (chapters 8–14) are described before the presentation of health-related and skill-related fitness tests (chapter 15, "Physical Fitness") so that the student will better understand these components. These chapters may be presented in a different sequence if the instructor wishes to do so. Functional fitness of the "Older Adult" is discussed in chapter 16. Chapter 17, "Special Populations"; chapter 18, "Sports Skills"; and chapter 19, "Affective Behavior," also may be presented in a different sequence by the instructor.

Approach

The statistics information is presented in a friendly and simplified manner so that it is nonintimidating. In addition, although the text information is sometimes presented in a "nuts-and-bolts" style, it is comprehensive as well as straightforward, accurate, and practical.

This book and related assignments can be completed without the use of a microcomputer, but the microcomputer can be applied in a variety of ways. College professors are not in agreement about the use of the computer in the teaching of fundamental statistics. Some professors advocate that the computer eliminates the need to understand certain statistical concepts (i.e., if the student knows the appropriate statistics to use, data can be entered into a computer and the correct answers produced). Other professors believe that the student should understand these concepts before using statistics software and the computer. Sometimes this means that the student should perform statistical procedures with pencil, paper, and a calculator. Either method, or both methods, can be used with this text.

Pedagogy

The following features of this book will assist the student in mastering the material:

- The text is readable and understandable.
- Specific objectives are stated at the beginning of each chapter.
- Key words are in bold print.
- Statistical procedures are provided in steps, or cookbook format, and examples related to physical education are provided.
- Reminders of chapter objectives are placed in the text in the form of "Are you able to do the following" questions.
- Review problems to reinforce the chapter objectives are provided at the conclusion of most chapters.

New to This Edition

The usual changes—updating of material and minor changes—are included in this edition. More significant changes and additions are as follows:

- A section on software available in chapter 1.
- Updated criterion-referenced standards in chapter 4.
- Expansion on the difference between the terms *assessment* and *evaluation* in chapter 6.
- Information on "Construction of Psychomotor Tests" and "Testing in the Psychomotor Domain" has been combined into one chapter (chapter 7).
- The PAR-Q & YOU questionnaire is now included in chapter 10.
- Information on the limitations of using height-weight tables in relation to body composition (chapter 13).

- New information on the FITNESSGRAM by the Cooper Institute for Aerobics Research in chapter 15.
- New information on the AAHPERD Health-Related Physical Fitness Test for College Students in chapter 15.
- New information on the ACSM Fitness Test in chapter 15.
- New information on the Canadian Physical Activity, Fitness and Lifestyle Appraisal: CSEPs Guide to Healthy Living—Health Related Fitness Appraisal in chapter 15.
- New information on the Amateur Athletic Union Physical Fitness Program in chapter 15.
- New chapter 16, "Older Adult," with information on functional fitness of the older adult.
- Information on the Brockport Physical Fitness Test in chapter 17.
- Additional exercises and examples throughout the chapters.
- New and updated tables and figures throughout the text.

Acknowledgments

I am grateful to the many students and colleagues who contributed to the development of the four editions of this text. The production of this text is possible because of your support. I also am thankful to the publishers who permitted use of their materials. To Lynda Huenefeld, and Mary Powers, and all other McGraw-Hill Higher Education staff members who contributed to the development of this edition, I say thanks for your patience, thoughtfulness, and guidance. It truly was a pleasure to work with you.

Second, Third, and Fourth Edition Reviewers

Dr. Chester "Chet" Sample
Sul Ross State University

Dr. Susan E. King
University of Kansas

Dr. William Russell
Catawba College

Dr. Layne Jorgensen
The University of Texas

Dr. Rebecca Brown
Keene State College

Dr. Steve Mitchell
Kent State University–Main Campus

Shirley Houzer
Alabama A & M University

Carol Haussermann
Dana College

Ann Sebren
Idaho State University

Michael J. Fratzke
Indiana Wesleyan University

John Dagger
UIC School of Kinesiology

Dr. Pat Floyd
Alabama State University

R. E. Stadulis
Kent State University

Robert O. Ruhling
George Mason University

Willie Lee Taylor
Greensboro College

Dr. Max Dobson
Oklahoma Christian University

Susan E. King
University of Kansas

Carol E. Plimpton
University of Toledo

Arthur W. Miller
University of Montana

Jim Helmer
Southwestern College

Charles Finke
Concordia University

1

Measurement, Evaluation, Assessment, and Statistics

Upon completion of this chapter, you should be able to

1. Define the term *statistics;*

2. Define the terms *test, measurement, evaluation,* and *assessment,* and give examples of each;

3. List and describe the reasons for measurement, evaluation, and

assessment by the physical educator; and

4. State why the ability to use statistics is important for the physical educator.

"Why statistics? I don't need statistics to be a good teacher." "I don't need statistics. I plan to work in a health fitness center."

Perhaps you have made comments similar to these or have heard some of your classmates make them. If you do not plan to perform your responsibilities as they should be performed, and you do not plan to continue your professional growth as a physical educator, you are correct in believing that you do not need statistics. However, if you want to be the best physical educator you can possibly be, the study of statistics should be included in your professional preparation.

Statistics involves the collection, organization, and analysis of numerical data. Statistical methods require the use of symbols, terminology, and techniques that may be new to you, but you should not fear these methods. The idea that statistics is a form of higher mathematics is incorrect. To successfully perform the statistics presented in this book, you need only a basic knowledge of arithmetic and some simple algebra. The most complex formula in statistics can be reduced to a series of logical

steps involving adding, subtracting, multiplying, and dividing. If you are willing to study the statistical concepts and perform the provided exercises, you will master the statistics presented to you.

Before finding an answer to "Why statistics?" you should understand the meaning of measurement and evaluation and the reasons for measurement by the physical educator. Measurement is not a new concept to you. You measured your height and weight throughout your growing years. You have read how fast athletes have run, how high some have jumped, and how far a baseball or a golf ball has been hit. All of these are examples of measurement. When you assume a position as a physical educator, you will perform measurement tasks. On many occasions this measurement will be administered in the form of a test, resulting in a score. For our purposes, a **test** is an instrument or a tool used to make a particular measurement. The tool may be written, oral, mechanical, or another variation. Examples of these tests are cardiorespiratory fitness tests, flexibility tests, and sports skills tests. On other occasions measurement may not involve a performance by a person but will consist of the measurement of a particular attribute. Anthropometric and body fat measurements are such examples. You should recognize that in all of the preceding examples, a number, or numbers, is obtained. So we can say that **measurement** is usually thought of as quantitative; it is the process of assigning a number to a performance or an attribute of a person. Sometimes when you measure, the score is a term or a phrase, but usually measurement will involve the use of numbers. Of course, objects are measured too, but as a physical educator you will be concerned primarily with people.

Once you have completed the measurement of a particular attribute of an individual, you must give meaning to it. For instance, if you administer a cardiorespiratory fitness test to participants of an adult fitness group, they will immediately want to know the status of their cardiorespiratory fitness. Without an interpretation of the quality of the test scores, the test has no meaning to the group. If you perform skinfold measurements in a physical education class, on athletes, or on members of a health club, the individuals will want to know what the sum of the measurements means in relation to body fat; otherwise, the measurements will have no meaning. The same can be said for written tests. There must be an interpretation of the test scores if they are to have meaning. This interpretation of measurement is **evaluation:** that is, a judgment about the measurement. For measurement to be effective, it must be followed by evaluation.

It is at this point that some physical educators stop. They measure an attribute, interpret the results to individuals, and go no further. They fail to use the results of their measurement and evaluation to identify performance and behavior problems and to prescribe how the problems can be corrected. This process—measure, evaluate, identify, and prescribe—is referred to as **assessment.** Let's again use the example of skinfold measurements. Assume that several individuals in the group that you measure are diagnosed as overfat as a result of your measurements. You should attempt to determine the eating and activity habits of the individuals and prescribe the proper diet and exercise program. The teaching of a skill involves the same approach. Through various methods, data are gathered about the skill level of the individuals, the data are interpreted, a diagnosis is made of any learning problems, and a prescription for correction of the learning problems is made. Assessment will be discussed again in a later chapter.

?ARE YOU ABLE TO DO THE FOLLOWING:

- define the term *statistics?*
- define the terms *test, measurement, evaluation,* and *assessment,* and give examples of measurement, evaluation, and assessment?

Reasons for Measurement, Evaluation, and Assessment by the Physical Educator

Now that you know what is meant by the terms *measurement, evaluation,* and *assessment,* let's look at ways you will use them in your profession.

Motivation

If used correctly, measurement can highly motivate most individuals. In anticipation of a test, students usually study the material or practice the physical tasks that are to be measured. This study or practice should improve performance. Skinfold measures might encourage overfat individuals in health fitness programs to lose body fat. A sports skills test administered to inform individuals of their ability in the sport might motivate them to improve their skills. This motivation is more likely to occur, however, if you as the instructor provide positive feedback. Always try to keep your evaluation and assessment positive rather than negative.

Finally, most everyone enjoys comparing past performances with current ones. Knowing that a second measurement will take place, students and adults often work to improve on the original score.

Diagnosis

Through measurement you can assess the weaknesses (needs) and strengths of a group or individuals. Measurement before the teaching of a sports skill, physical fitness session, or other events you teach as a physical educator may cause you to alter your initial approach to what you are teaching. For example, you may discover that, before you do anything else in a softball class, you need to teach the students how to throw properly. You also may find that some individuals need more or less attention than others in the group. Identifying those students who can throw with accuracy and good form will enable you to devote more time to the students who cannot perform the skill. If you serve as an adult fitness leader, the identification of individuals with a higher level of fitness than the rest of the group will enable you to begin their program at a different level.

In certain settings, you may be able to prescribe personal exercises or programs to correct the diagnosed weaknesses. Exercise prescription is a popular term in fitness programs, but appropriate activities may be prescribed in other programs as well. Diagnostic measurement is valuable also after a group has participated in a class for several weeks. If some students are not progressing as you feel they should, testing may help you determine why they are not.

Classification

There may be occasions when you would like to classify students into similar groups for ease of instruction. In addition, individuals usually feel more comfortable when performing with others of similar skill. Sometimes, even in so-called noncontact sports, homogeneous grouping should be done for safety reasons. Also, homogeneous grouping is occasionally necessary in aerobic and fitness classes so that individuals with a low level of fitness will not attempt to perform at the same intensity as individuals with a high level of fitness.

Achievement

The most common reason for measurement and assessment is to determine the degree of achievement of program objectives and personal goals. Students certainly like to know how far they have progressed in a given period of time, and you need to know their achievement to better evaluate the effectiveness of your instruction. Individuals in wellness programs want to know the progress toward their health goals, and measurement can often best provide this information.

Achievement often is used to determine grades in physical education. If administered properly, performance tests and knowledge tests are appropriate for grad-

ing, and they serve to decrease the need of subjective grading of the students. Many physical education teachers, however, mistakenly use tests only for determining grades. The assigning of grades will be discussed at length in chapter 6.

Evaluation of Instruction and Programs

With any responsibility you assume as a physical educator, occasionally you will have to justify the effectiveness of your instruction or program to your employer. For instance, when budget cuts are anticipated in the public schools, physical education and the arts are often the first programs considered for elimination. It also is necessary to justify a program when budget increases are requested. Furthermore, school accreditation studies require assessment of instruction and programs. If measurement and evaluation identify instructional or program problems, correctional procedures are stated. Standardized forms are available for program evaluation, but if program content is professionally sound, the success and effectiveness of instruction and programs are best determined by how well the participants fulfill program objectives. This statement is true for school programs, fitness and wellness programs, and all other professional programs in which you may have responsibilities. You must be able to measure and assess instruction and programs.

Assessment of each student's skill at the beginning of an activity unit helps you determine the effectiveness of previous instruction and programs and at what point you should begin your instruction. If the students do not know basic rules and cannot demonstrate the elementary playing skills of an activity, it will be necessary to begin instruction at that level. In addition, there may be times when you want to compare different methods of teaching sports skills or fitness. If you can be confident that the different groups are of equal initial ability, it is possible to compare the results of test scores at the conclusion of instruction and determine if one method of teaching is better than another. This procedure will be discussed in greater detail in chapter 3.

Prediction

Measurement to predict future performance in sport has increased in popularity, but this type of testing usually requires expertise in exercise physiology and psychology.

Maximum oxygen uptake, muscle biopsies, and anxiety level are examples of tests that are used to predict future performance in sport.

Research

Research is used to find meaningful solutions to problems and as a means to expand a body of knowledge. It is of value for program evaluation, instructor evaluation, and improvement in performance, as well as other areas related to physical education. Many opportunities exist for physical educators who wish to perform research.

Now that you are aware of the primary reasons for measurement, evaluation, and assessment in physical education, you are ready to answer the question "Why statistics?"

?ARE YOU ABLE TO DO THE FOLLOWING:

- list and describe the reasons for measurement, evaluation, and assessment by the physical educator?

Why Statistics?

Whether you teach, instruct in a fitness center, administrate, or have responsibilities in a corporate setting, the ability to use statistics will be of value to you. Although no attempt will be made in this book to provide an extensive coverage of statistics, after you have completed chapters 2 and 3, you should have the skill to do the following.

Analyze and Interpret Data

The data gathered for any of the measurement reasons described should be statistically analyzed and interpreted. It is a mistake to gather data and make important decisions about individuals without this analysis. Decisions regarding improvement in group performance and differences in teaching methodology should not be made without statistical analysis. Also, if you are willing to sta-

tistically analyze and interpret test scores, you can better inform all participants of the test results than you can with a routine analysis of the scores. So, using statistical analysis and interpretation, you can provide a more meaningful evaluation of your measurement.

Interpret Research

As a physical educator you should read research published in professional journals. After completion of this book you will not understand all statistical concepts, but you will understand enough to accurately interpret the results and conclusions of many studies. This ability will enable you to put into practice the conclusions of research. Too many physical educators fail to use research findings because they do not understand them. If you are to continue your professional growth, it is essential that you be able to interpret research related to physical education.

Standardized Test Scores

Many measurements performed by the physical educator will be in different units; for example, feet, seconds, and numbers. To compare such measurements, it is best to convert the scores to standardized scores. A popular form of standardized scores is percentile scores (as reported SAT scores).

Determine the Worth (Validity and Reliability) of a Test

Validity and reliability of a test may not mean much to you now, but by knowing how to interpret statements about these characteristics, you are more likely to select the appropriate test to administer to your students, clients, or customers. In addition, you will be able to estimate the validity and reliability of tests that you construct.

?ARE YOU ABLE TO DO THE FOLLOWING:

- state why the ability to use statistics is important to the physical educator?

---

2 Describing and Presenting a Distribution of Scores

Upon completion of this chapter, you should be able to

1. Define all statistical terms that are presented;

2. Describe the four scales of measurement, and give examples of each;

3. Describe a normal distribution and four curves for distributions that are not normal;

4. Define the terms *measures of central tendency* and *measures of variability;*

5. Define the three measures of central tendency; identify the symbols used to represent them; describe their characteristics; calculate them with ungrouped and grouped data; and state how they can be used to interpret data;

6. Define the four measures of variability; identify the symbols used to represent them; describe their characteristics; calculate them with ungrouped and grouped data; and state how they can be used to interpret data;

7. Define *percentile* and *percentile rank;* identify the symbols used to represent them; calculate them with ungrouped and grouped data; and state how they can be used to interpret data;

8. Describe a histogram and a frequency polygon; and

9. Define standard scores; calculate z-scores and T-scores, and interpret their meanings.

Regardless of your employment site, as a physical educator you often will test individuals. You may test for health fitness, sport fitness or skills, subject knowledge, or other areas. After the administration of a test, you will be expected to analyze the test scores and present your analysis to the test takers. The analysis of a set of test scores is referred to as descriptive statistics.

Statistical Terms

Before you begin to develop the skills to use descriptive statistics, become familiar with the following terms. Understanding these terms will be valuable to you in chapter 3 also.

Data. The result of measurement is called data. The term *data* usually means the numerical result of measurement but can also mean verbal information.

Variable. A variable is a trait or characteristic of something that can assume more than one value. Examples of variables are cardiovascular endurance, percent body fat, flexibility, and muscular strength. Their values will vary from one person to another, and they may not always be the same for one individual.

Population. A population includes all subjects (members) within a defined group. All subjects of the group have some measurable or observable characteristic. For example, if you wanted to determine the physical fitness of twelfth-grade students in a particular high school, the population would be all students in the twelfth grade.

Sample. A sample is a part or subgroup of the population from which the measurements are actually obtained. Rather than collect physical fitness data on all students in the twelfth grade, you could choose a smaller number to represent the population.

Random Sample. A random sample is one in which every subject in the population has an equal chance of being included in the sample. A sample could be formed by randomly selecting a group to represent all twelfth graders. The selection could be done by placing the names of all twelfth-grade students in a container and randomly drawing the names out of it or by using a table of random numbers.

Parameter. A parameter is a value, a measurable characteristic, that refers to a population. The population mean (the average) is a parameter.

Statistic. A statistic is a value, a measurable characteristic, that refers to a sample. The sample mean is a statistic. Statistics are used to estimate the parameters of a defined population. (*Note:* When used in this manner the word *statistics* is plural. If used to denote a subject or a body of knowledge, the word *statistics* is singular.)

Descriptive Statistics. When every member of a group is measured and no attempt is made to generalize to a larger group, the methods used to describe the group are called descriptive statistics. Conclusions are reached only about the group being studied.

Inferential Statistics. When a random sample is measured and projections or generalizations are made about a larger group, inferential statistics

are used. The correct use of inferential statistics permits you to use the data generated from a sample to make inferences about the entire population. Suppose you were in charge of a physical fitness program at a wellness center and wanted to estimate the physical fitness of all three hundred female adults in the program. You could randomly select thirty of the females, test them, and through the use of inferential statistics, estimate the physical fitness of the three hundred females.

Discrete Data. Discrete data are measures that can have only separate values. The values are limited to certain numbers, usually whole numbers, and cannot be reported as fractions. Examples of discrete data are the sex of the individual, the number of team members, the number of shots made, and the number of hits in a softball game.

Continuous Data. Continuous data are measures that can have any value within a certain range. The values can be reported as fractions. Running and swimming events (time) and throwing events (distance) are examples of continuous data.

Ungrouped Data. Ungrouped data are measures not arranged in any meaningful manner. The raw scores as recorded are used for calculations.

Grouped Data. Grouped data are measures arranged in some meaningful manner to facilitate calculations.

?ARE YOU ABLE TO DO THE FOLLOWING:

- define statistical terms?

Scales of Measurement

Variables may be grouped into four categories of scales depending on the amount of information given by the data. Different rules apply at each scale of measurement, and each scale dictates certain types of statistical procedures. As measurement moves from the lowest to the highest scale, the result of measurement is closer to a pure measure of a count of quantity or amount. The lower the level of the data, the less information the data provide.

Nominal Scale

The **nominal scale** is the lowest and most elementary scale. It is used to identify and report the frequency of objects or persons. Names are given to the variables, and categories are exclusive of each other; no comparisons of the categories can be made, and each category is assumed to be as valuable as the others. Some nominal scales have only two categories, but others may have more. Positions on sports teams, level of education, and state of residence are examples of the nominal scale. Numbers may be used to represent the variables, but the numbers do not have numerical value or relationship. For example, 0 may be used to represent the male classification and 1 the female classification.

Ordinal Scale

The **ordinal scale** provides some information about the order or rank of the variables, but it does not indicate how much better one score is than another. No determination can be made of the relative differences from rank to rank. For example, the order of finish in a 10-kilometer race provides information about who is fastest, but it does not indicate how much faster the number 1 finisher is than the number 2 finisher, or any of the other runners. Examples of the ordinal

scale are the ranking of the tennis team members from best to worst, class rank in a high school graduating class, team standings in an athletic conference, body frames (large, medium, small), and body fat (lean, normal, overfat).

Interval Scale

An **interval scale** provides information about the order of the variables, using equal units of measurement. The distance between divisions of the scale is always the same, so it is possible to say how much better one number is than another. However, the interval scale has no true zero point. A good example of an interval scale is temperature. It is possible to say that 90°F is 10° warmer than 80°F and that 55°F is 10° warmer than 45°F, but it cannot be said that 90° is twice as hot as 45°. Since 0°F does not mean the complete absence of heat, there is no true zero point. Many measurements in physical education are in the interval scale. Surveys regarding sportsmanship and attitude toward physical activity are examples of the interval scale. In surveys of these types, a zero score does not mean that a person has absolutely no sportsmanship or no attitude toward activity.

Ratio Scale

A **ratio scale** possesses all the characteristics of the interval scale and has a true zero point. Examples of ratio scales are height, weight, time, and distance. Ten feet is

TABLE 2.1 Scales of Measurement

Scale	Characteristics	Examples
Nominal	Numbers represent categories. Numbers do not distinguish groups and do not reflect differences in magnitude.	Divisions by sex, race, or eye color
Ordinal	Numbers indicate rank order of measurements, but they do not indicate the magnitude of the interval between the measures.	Order of finish in races, grades for achievement
Interval	Numbers represent equal units between measurements. It is possible to say how much better one measure is than another, but there is no true zero point.	Temperature, year, IQ
Ratio	Numbers represent equal units between measurements, and there is an absolute zero point.	Height, weight, distance, time

Describing and Presenting a Distribution of Scores **7**

twice as long as 5 feet; 9 minutes is three times as long as 3 minutes; and 20 pounds is four times as heavy as 5 pounds. (Table 2.1 summarizes the major differences among these four scales of measurement.)

? ARE YOU ABLE TO DO THE FOLLOWING:

- define the four scales of measurement, and give examples of each?

Normal Distribution

Most of the statistical methods used in descriptive and inferential statistics are based on the assumptions that a distribution of scores is normal and that the distribution can be graphically represented by the normal (bell-shaped) curve as shown in figure 2.1. For example, the distribution of the college entrance test scores of all test takers nationally would be normal. The test scores for a particular high school or group of students, however, may not have a normal distribution. Individuals in the school or group may score exceptionally high or low, causing the curve to be skewed. This concept will be discussed later in the chapter. As they are on all graphic representations of frequency distributions, the score values are placed on the horizontal axis, and the frequency of each score is plotted with reference to the vertical axis. The two ends of the curve are symmetrical and represent the scores at the extremes of the distribution.

The normal distribution is theoretical and is based on the assumption that the distribution contains an infinite number of scores. You will not measure groups of infinite size, so you should not be surprised when distributions do not conform to the normal curve. If the distribution is based on a large number of scores, however, it will be close to normal distribution. You can have a large number of scores if you administer the same test to several groups or if you combine your test scores from several years of testing into one distribution. A normal distribution has the following characteristics:

1. A bell-shaped curve
2. Symmetrical distribution about the vertical axis of the curve; whatever happens on one side of the curve is mirrored on the other
3. Greatest number of scores found in the middle of the curve, with fewer and fewer found toward the ends of the curve

FIGURE 2.1 Normal curve.

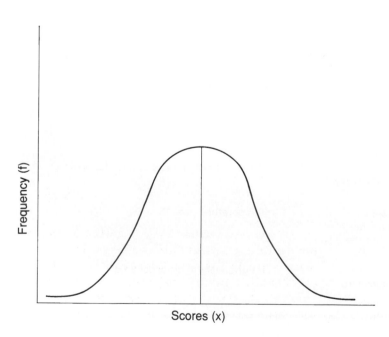

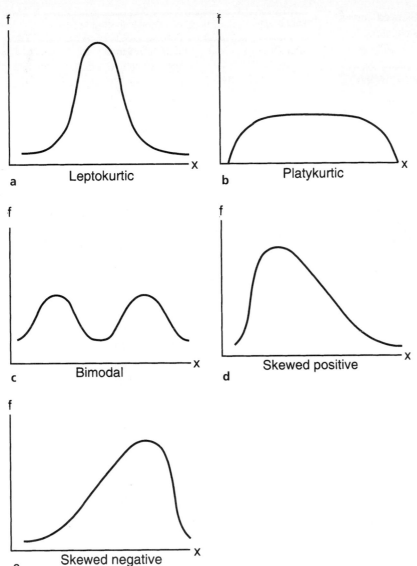

FIGURE 2.2 (a) Leptokurtic,
(b) platykurtic, (c) bimodal,
(d) positively skewed, and
(e) negatively skewed curves.

a Leptokurtic

b Platykurtic

c Bimodal

d Skewed positive

e Skewed negative

4. All measures of central tendency (mean, median, mode) at the vertical axis

Note: Distributions that are not close to normal have different curves, as shown in figure 2.2. The curve, called **leptokurtic,** for a very homogeneous group that has similar scores is pointed. The curve, called **platykurtic,** for a very heterogeneous group that has a wide distribution of different scores is flat. If a group of scores has two modes, the curve called **bimodal** has two high points. Some distributions of scores may have more than two modes, producing a curve with more than two high points. The curve in which the scores are clustered at one end is **skewed.** Skewed curves will be described in greater detail later in this chapter.

☝ARE YOU ABLE TO DO THE FOLLOWING:

- describe a normal distribution and four curves for distributions that are not normal?

Analysis of Ungrouped Data

Imagine that you have given a volleyball knowledge test to a group of 30 seventh-grade students, and you want to have a better understanding of the test results as well as interpret the scores to the students. With the aid of an inexpensive calculator, you can fulfill both of those objectives. This portion of the chapter shows you how to use descriptive statistics to analyze and interpret the volleyball knowledge test scores as well as other ungrouped data. A test with high scores has intentionally been selected as an example to demonstrate that the procedures are not difficult. Tables 2.2, 2.3, and 2.4 report the results of the volleyball knowledge test analysis.

Score Rank

Although you can perform statistical analysis without putting the scores in rank order, you may first want to carry out this procedure, which provides you with information about each person's rank in the score distribution. Be careful how you use the rank of scores. Sometimes, all the scores will be above what you consider a satisfactory score. Because someone has to be at the bottom when scores are ranked, you may not want to share this information with the group. Do not create alarm or embarrassment when there is no need. Table 2.2 has the ranking of the thirty volleyball knowledge test scores. The steps for ranking the scores are as follows:

1. List the scores in descending order.
2. Number the scores. The highest score is number 1, and the last score is the number of the total number of scores. (Table 2.2 has thirty scores, so the last score is number 30.)
3. Because identical scores should have the same rank, average the rank, or determine the midpoint, and assign them the same rank.

TABLE 2.2   Rank of Volleyball Knowledge Test Scores

Rank		Score
1		96
2		95
3		93
4	4.5	92
5		92
6		91
7	6.5	91
8		90
9	9	90
10		90
11		89
12	12	89
13		89
14		88
15		88
16	16	88
17		88
18		88
19		87
20	20	87
21		87
22		86
23	22.5	86
24		85
25	24.5	85
26		84
27	26.5	84
28		83
29		82
30		81

Measures of Central Tendency

Measures of central tendency are descriptive statistics that describe the middle characteristics of a distribution of scores. The most widely used statistics, they represent scores in a distribution around which other scores seem to center. Measures of central tendency are the mean, median, and mode.

The Mean. With any test, the first question usually asked by the students upon knowing their individual score is, "What is the class average?" The **mean,** the most generally used measure of central tendency, is the arithmetic average of a distribution of scores. It is calculated by summing all the scores and dividing by the total number of scores. The following are some important characteristics of the mean:

1. It is the most sensitive of all the measures of central tendency. It will always reflect any change within a distribution of scores.
2. It is the most appropriate measure of central tendency to use for ratio data and may be used on interval data.
3. It considers all information about the data and is used to perform other important statistical calculations.
4. It is influenced by extreme scores, especially if the distribution is small. For example, when one or more scores are high in relation to the other scores, the mean is pulled in that direction. This characteristic is the chief disadvantage of the mean.

The symbols used to calculate the mean and other statistics are as follows:

$\overline{X}$ = the mean (called X-bar)

Σ (Greek letter sigma) = "the sum of"

X = individual score

N = the total number of scores in a distribution

The formula for calculating the mean is

$$\overline{X} = \frac{\Sigma X}{N}$$

Simply, to calculate the mean, you add all the scores in a distribution and divide by the number of scores you have. The calculation of $\overline{X}$ from the distribution in table 2.3 is

$$\overline{X} = \frac{2644}{30} = 88.1$$

You probably would report the scores to the students in whole numbers, so you should round the mean to 88.

?ARE YOU ABLE TO DO THE FOLLOWING:

- define the term *measures of central tendency?*
- identify the symbol for the mean?
- define the mean?
- describe the characteristics of the mean?
- calculate the mean with ungrouped data and use it to interpret the data?

The Median. The **median** is the score that represents the exact middle in the distribution. It is the fiftieth percentile, the score that 50% of the scores are above and 50% of the scores are below. The following are some important characteristics of the median:

1. It is not affected by extreme scores; it is a more representative measure of central tendency than the mean when extreme scores are in the distribution. As an example of this fact, consider the height of five individuals. If the heights are 71", 72", 73", 74", and 75", the mean height of the five people is 73", and the median height is 73". Now imagine that we exchange the individual who is 75" in height for an individual who is 85" in height. The mean is now 75", but the median remains at 73".
2. It is a measure of position; it is determined by the number of scores and their rank order. It is appropriately used on ordinal or interval data.
3. It is not used for additional statistical calculations.

The median may be represented by Mdn or P_{50}. The steps for calculation of P_{50} are as follows:

1. Arrange the scores in ascending order.
2. Multiply N by .50 to find 50% of the distribution.
3. If the number of scores is odd, P_{50} is the middle score of the distribution.
4. If the number of scores is even, P_{50} is the arithmetic average of the two middle scores of the distribution.

The calculation of P_{50} from the distribution in table 2.3 is as follows:

TABLE 2.3 Measures of Central Tendency and Variability and Percentiles (Deciles) Computed from Ungrouped Volleyball Knowledge Test Scores (N = 30)

Score	X²	cf	Percentile
96	9216	30	
95	9025	29	
93	8649	28	
92	8464	27	90
92	8464	26	
91	8281	25	
91	8281	24	80
90	8100	23	
90	8100	22	
90	8100	21	70
89	7921	20	
89	7921	19	
89	7921	18	60
88	7744	17	
88	7744	16	
88	7744	15	50
88	7744	14	
88	7744	13	
87	7569	12	40
87	7569	11	
87	7569	10	
86	7396	9	30
86	7396	8	
85	7225	7	
85	7225	6	20
84	7056	5	
84	7056	4	
83	6889	3	10
82	6724	2	
81	6561	1	
ΣX = 2644	ΣX² = 233,398		

$R = 96 - 81 = 15$

$\overline{X} = \dfrac{\Sigma X}{N} = \dfrac{2644}{30} = 88.1 \qquad Q = \dfrac{Q_3 - Q_1}{2} = \dfrac{90 - 85.5}{2} = 2.25$

$P_{50} = 88 \qquad\qquad s = \sqrt{\dfrac{N\Sigma X^2 - (\Sigma X)^2}{N(N-1)}} = \sqrt{\dfrac{30(233,398) - (2644)^2}{30(30-1)}}$

$Mo = 88 \qquad\qquad s = 3.6$

1. $.50(30) = 15$
2. The fifteenth and sixteenth scores (middle scores of distribution) are 88.
3. $P_{50} = 88$

Because you will be using this same procedure to calculate any percentile, you may want to place a cumulative frequency (cf) column with the ascending listing of scores. The cumulative frequency is an accumulation of frequencies beginning with the bottom score. In the cf column the highest score will have the same number as N.

? ARE YOU ABLE TO DO THE FOLLOWING:

- identify the symbol for the median?
- define the median?
- describe the characteristics of the median?
- calculate the median with ungrouped data and use it to interpret the data?

The Mode. The **mode** is the score that occurs most frequently. In a normal distribution, the mode is representative of the middle scores. In some distributions, however, the mode may be an extreme score. If a distribution has two modes, it is bimodal, and it is possible for a distribution to be multimodal or to have no mode at all. Because no symbol is used to represent the mode, Mo is sometimes used. Some characteristics of the mode are as follows:

1. It is the least used measure of central tendency. It might be useful when estimating what sizes to order in equipment, such as helmets, caps, pants, or shirts. If you did not know how many of each size to order, you could order more of the most popular size.
2. It is not used for additional statistical calculations.
3. It is not affected by extreme scores, the total number of scores, or their distance from the center of the distribution.

The mode of the distribution in table 2.3 is 88.

? ARE YOU ABLE TO DO THE FOLLOWING:

- define the mode?
- describe the characteristics of the mode?
- calculate the mode with ungrouped data and use it to interpret the data?

Which Measure of Central Tendency Is Best for Interpretation of Test Results?

You have studied the definitions of the three measures of central tendency, calculation procedures, and some characteristics of each. Do you know which of the three is best for interpreting test results to any group that you might be testing? In making your decision, you should consider the following:

1. The mean, median, and mode are the same for a normal distribution (symmetrical curve), but you often will not have a normal curve.
2. The farther away from the mean and median the mode is, the less normal the distribution (i.e., the curve is skewed). Figure 2.3 shows the relationship of these measures to a symmetrical curve, a positively skewed curve, and a negatively skewed curve. In a positively skewed curve the scores are clustered at the lower end of the scale; the longer tail of the curve is to the right, and the mean is higher than the median. In a negatively skewed curve the scores are clustered at the upper end of the scale; the longer tail of the curve is to the left, and the mean is lower than the median. An extremely difficult test, on which most of the scores are low but a few high scores increase the mean, often results in a positively skewed curve. An easy test, on which most of the scores are high but a few low scores decrease the mean, usually results in a negatively skewed curve.
3. The mean and median are both useful measures. If the curve is badly skewed with extreme scores, you may want to use only the median. You must decide how important the extreme scores are. If the curve is approximately normal, use the mean and median.

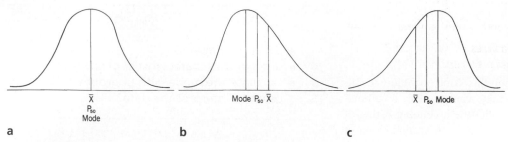

FIGURE 2.3   (a) Normal curve, (b) positively skewed curve, and (c) negatively skewed curve.

4. In most testing, the mean is the most reliable and useful measure of central tendency. It also is used in many other statistical procedures.

- use the three measures of central tendency to interpret test results to a group?

Measures of Variability

You now are prepared to use the mean, median, and mode to interpret data in relation to a central grouping of scores. However, to provide a more meaningful interpretation you also need to know how the scores spread, or scatter. For example, it is possible for two classes to have the same mean on a skills test, but the spread of the scores can be entirely different. To illustrate this point, consider the following two sets of scores:

Group A: 80, 82, 83, 84, 86 $\overline{X} = 83$
Group B: 65, 75, 90, 90, 95 $\overline{X} = 83$

Both groups have a mean of 83, but the spreads of the scores are very different. The spread, or scatter, of scores is referred to as **variability.** When groups of scores are compared, measures of variability should be considered as well as measures of central tendency. By knowing the measures of variability, you can determine the amount that the scores spread, or deviate, from the measures of central tendency. The measures of variability are the range, quartile deviation, mean deviation, and standard deviation.

The Range.   The **range** is determined by subtracting the lowest score from the highest score. It is the easiest measure of variability to compute, but because it represents only the extreme scores and provides no distribution information, it is also the least useful. Two groups of data may have the same range but have very different distributions. Consider the following scores:

Group A: 97, 95, 89, 87, 86, 85, 83, 80, 75, 72
Group B: 81, 77, 75, 73, 70, 68, 64, 61, 58, 56

Both groups have a range of 25, but the distributions are not similar. It is possible for you to have completely different distributions when you administer the same knowledge or physical performance test to different groups.

Some characteristics of the range are as follows:

1. It is dependent on the two extreme scores.
2. Because it indicates nothing about the variability of the scores between the two extreme scores, it is the least useful measure of variability.

The formula for determining the range (R) is

$$R = \text{High score} - \text{Low score}$$

You may see this formula also:

$$R = H_x - L_x$$

The range for the distribution in table 2.3 is R = 96 − 81 = 15.

- define the term *measures of variability?*
- identify the letter used to represent the range?
- define the range?
- describe the characteristics of the range?
- calculate the range with ungrouped data and use it to interpret the data?

The Quartile Deviation. Sometimes called the semi-quartile range, the **quartile deviation** is the spread of the middle 50% of the scores around the median. The quartile deviation is not reported often, but it is of value if the distribution is on the ordinal scale. The extreme scores will not affect the quartile deviation; thus, it is more stable than the range. Much like the other measures of variability, the quartile deviation is useful when comparing groups.

The following are some characteristics of the quartile deviation:

1. It uses the seventy-fifth percentile and twenty-fifth percentile to determine the deviation. The difference between these two percentiles is referred to as the interquartile range.
2. It indicates the amount that needs to be added to, and subtracted from, the median to include the middle 50% of the scores.
3. It usually is not used in additional statistical calculations. The symbols used to calculate the quartile deviation are
   Q = quartile deviation
   Q_1 = twenty-fifth percentile or first quartile (P_{25} may be used also) = score in which 25% of the scores are below and 75% of the scores are above
   Q_3 = seventy-fifth percentile, or third quartile (P_{75} may be used also) = score in which 75% of the scores are below and 25% of the scores are above

The steps for calculation of Q_3 are as follows:

1. Arrange the scores in ascending order.
2. Multiply N by .75 to find 75% of the distribution.

3. Count up from the bottom score to the number determined in step 2. Approximation and interpolation may be required to calculate Q_3 and Q_1 as well as other percentiles. Interpolation is necessary in the calculation of Q_1 from the distribution in table 2.3.

The steps for calculation of Q_1 are as follows:

1. Multiply N by .25 to find 25% of the distribution.
2. Again count up from the bottom score to the number determined in step 1.

To calculate Q, substitute the values in the formula

$$Q = \frac{Q_3 - Q_1}{2}$$

The calculation of Q from the distribution in table 2.3 is as follows:

1. .75(30) = 22.5
   The twenty-second score from the bottom is 90, and the twenty-third score is 90. Midway between these two scores would be the same score, so the score of 90 is at the 75%.
2. .25(30) = 7.5
   The seventh score from the bottom is 85, and the eighth score is 86. Since 7.5 is midway between these two scores, the score of 85.5 is at the 25%. Calculating the average of 85 and 86 would serve the same purpose.
3. $Q = \frac{90 - 85.5}{2} = \frac{4.5}{2} = 2.25$

Now what does 2.25 mean? Remember we said that the quartile deviation is used with the median. So now add 2.25 to 88 (the median in table 2.3) and subtract 2.25 from 88.

$$88 + 2.25 = 90.25$$
$$88 - 2.25 = 85.75$$

Theoretically, the middle 50% of the scores in the distribution should fall between the values 85.75 and 90.25. With thirty scores there should be fifteen scores between 85.75 and 90.25, but you will discover that sixteen scores fall between these two values. The difference is explained in the fact that the distribution in table 2.3 does not fulfill all requirements of normalcy. However, it is similar enough to use Q for interpretation purposes. Most of the test distributions you will use in your professional responsibilities will be similar enough to normalcy.

? ARE YOU ABLE TO DO THE FOLLOWING:

- identify the symbol for the quartile deviation?
- define the quartile deviation?
- describe the characteristics of the quartile deviation?
- calculate the quartile deviation with ungrouped data and use it to interpret the data?

The Mean Deviation. The **mean deviation,** sometimes called the average deviation, is another way to determine the variability of a distribution. To calculate the mean deviation, you must consider the deviation of each score from the mean of the distribution. A deviation is defined as the distance any score is from the mean of the distribution. This deviation score is represented by a small *d* or a small *x*.

The deviation score always has a plus or a minus sign. If the score is above the mean, a plus sign is used, and if the score is below the mean, a minus sign is used. In any distribution, the sum of the deviation scores from the mean is equal to zero. With a sum of zero, no average deviation can be found unless the procedure is changed. So, in determining the mean deviation, you ignore the plus and minus signs and simply sum all the deviations and divide by N. In a normal distribution, the scores between the range of the mean plus one mean deviation and the mean minus one mean deviation will include the middle 57.5% of the scores.

The following are some characteristics of the mean deviation:

1. It is a more meaningful measure of variability than the range and the quartile deviation because it considers all scores rather than just the two extreme scores or the seventy-fifth and twenty-fifth percentiles.
2. It indicates the value that needs to be added to and subtracted from the mean to include the middle

57.5% of the scores. It includes 7.5% more scores than does the quartile deviation.
3. Although it is usually not used to analyze data, it does form the basis of the standard deviation.

The following symbols are used to calculate the mean deviation:

$$MD = \text{mean deviation}$$
$$\Sigma = \text{sum of}$$
$$d \text{ or } x = \text{deviation score } (X - \overline{X})$$
$$X = \text{individual score}$$
$$\overline{X} = \text{mean}$$
$$N = \text{number of scores}$$

The formula used to calculate the mean deviation is

$$MD = \frac{\Sigma d}{N}$$

The steps for calculation of MD are as follows:

1. Arrange the scores into a series.
2. Determine d for each score.
3. Determine Σd.
4. Substitute values in the formula.

Table 2.4 includes the deviations of the volleyball knowledge test scores found in table 2.3. The calculation of MD from the distribution in table 2.4 is as follows:

1. $\Sigma d = 82.4$
2. $MD = \dfrac{82.4}{30}$

   $= 2.74$

   $MD = 2.7$

To determine the middle 57.5% of the scores, you now add 2.7 to $\overline{X}$ and subtract 2.7 from $\overline{X}$.

$$\overline{X} + 2.7 = 88.1 + 2.7 = 90.8$$
$$\overline{X} - 2.7 = 88.1 - 2.7 = 85.4$$

If the distribution were normal, the middle 57.5% of the scores would be between the values 85.4 and 90.8. Again, though the distribution is not normal, it is similar enough to use MD for interpretation of the scores.

TABLE 2.4 Mean Deviation and Standard Deviation Computed from Volleyball Knowledge Test Scores, Deviations, and Squared Deviations (N = 30)

Score	d	d²	Score	d	d²
96	7.9	62.41	88	−0.1	0.01
95	6.9	47.61	88	−0.1	0.01
93	4.9	24.01	87	−1.1	1.21
92	3.9	15.21	87	−1.1	1.21
92	3.9	15.21	87	−1.1	1.21
91	2.9	8.41	86	−2.1	4.41
91	2.9	8.41	86	−2.1	4.41
90	1.9	3.61	85	−3.1	9.61
90	1.9	3.61	85	−3.1	9.61
90	1.9	3.61	84	−4.1	16.81
89	0.9	0.81	84	−4.1	16.81
89	0.9	0.81	83	−5.1	26.01
89	0.9	0.81	82	−6.1	37.21
88	−0.1	0.01	81	−7.1	50.41
88	−0.1	0.01	Σx = 2644	Σd = 82.4	Σd² = 373.50
88	−0.1	0.01			

$\overline{X} = 88.1$

$$MD = \frac{\Sigma d}{N} = \frac{82.4}{30} = 2.7$$

$$s = \sqrt{\frac{\Sigma d^2}{N-1}} = \sqrt{\frac{373.5}{29}} = 3.6$$

❓ARE YOU ABLE TO DO THE FOLLOWING:

- identify the symbol for the mean deviation?
- define the mean deviation?
- describe the characteristics of the mean deviation?

- calculate the mean deviation with ungrouped data and use it to interpret data?

The Standard Deviation. The **standard deviation** is the most useful and sophisticated measure of variability.

It describes the scatter of scores around the mean. The standard deviation is a more stable measure of variability than the range or quartile deviation because it depends on the weight of each score in the distribution.

The lowercase Greek letter sigma (σ) is used to indicate the standard deviation of a population, and the letter *s* is used to indicate the standard deviation of a sample. Because you generally will be working with small groups (or samples), the formula for determining the standard deviation will include (N – 1) rather than N. This adjustment produces a standard deviation that is closer to the population standard deviation.

Some characteristics of the standard deviation are as follows:

1. It is the square root of the variance, which is the average of the squared deviations from the mean. The variance is used in other statistical procedures. The population variance is represented as σ^2 and the sample variance is represented as s^2.
2. It is applicable to interval and ratio level data, includes all scores, and is the most reliable measure of variability.
3. It is used with the mean. In a normal distribution, one standard deviation added to the mean and one standard deviation subtracted from the mean includes the middle 68.26% of the scores.
4. With most data, a relatively small standard deviation indicates that the group being tested has little variability; it has performed homogeneously. A relatively large standard deviation indicates the group has much variability; it has performed heterogeneously.
5. It is used to perform other statistical calculations. The standard deviation is especially important for comparing differences between means. Techniques for making these comparisons will be presented later in this chapter.

The symbols used to determine the standard deviation are as follows:

$$s = \text{standard deviation}$$
$$\overline{X} = \text{mean}$$
$$\Sigma = \text{sum of}$$
$$d = \text{deviation score } (X - \overline{X})$$

$$X = \text{individual score}$$
$$N = \text{number of scores}$$

Two methods for determining the standard deviation will be presented. The first method requires only the use of the individual scores and a calculator. The calculator should be able to compute the square root of a number, or you should be able to figure the square root by hand. An example of computing the square root by hand is provided in appendix A. The second method requires the use of the squared deviations. The two methods obtain the same results.

Calculation with ΣX^2

1. Arrange the scores into a series.
2. Find ΣX.
3. Square each of the scores and add to determine the ΣX^2.
4. Insert the values into the formula

$$s = \sqrt{\frac{N\Sigma X^2 - (\Sigma X)^2}{N(N-1)}}$$

The calculation of s from the distribution in table 2.3 is as follows:

1. Scores are in a series.
2. $\Sigma X = 2644$
3. $\Sigma X^2 = 233,398$

4. $$s = \sqrt{\frac{30(233,398) - (2644)^2}{30(30-1)}}$$
$$= \sqrt{\frac{7,001,940 - 6,990,736}{30(29)}}$$
$$= \sqrt{\frac{11,204}{870}}$$
$$= \sqrt{12.8781}$$
$$= 3.59$$
$$s = 3.6$$

Calculation with Σd^2

1. Arrange the scores into a series.
2. Calculate $\overline{X}$.
3. Determine d and d^2 for each score; then calculate Σd^2.

4. Insert the values into the formula

$$s = \sqrt{\frac{\Sigma d^2}{N-1}}$$

The calculation of s from the distribution in table 2.4 is as follows:

1. Scores are in a series.
2. $\overline{X} = 88.1$
3. $\Sigma d^2 = 373.5$
4. $s = \sqrt{\dfrac{373.5}{30-1}}$

$= \sqrt{\dfrac{373.5}{29}}$ *Note:* The s value should be the

$= \sqrt{12.8793}$ same value as found in the ΣX^2 method, but owing to the rounding

$s = 3.6$ off of $\overline{X}$, there is a slight difference.

To determine the middle 68.26% of the scores, you now add 3.6 to $\overline{X}$ and subtract 3.6 from $\overline{X}$.

$$\overline{X} + 3.6 = 88.1 + 3.6 = 91.7$$
$$\overline{X} - 3.6 = 88.1 - 3.6 = 84.5$$

If the distribution were normal, the middle 68.26% of the scores would be between the values 84.5 and 91.7.

Because each score must be subtracted from the mean, and the mean is often not a whole number, this method can be time-consuming. However, if you have already calculated the mean deviation, much of the necessary work has been completed.

Relationship of Standard Deviation and Normal Curve

The use of the standard deviation has more meaning when it is related to the normal curve. On the basis of the probability of a normal distribution, there is an exact relationship between the standard deviation and the proportion of area and scores under the curve. The standard deviation marks off points along the base of the curve. An equal percentage of the curve will be found between the mean plus one standard deviation and the mean minus one standard deviation. The same is true for plus and minus 2.0 or 3.0 standard deviations.

The following observations can be made about the standard deviation and the areas under a normal curve:

1. 68.26% of the scores will fall between +1.0 and −1.0 standard deviations.
2. 95.44% of the scores will fall between +2.0 and −2.0 standard deviations.
3. 99.73% of the scores will fall between +3.0 and −3.0 standard deviations. Generally, scores will not exceed +3.0 and −3.0 standard deviations from the mean. Figure 2.4 shows these observations.

The relationship of the standard deviation and the normal curve provides you a meaningful and consistent way to compare the performance of different groups using the same test and to compare the performance of one individual with the group. In addition, by knowing the value of the mean and of the standard deviation, you can express the percentile rank of the scores. To illustrate how these procedures can be done, consider the following example.

As part of a physical fitness test, a fitness instructor administered a 60-second sit-up test to two fitness classes. She found the mean and the standard deviation for each class to be as follows:

Class 1 Class 2
$\overline{X} = 32$ $\overline{X} = 28$
$s = 2$ $s = 4$

Figure 2.5 compares the spread of the two distributions. You can see that Class 1 is a more homogeneous group.

Now consider individual A in class 1, who completed thirty-four sit-ups, and individual B in class 2, who also completed thirty-four sit-ups. Though the two individuals have the same score, figure 2.6 shows that they do not have the same relationship to their respective class means and standard deviations. Individual A is 1 standard deviation above the Class 1 mean, and individual B is 1.5 standard deviations above the Class 2 mean. Table 2.5 shows that +1 standard deviation above the mean includes approximately 84% of the curve and that +1.5 standard deviations above the mean include approximately 93% of the curve. Though the two scores are the same, they do not have the same percentile score.

The steps for calculating the percentile rank through use of the mean and the standard deviation are as follows.

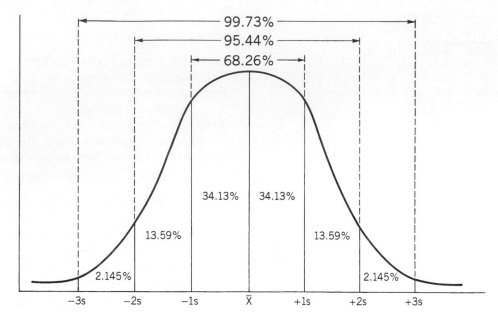

FIGURE 2.4 Characteristics of normal curve.

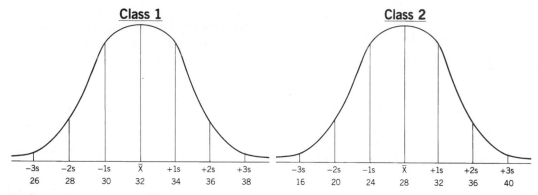

FIGURE 2.5 Comparison of $\overline{X}$ and s for sit-up test.

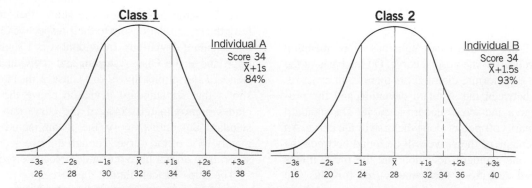

FIGURE 2.6 Comparison of individual performances for sit-up test.

TABLE 2.5 Percentile Scores Based on the Mean and Standard Deviation Units

X̄ and s Units	Percentile Rank	T-score	X̄ and s Units	Percentile Rank	T-score
X̄ + 3.0s	99.87	80	X̄ − 0.1s	46.02	49
X̄ + 2.9s	99.81	79	X̄ − 0.2s	42.07	48
X̄ + 2.8s	99.74	78	X̄ − 0.3s	38.21	47
X̄ + 2.7s	99.65	77	X̄ − 0.4s	34.46	46
X̄ + 2.6s	99.53	76	X̄ − 0.5s	30.85	45
X̄ + 2.5s	99.38	75	X̄ − 0.6s	27.43	44
X̄ + 2.4s	99.18	74	X̄ − 0.7s	24.20	43
X̄ + 2.3s	98.93	73	X̄ − 0.8s	21.19	42
X̄ + 2.2s	98.61	72	X̄ − 0.9s	18.41	41
X̄ + 2.1s	98.21	71	X̄ − 1.0s	15.87	40
X̄ + 2.0s	97.72	70	X̄ − 1.1s	13.57	39
X̄ + 1.9s	97.13	69	X̄ − 1.2s	11.51	38
X̄ + 1.8s	96.41	68	X̄ − 1.3s	9.68	37
X̄ + 1.7s	95.54	67	X̄ − 1.4s	8.08	36
X̄ + 1.6s	94.52	66	X̄ − 1.5s	6.68	35
X̄ + 1.5s	93.32	65	X̄ − 1.6s	5.48	34
X̄ + 1.4s	91.92	64	X̄ − 1.7s	4.46	33
X̄ + 1.3s	90.32	63	X̄ − 1.8s	3.59	32
X̄ + 1.2s	88.49	62	X̄ − 1.9s	2.87	31
X̄ + 1.1s	86.43	61	X̄ − 2.0s	2.28	30
X̄ + 1.0s	84.13	60	X̄ − 2.1s	1.79	29
X̄ + 0.9s	81.59	59	X̄ − 2.2s	1.39	28
X̄ + 0.8s	78.81	58	X̄ − 2.3s	1.07	27
X̄ + 0.7s	75.80	57	X̄ − 2.4s	0.82	26
X̄ + 0.6s	72.57	56	X̄ − 2.5s	0.62	25
X̄ + 0.5s	69.15	55	X̄ − 2.6s	0.47	24
X̄ + 0.4s	65.54	54	X̄ − 2.7s	0.35	23
X̄ + 0.3s	61.79	53	X̄ − 2.8s	0.26	22
X̄ + 0.2s	57.93	52	X̄ − 2.9s	0.19	21
X̄ + 0.1s	53.98	51	X̄ − 3.0s	0.13	20
X̄ + 0.0s	50.00	50			

1. Calculate the deviation of the score from the mean:

$$d = (X - \overline{X})$$

2. Calculate the number of standard deviation units the score is from the mean. Some textbooks refer to

these units as z-scores. The use and interpretation of z-scores are described on page 30.

$$\text{No. of standard deviation units from the mean} = \frac{d}{s}$$

Describing and Presenting a Distribution of Scores **21**

3. Use table 2.5 to determine where the percentile rank of the score is on the curve. On occasions it may be necessary to approximate the percentile rank. *Note:* If a negative value is found in step 1, the percentile rank will always be less than 50. If a positive value is found in step 1, the percentile rank will always be more than 50.

℘ARE YOU ABLE TO DO THE FOLLOWING:

- identify the symbol for the standard deviation?
- define the standard deviation?
- describe the characteristics of the standard deviation?
- calculate the standard deviation with ungrouped data and use it to interpret the data?
- describe the normal curve?

Which Measure of Variability Is Best for Interpretation of Test Results?

You have studied the definitions of the four measures of variability, how to calculate them, and some characteristics of each. In deciding which of the four is best for interpreting test results of a group you might be testing, you should consider the following:

1. The range is the least reliable of the four, but it is used when a fast method is needed.
2. The quartile deviation is more meaningful than the range, but it considers only the middle 50% of the scores.
3. The mean deviation considers every score but it is not mathematically sound (negative signs are ignored).
4. The standard deviation considers every score, is the most reliable, and is the most commonly used measure of variability.

℘ARE YOU ABLE TO DO THE FOLLOWING:

- properly use the four measures of variability to interpret test results to a group?

Percentiles and Percentile Ranks

Though you have learned to calculate percentiles and percentile rank, it will be beneficial to discuss them in greater detail. **Percentile** refers to a point in a distribution of scores below which a given percentage of the scores fall. For example, the sixtieth percentile is the point where 60% of the scores in a distribution are below and 40% of the scores are above. To calculate a percentile, you first multiply N by the desired percentage. You then determine the score that is at that percentile in a distribution. In table 2.3 (page 12), the sixtieth percentile score is 89.

The **percentile rank** of a given score in a distribution is the percentage of the total scores that fall below the given score. A percentile rank, then, indicates the position of a score in a distribution in percentage terms. Percentile ranks are determined by beginning with the raw scores and calculating the percentile ranks for the scores. In table 2.3, the score of 89 has a percentile rank of 60.

Although percentiles are of value for interpretation of data, they do have weaknesses. The relative distances between percentile scores are the same, but the relative distances between the observed scores are not. Because percentiles are based on the number of scores in a distribution rather than on the size of the raw score obtained, it is sometimes more difficult to increase a percentile score at the ends of the scale than in the middle. The average performers, whose raw scores are found in the middle of the scale, need only a small change in their raw scores to produce a large change in their percentile scores. However, the below-average and above-average performers, whose raw scores are found at the ends of the scale, need a large change in their raw scores to produce even a small change in their percentile scores. This weakness is usually found in all percentile scores.

If you do not remember how to calculate percentiles, you should refer to the sections on the median and quartile deviation. In table 2.3 the percentile scale is divided into deciles (ten equal parts). Deciles are represented as D_1 (tenth percentile), D_2 (twentieth percentile), D_3 (thirtieth percentile), on up to D_9 (ninetieth percentile).

℘ARE YOU ABLE TO DO THE FOLLOWING:

- identify the symbols for percentiles, quartiles, and deciles?

- define percentile and percentile rank?
- calculate percentiles and use them to interpret the data?

You now should be able to statistically analyze ungrouped data. Practice using that ability by completing the following review problems.

REVIEW PROBLEMS

1. Mrs. Block completed the volleyball unit with her 2 ninth-grade classes by administering the same volleyball skills test to both classes. One of the test items was the volleyball serve. Calculate the range, $\overline{X}$, P_{50}, mode, Q, MD, s, and deciles for the two groups of scores. Were the performances of the classes different in any way? Was one class more homogeneous?

   Class A
   42, 50, 57, 45, 56, 69, 45, 43, 46, 51, 61, 55, 40, 47, 59, 47, 46, 30, 48, 53, 40, 40, 64, 48, 41

   Class B
   51, 43, 43, 37, 33, 53, 44, 44, 38, 34, 37, 51, 20, 24, 39, 34, 38, 50, 10, 37, 39, 27, 25, 29, 23

2. Calculate the $\overline{X}$ and s for these 2-minute sit-up test scores:

   42, 41, 53, 60, 84, 49, 57, 65, 61, 48, 33, 57, 55, 50, 65, 54, 55, 57, 65, 45, 58, 54, 52, 40, 55

3. Given the following information, use the normal curve and determine the percentile rank for the three observed scores.

$$\overline{X} = 33$$
$$s = 2$$
$$X_1 = 36$$
$$X_2 = 29$$
$$X_3 = 32$$

Analysis of Grouped Data

The widespread availability of calculators and microcomputers has made the grouping of data less prevalent than it once was. However, you may have occasions when you want to analyze a large number of scores. Even with a calculator, it is difficult to work with the data unless they are arranged in a more convenient form.

A frequency distribution is one method for arranging the data in a more convenient form. Frequency distributions can be either simple or grouped. In a simple frequency distribution all scores are listed in descending order, and the number of times each individual score occurs is indicated in a frequency column. Table 2.6 shows a simple frequency distribution.

If the scores are spread over a wide range, however, a simple frequency distribution is long and bulky. There may be gaps in the range where no scores occur or so few scores fall at each score value that the group pattern is not very clear. In such instances, it is more convenient to represent the scores in a grouped frequency distribution rather than individually.

To help you understand the procedures for arranging data into a grouped frequency distribution, the following example will be used.

Mrs. Wren administered a tennis serve test to 3 tenth-grade physical education classes (N = 75) and grouped the scores into a frequency distribution for analysis purposes. The scores were as follows:

88 83 75 81 56 82 86 62 87 79 93 58 61 61 75
73 94 48 79 72 81 85 52 73 62 80 73 84 63 61
67 63 75 73 67 72 73 72 77 73 85 82 70 57 58
54 79 68 54 70 77 81 68 83 65 77 90 52 75 62
84 69 56 68 69 63 70 91 70 80 65 70 88 72 63

Table 2.7 shows the frequency distribution for the scores. Mrs. Wren used the following steps to construct the frequency distribution:

1. Determine the range.
   Note: Some textbooks define the range as the highest score minus the lowest score plus one, when grouping the scores. R for the table 2.7: 94 − 48 = 46
2. Determine the number of class intervals. The number of intervals depends on the number of

TABLE 2.6 Simple Frequency Distribution of Push-Up Scores

X	t	f
51	1	1
50	11	2
49	111	3
48	TH⅃	5
47	TH⅃ 1	6
46	TH⅃ 1	6
45	TH⅃ 1	6
44	TH⅃ 11	7
43	TH⅃ 11	7
42	TH⅃ 111	8
41	TH⅃ 111	8
40	TH⅃ TH⅃	10
39	TH⅃ 1111	9
38	TH⅃ 1	6
37	TH⅃ 1	6
36	TH⅃ 11	7
35	TH⅃	5
34	1111	4
33	1111	4
32	TH⅃	5
31	1111	4
30	11	2
29	11	2
28	1	1
27	1	1
		N = 125

scores, the range of the scores, and the purpose of organizing the frequency table. If a frequency table has too few intervals (fewer than ten), the frequency of scores in each interval may be quite large, making it difficult to observe the essential characteristics of the distribution. If too many intervals are included (more than twenty), several intervals may not contain any scores and too much work is required to complete the table. Generally it is best to have between ten and twenty intervals. Fifteen intervals is usually a good number of intervals.

Once the approximate number of intervals has been decided, the size of the class interval (i) must be determined. An estimate of i can be found by dividing the range of the scores by the number of intervals wanted. If the range of a distribution happens to be 54, i could be found as follows:

$$\frac{54}{15} = 3.6$$

It is easier to work with whole numbers, so we have the choice of using 3 or 4 for i. When i is smaller than 10, the numbers 2, 3, 5, 7, and 9 are usually used. Even numbers other than the number 2 may be used, however. The advantage of odd numbers is that the midpoint of the intervals will be a whole number, and it is often necessary to find the midpoint of intervals. When i is larger than 10, multiples of 5 (10, 15, 20, etc.) are generally used.

You also may determine the number of class intervals by dividing the range by what you feel would be an appropriate i. In the above example the procedure would be as follows:

$$\frac{54}{3} = 18 \text{ or } \frac{54}{5} = 11$$

The number of intervals may be 18 or 11, which of course means that i = 3 or 5 is acceptable.

Class intervals and i for table 2.7 could be found as follows:

$$\frac{46}{15} = 3.06$$

Note: With i = 3, there will be sixteen intervals.

TABLE 2.7 Frequency Distribution and Measures of Central Tendency and Variability for Tennis Serve Scores

Class Interval	t	f	cf	d	fd	fd²
93–95	11	2	75	7	14	98
90–92	11	2	73	6	12	72
87–89	111	3	71	5	15	75
84–86	ͳ̶ͳ̶ͳ̶1	5	68	4	20	80
81–83	ͳ̶ͳ̶ͳ̶1 11	7	63	3	21	63
78–80	ͳ̶ͳ̶ͳ̶1	5	56	2	10	20
75–77	ͳ̶ͳ̶ͳ̶1 11	7	51	1	7	7
72–74	ͳ̶ͳ̶ͳ̶1 ͳ̶ͳ̶ͳ̶1	10	44	0	0	0
69–71	ͳ̶ͳ̶ͳ̶1 11	7	34	−1	−7	7
66–68	ͳ̶ͳ̶ͳ̶1	5	27	−2	−10	20
63–65	ͳ̶ͳ̶ͳ̶1 1	6	22	−3	−18	54
60–62	ͳ̶ͳ̶ͳ̶1 1	6	16	−4	−24	96
57–59	111	3	10	−5	−15	75
54–56	1111	4	7	−6	−24	144
51–53	11	2	3	−7	−14	98
48–50	1	1	1	−8	−8	64
		N = 75			Σfd = −21	Σfd² = 973

$$R = 94 - 48 = 46$$

$$Mo = LL + 1/2(i) = 71.5 + 1/2(3) = 73$$

$$\overline{X} = AM + i\left(\frac{\Sigma fd}{N}\right) = 73 + 3\left(\frac{-21}{75}\right) = 72.16$$

$$P_{50} = LL + i\left(\frac{\%(N) - cf_b}{f_w}\right) = 71.5 + 3\left(\frac{.50(75) - 34}{10}\right) = 72.55$$

$$Q = \frac{Q_3 - Q_1}{2} = \frac{80.61 - 63.87}{2} = 8.37$$

$$s = i\sqrt{\frac{\Sigma fd^2}{N} - \left(\frac{\Sigma fd}{N}\right)^2} = 3\sqrt{\frac{973}{75} - \left(\frac{-21}{75}\right)^2} = 10.77$$

3. Determine the limits of the bottom class interval. A general practice is to begin the bottom interval with a number that is a multiple of the interval size. It is acceptable, however, to begin the bottom interval with the lowest score or to make the lowest score the midpoint of the interval.

   Bottom interval for table 2.7: 48 to 50

4. Construct the table. The remaining intervals are formed by increasing each interval by the size of i until an interval is reached that includes the highest score.

   Note: There is a difference in the "apparent limits" and "real limits" of the intervals. It can be observed in table 2.7 that there is a one-point gap between the end of one interval and the beginning of the next interval. This gap is avoided if the real limits of the bottom interval are 47.50 to 50.4999. The real limits of the next interval are 50.50 to 53.4999, and so forth.

5. Tally the scores. The scores are counted one at a time, and a tally mark is placed to the right of the appropriate interval.
6. Record the tallies under the column headed f (which stands for frequencies). Sum the frequencies ($\Sigma f = N$).

🔊 ARE YOU ABLE TO DO THE FOLLOWING:

- group scores into a frequency distribution?

Measures of Central Tendency

Observing table 2.7, you notice that columns other than the f column are included. These columns are used to calculate the measures of central tendency and variability. Because the definitions (with the exception of the mode), characteristics, and uses for these measures are the same as when they are calculated with ungrouped data, they will not be repeated.

The Mode. The mode for grouped data is defined as the midpoint of the interval that has the largest number of frequencies. The midpoint of an interval is calculated by adding one-half of i to the real lower limit of the interval. One symbol used in the formula for this calculation is new to you:

LL = real lower limit of interval with largest number of scores

The mode in table 2.7 is

$$Mo = LL \text{ of interval} + 1/2 \text{ (i)}$$
$$= 71.5 + 1/2 (3)$$
$$= 71.5 + 1.5$$
$$Mo = 73$$

The Mean. Two symbols used in the formula for calculation of the mean of grouped data are new to you:

AM = assumed mean; midpoint of the interval you assume the mean to be

Σfd = sum of $f \times d$

The steps for calculation of the mean are as follows:

1. Label a column d. In the interval in which you assume (guess) the mean is located, place a 0. If the distribution is approximately normal, the mean will be close to the middle of the distribution. Do not be concerned about guessing the correct interval because the value of the mean will be the same regardless of where you assume the mean.
2. Indicate the deviation of each interval from the assumed mean by numbering consecutively above and below the interval of the assumed mean. Positive values are above the mean, and negative values are below.
3. Label a column fd. Multiply f times d for each interval.

   Note: Be aware that you will have positive values above the interval of the assumed mean and negative values below.
4. Calculate Σfd.

   Note: Be aware that you are summing positive and negative numbers. The Σfd is a correction factor. A negative value for fd indicates that you have assumed the mean to be higher than it actually is, and a positive value for fd indicates the opposite.
5. Substitute the values in the formula

$$\overline{X} = AM + i\left(\frac{\Sigma fd}{N}\right)$$

The calculation of the mean from the distribution in table 2.7 (page 25) is

$$\overline{X} = 73 + 3\left(\frac{-21}{75}\right)$$
$$= 73 + 3(-.28)$$
$$= 73 - .84$$
$$\overline{X} = 72.16$$

The Median. The following symbols are used in the formula to calculate the median and other percentiles for grouped data:

LL = the real lower limit of the interval containing the percentile of interest

% = the percentile you wish to determine

cf_b = the cumulative frequency in the interval below the interval of interest

f_w = the frequency of scores in the interval of interest

The steps for calculation of the median are as follows:

1. Label a column cf and determine the cumulative frequency for each interval.
2. Multiply .50(N) and determine in which interval P_{50} is located.
3. Identify cf_b and f_w.
     Note: The cf_b value will not exceed the number found in step 2.
4. Substitute the values in the formula

$$P_{50} = LL + i\left(\frac{\%(N) - cf_b}{f_w}\right)$$

The calculation of the median from the distribution in table 2.7 is

$$.50(75) = 37.5$$

$$P_{50} = 71.5 + 3\left(\frac{37.5 - 34}{10}\right)$$

$$= 71.5 + 3\left(\frac{3.5}{10}\right)$$

$$= 71.5 + 3(.35)$$

$$= 71.5 + 1.05$$

$$P_{50} = 72.55$$

☝ ARE YOU ABLE TO DO THE FOLLOWING:

- calculate the measures of central tendency and percentiles with data grouped into a frequency distribution?

Measures of Variability

Calculation of the range for grouped data was described previously. Calculation of the quartile deviation and standard deviation will be covered now.

The Quartile Deviation. The formula for the quartile deviation is the same for grouped and ungrouped data, and the technique and formula for calculating Q_3, Q_1, and other percentiles are the same as described for calculation of the median.

The calculation of Q from the distribution in table 2.7 is

Q_3	Q_1
$.75(75) = 56.25$	$.25(75) = 18.75$

$$Q_3 = 80.5 + 3\left(\frac{56.25 - 56}{7}\right) \qquad Q_1 = 62.5 + 3\left(\frac{18.75 - 16}{6}\right)$$

$$= 80.5 + 3\left(\frac{.25}{7}\right) \qquad\qquad = 62.5 + 3\left(\frac{2.75}{6}\right)$$

$$= 80.5 + 3(.036) \qquad\qquad = 62.5 + 3(.458)$$

$$= 80.5 + .11 \qquad\qquad = 62.5 + 1.37$$

$$Q_3 = 80.61 \qquad\qquad Q_1 = 63.87$$

$$Q = \frac{Q_3 - Q_1}{2}$$

$$= \frac{80.61 - 63.87}{2}$$

$$= \frac{16.74}{2}$$

$$Q = 8.37$$

The Standard Deviation. One symbol used in the formula for calculation of the standard deviation for grouped data is new to you:

$$\Sigma fd^2 = \text{sum of } d \times fd$$

The steps for calculation of the standard deviation are as follows:

1. Label a column fd^2 and determine fd^2 for each interval.
     Note: You are to multiply $d \times fd$.
2. Calculate Σfd^2.
3. Substitute the values in the formula

$$s = i\sqrt{\frac{\Sigma fd^2}{N} - \left(\frac{\Sigma fd}{N}\right)^2}$$

The calculation of s in the distribution in table 2.7 is

$$s = 3\sqrt{\frac{973}{75} - \left(\frac{-21}{75}\right)^2}$$

$$= 3\sqrt{12.9733 - (.28)^2}$$

$$= 3\sqrt{12.9733 - .0784}$$

$$= 3\sqrt{12.8949}$$
$$= 3(3.59)$$
$$s = 10.77$$

- calculate the quartile deviation and standard deviation with data grouped into a frequency distribution?

To test your ability to group data into a frequency distribution and to calculate the measures of central tendency and variability, complete the following review problems.

REVIEW PROBLEMS

1. Mr. Bird administered a badminton clear test to sixty students. Group the scores into a frequency distribution and determine the range, mode, median, mean, quartile deviation, and standard deviation. The scores are as follows:

74 75 64 86 73 74 75 70 69 67
80 78 61 81 77 78 65 65 70 69
85 84 83 62 84 74 75 81 66 74
63 73 77 64 66 72 80 77 80 70
66 69 72 83 69 67 73 72 75 75
70 67 65 73 73 72 72 73 74 73

2. Dr. Grade administered a test to his two measurement and evaluation classes (N = 80). Group the scores and determine the mean, median, and standard deviation. The scores are as follows:

60 69 81 84 93 96
67 65 79 77 82 80
79 74 71 78 89 97
61 62 70 75 80 94
88 78 81 69 76 76
76 80 89 93 73 82

73 68 92 85 84 89
84 67 68 71 99 95
97 93 84 81 71 90
83 79 61 55 90 70
95 79 70 72 76 68
82 77 76 66 96 78
75 62 95 88 60 64
83 75

Graphs

Data are often presented in a graphic form. Well-prepared graphs enable individuals to interpret data without reading the raw data or tables. Computer programs include different types of graphs, but only the histogram and the frequency polygon will be described here. The following guidelines should be used when constructing these graphs:

1. The length of the vertical axis (Y), called the *ordinate,* is about two-thirds to three-fourths the length of the horizontal axis (X), called the *abscissa.*
2. The vertical axis begins with zero.
3. The score values are recorded from low to high, left to right.
4. A space of one-half to one column is left between the vertical axis and the first column and between the last column and the end of the horizontal axis.
5. The graph is given a title.

Histogram

A **histogram** is a bar graph in which the score frequencies are represented by a series of columns. The width of each column corresponds to the interval size, and the height of each column corresponds to the frequencies in each interval. The midpoint of each interval is in the middle of the column. Figure 2.7 is a histogram of the data in table 2.7 (page 25).

Frequency Polygon

A **frequency polygon** is a line graph in which the midpoints of the intervals are plotted at a point corresponding

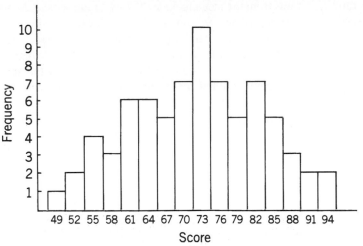

FIGURE 2.7 Histogram of tennis serve scores made by 75 students.

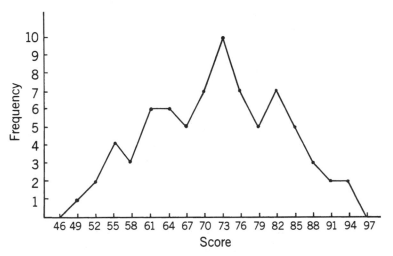

FIGURE 2.8 Frequency polygon of tennis serve scores made by 75 students.

to the frequency of the interval and connected with straight lines. At each end of the polygon, a line is drawn back to zero. Figure 2.8 is a frequency polygon of the data in table 2.7.

❓ARE YOU ABLE TO DO THE FOLLOWING:

- define histogram and frequency polygon and state when they may be used appropriately?

Standard Scores

After collecting scores for different performances, you may want to combine or compare scores, but, because the scores have no similarities, you cannot perform these functions. For example, suppose you are teaching a physical fitness unit to a high school class, and at the conclusion of the unit you administer a 2-minute sit-up test, the sit-and-reach test, a 2-mile run, and a physical fitness knowledge test. How do you average the scores of the four tests? You certainly cannot add the scores and divide by four. How do you compare a student's performance on

Describing and Presenting a Distribution of Scores **29**

the sit-up test with her performance on the 2-mile run? You cannot tell her that fifty-five sit-ups is a better score than a time of 15:10—unless you have a procedure to convert the raw scores into standard scores. Procedures to make such conversions follow.

z-Scores

A **z-score** represents the number of standard deviations a raw score deviates from the mean. After calculation of the mean and standard deviation of a distribution, it is possible to determine the z-score for any raw score in the distribution through the use of this formula:

$$z = \frac{X - \overline{X}}{s}$$

Consider the example of Mrs. Wren's tennis serve test described on page 23. If Mrs. Wren wanted to convert the tennis serve test scores into z-scores, she would substitute each individual score in the formula. For the scores of 88 and 54 the z-scores would be

$$z = \frac{88 - 72.2}{10.8} \qquad z = \frac{54 - 72.2}{10.8} \qquad \left(\overline{X} \text{ and s are rounded to one decimal place}\right)$$

$$= \frac{15.8}{10.8} \qquad = \frac{-18.2}{10.8}$$

$$z = 1.46 \qquad z = -1.69$$

How are these z-scores interpreted? The z-scale has a mean of 0 and a standard deviation of 1, and it normally extends from −3 to +3 (plus and minus 3 standard devia-

tions from the mean include 99.73% of the scores). In observing figure 2.9, you see that a z-score of 1.46 is approximately 1.5 standard deviations above the mean, and a z-score of −1.69 is more than 1.5 standard deviations below the mean. Knowing the relationship of the standard deviation and the normal curve, we can state that 1.46 is an excellent z-score and −1.69 is a poor z-score. Also, by referring to table 2.5 (page 21), we see that 1.5 standard deviations above the mean has a percentile rank of 93, and 1.7 deviations below the mean has a percentile rank of 4.

If Mrs. Wren had administered other tennis skills tests (e.g., forehand, backhand, and lob tests) with similar distributions, she could convert the scores to z-scores and average them for one tennis skill score. She also could compare each student's z-scores for the four tests and determine the strongest and weakest skills of each student.

All standard scores are based on the z-score. Because z-scores are expressed in small numbers, involve decimals, and may be positive or negative, many testers do not use them.

T-Scores

The **T-scale** has a mean of 50 and a standard deviation of 10. T-scores may extend from 0 to 100, but it is unlikely that any T-score would be beyond 20 or 80, since this range includes plus and minus 3 standard deviations. Figure 2.9 shows the relationship of z-scores, T-scores, and the normal curve. The z-score is part of the formula for conversion of raw scores into T-scores. The formula is

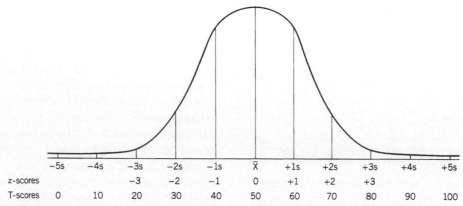

	−5s	−4s	−3s	−2s	−1s	X̄	+1s	+2s	+3s	+4s	+5s
z-scores			−3	−2	−1	0	+1	+2	+3		
T-scores	0	10	20	30	40	50	60	70	80	90	100

FIGURE 2.9 z-scores and T-scores plotted on a normal curve.

$$\text{T-score} = 50 + 10\left(\frac{(X - \overline{X})}{s}\right) = 50 + 10\,z$$

Again, consider the scores of 88 and 54 for Mrs. Wren's tennis serve test. The T-scores are

$$T_{88} = 50 + 10(1.46) \qquad T_{54} = 50 + 10(-1.69)$$
$$= 50 + 14.6 \qquad\qquad = 50 + (-16.9)$$
$$= 64.6 = 65 \qquad\qquad = 33.1 = 33$$

Note: T-scores are reported as whole numbers.

T-scores may be used in the same way as z-scores. However, because only positive whole numbers are reported and the range is 0 to 100, the T-scale is easier to interpret. However, it is sometimes confusing to the individuals being tested when they are told that a T-score of 60 or above is a good score. If you use T-scores, you should be prepared to fully explain their meanings. Table 2.5 (page 21) shows the relationship of the mean and standard deviation, percentile rank, and T-scores.

You may prefer to convert the raw scores in a distribution to T-scores through the following procedure:

1. Number a column of T-scores from 20 to 80.
2. Place the mean of the distribution of the scores opposite the T-score of 50.
3. Divide the standard deviation of the distribution by 10. The standard deviation for the T-scale is 10, so each T-score from 0 to 100 is one-tenth of the standard deviation.
4. Add the value found in step 3 to the mean and each subsequent number until you reach the T-score of 80.
5. Subtract the value found in step 3 from the mean and each decreasing number until you reach the number 20.
6. Round off the scores to the nearest whole number.

   Note: For some measurements, lower scores are better (e.g., timed events and heart rate). When you are working with such scores, you should subtract the t-values toward 80 and add the values toward 20. Table 2.8 shows the conversion of Mrs. Wren's tennis serve scores to T-scores. For illustration purposes, only the T-scores 40 to 60 are included in the table. The value found in dividing the standard deviation by 10 (1.077) is rounded to 1.1.

TABLE 2.8 Conversion of Tennis Serve Scores to T-Scores

T-score	Observed Score
60	83.2 = 83
59	82.1 = 82
58	81.0 = 81
57	79.9 = 80
56	78.8 = 79
55	77.7 = 78
54	76.6 = 77
53	75.5 = 76
52	74.4 = 74
51	73.3 = 73
50	72.2 = 72
49	71.1 = 71
48	70.0 = 70
47	68.9 = 69
46	67.8 = 68
45	66.7 = 67
44	65.6 = 66
43	64.5 = 65
42	63.4 = 63
41	62.3 = 62
40	61.2 = 61

$\overline{X} = 72.2$

$s = 10.77$

$$\frac{s}{10}\left(\begin{array}{l}\text{value added to and}\\\text{subtracted from }\overline{X}\end{array}\right) = \frac{10.77}{10} = 1.077 = 1.1$$

Percentiles

Percentile scores are also standard scores and may be used to compare scores of different measurements. Because they change at different rates (remember the comparison of low and high percentile scores with middle percentiles), they should not be averaged to determine one score for several different tests. For this reason, you may prefer to use the T-scale when converting raw scores to standard scores. The calculation of percentiles was previously described, so it will not be described here.

Describing and Presenting a Distribution of Scores   **31**

Statistics Software

Numerous statistics software programs—varying in cost, statistical procedures, computer requirements, and ease of use—may be purchased. In addition, student versions of many of these programs are available. Statistical Package for Social Science (SPSS), available with this text, is one such program. You should become familiar with a statistical software program during your college experience. Use of the microcomputer and statistics software will significantly reduce the time needed to perform statistical procedures, and you will feel more confident in the results of your work than if you performed the calculations yourself. The use of statistics software will be especially helpful in regard to the statistics presented in chapter 3. Another reason for developing the ability to use statistics software is that potential employers may expect you to have this skill.

Information about statistics programs is available in campus computing centers or bookstores and from computer software retailers. In addition, most statistics software producers have a Web home page.

ARE YOU ABLE TO DO THE FOLLOWING:

- describe the purposes of standard scores?
- convert raw scores into z-scores and T-scores and interpret them?

REVIEW PROBLEM

1. To test your ability to convert raw scores to standard scores, convert the scores in the review problems on page 28 to T-scores.

3

Investigating the Relationship of and Differences in Scores

Upon completion of this chapter, you should be able to

1. Define *correlation,* interpret the correlation coefficient, and use the rank-difference and product-moment methods to determine the relationship between two variables;

2. Construct a scattergram and interpret it;

3. Define and give examples of null hypothesis, degrees of freedom, level of significance, standard error of the mean, and standard error of the difference between means;

4. Define Type I and Type II errors;

5. Use and interpret the t-test for independent groups and the t-test for dependent groups;

6. Use and interpret analysis of variance for independent groups and analysis of variance for repeated measures; and

7. Use Tukey's honestly significant difference test (HSD).

In chapter 2, descriptive statistics were presented. Although it is important that you have the skills to use these statistics, your professional responsibilities will require that you be knowledgeable of other statistical procedures. You also should be able to demonstrate the relationship of scores and to determine if there is a significant difference in the means of different sets of scores. Skills in these procedures will enable you to better interpret professional literature and to conduct beneficial research.

Correlation

Correlation is a statistical technique used to express the relationship between two sets of scores (two variables). For example, is there a relationship between athletic participation and academic achievement? Do individuals with a high level of physical fitness earn higher academic grades? Is there a relationship between arm strength and golf driving distance? Is there a relationship between percent body fat and the ability to run 2 miles? Also, correlation techniques are used to determine the validity, reliability, and objectivity of tests. These techniques will be described in chapter 4.

The number that represents the correlation is called the **correlation coefficient.** Two techniques for determining the correlation coefficient will be presented here. Regardless of the technique used, correlation coefficients have several common characteristics. (Statements 2 and 3 are general statements; the size and significance of coefficient must be considered.)

1. The values of the coefficient will always range from +1.00 to −1.00. It is rare that the coefficients of +1.00, −1.00, and .00 are found, however.

2. A positive coefficient indicates direct relationship; for example, an individual who scores high on one variable is likely to score high on the second variable, and an individual who scores low on one variable is likely to score low on the second variable.

3. A negative coefficient indicates inverse relationship. The individual who scores low on one variable is likely to score high on the second variable, and the individual who scores high on the first variable is likely to score low on the second.

4. A correlation coefficient near .00 indicates no relationship. An individual who scores high or low on one variable may have any score on the second variable.

5. The number indicates the degree of *relationship,* and the sign indicates the type of relationship. The number +.88 indicates the same degree of relationship as the number −.88. The signs indicate that the directions of the relationship are different.

6. A correlation coefficient indicates relationship. After determining a correlation coefficient, you cannot infer that one variable causes something to happen to the other variable. If a high, positive correlation coefficient is found between participation in school sports and high academic grades, it cannot be said that participation in school sports causes a person to earn good grades. It can only be said that there is a high, positive relationship.

Scattergram

A **scattergram** is a graph used to illustrate the relationship between two variables. To prepare a scattergram, perform the following steps:

1. Determine the range for each variable.
2. Designate one variable as the X score and the other variable as the Y score.
3. Draw and label the axes. Represent the X scores on the horizontal axis and the Y scores on the vertical axis. Begin with the lower X scores at the left portion of the X axis and the lower Y scores at the lower portion of the Y axis.
4. Plot each pair of scores on the graph by placing a point at the intersection of the two scores.

Figure 3.1 is a scattergram of the relationship between isometric and isotonic strength scores.

The scattergram can indicate a positive relationship, a negative relationship, or a zero relationship. If a positive relationship exists, the points will tend to cluster along a

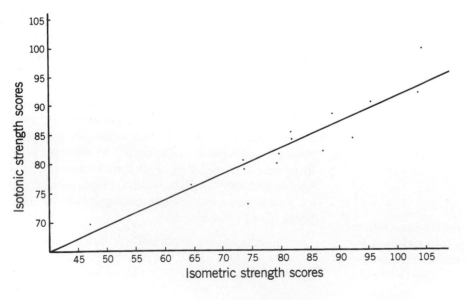

FIGURE 3.1 Scattergram of relationship between isometric and isotonic strength scores.

diagonal line that runs from the lower left-hand corner of the scattergram to the upper right-hand corner. In a negative relationship, the points tend to do the opposite; they move from the upper left-hand corner to the lower right-hand corner. With a positive or negative line, the closer the points cluster along the diagonal line, the higher the correlation. In a zero relationship the points are scattered throughout the scattergram. Figure 3.2 illustrates the three types of relationships.

Spearman Rank-Difference Correlation Coefficient

The **Spearman rank-difference correlation coefficient,** also called rank-order, is used when one or both variables are ranks or ordinal scales. The difference (D) between the ranks of the two sets of scores is used to determine the correlation coefficient. The following examples are relationships that could be determined through utilization of the rank-difference correlation coefficient:

- the ranking of participants in a badminton class and their order of finish in tournament play;
- the ability to serve well and the order of finish in a tennis tournament; and
- vertical jump scores and speed in the 100-meter run.

Of course, many other relationships can be determined with the rank-difference correlation coefficient.

The symbol for the rank-difference coefficient is the Greek rho (ρ) or $r_{\rho\eta o}$. To determine ρ, perform the following steps:

1. List each set of scores in a column.
2. Rank the two sets of scores.

Note: This procedure was described for you earlier in the chapter.
3. Place the appropriate rank beside each score.
4. Head a column D and determine the difference in rank for each pair of scores.

Note: The sum of the D column should always be 0. If it is not, check your work.
5. Square each number in the D column and sum the values (ΣD^2).
6. Calculate the correlation coefficient by substituting the values in the formula

$$\rho = 1.00 - \frac{6(\Sigma D^2)}{N(N^2 - 1)}$$

Table 3.1 illustrates the calculation of the rank-difference correlation coefficient for sit-up and push-up scores.

Pearson Product-Moment Correlation Coefficient

The **Pearson product-moment correlation coefficient,** also called Pearson r, is used when measurement results are reported in interval or ratio scale scores. The Spearman correlation coefficient actually is a Pearson r computed on the ranks. The Pearson r gives a more precise estimate of relationship because the actual scores, rather than the ranks of the scores, are taken into account. (This popular correlation coefficient has many variations, but only one method will be described.) The symbol for the product-moment correlation coefficient is r.

Observed scores are used with this calculation method of the product-moment correlation coefficient. The steps for calculation are as follows:

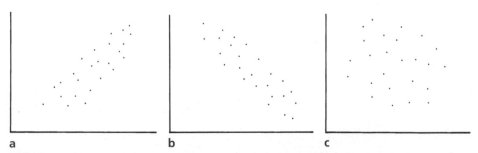

a   b   c

FIGURE 3.2   Scattergrams showing (a) positive, (b) negative, and (c) zero correlation between two variables.

TABLE 3.1   Rank-Difference Correlation Coefficient for Sit-Up and Push-Up Scores

Student	Sit-Up Score	Rank of S-U Score	Push-Up Score	Rank of P-U Score	D	D²
A	28	19.5	19	18.0	1.5	2.25
B	31	16.5	22	15.5	1.0	1.00
C	32	13.5	25	11.0	2.5	6.25
D	35	7.0	23	13.5	−6.5	42.25
E	32	13.5	27	8.5	5.0	25.00
F	40	1.0	35	1.0	0.0	0.00
G	33	10.0	29	4.5	5.5	30.25
H	35	7.0	28	6.5	0.5	0.25
I	32	13.5	26	10.0	3.5	12.25
J	36	4.5	29	4.5	0.0	0.00
K	35	7.0	31	3.0	4.0	16.00
L	31	16.5	33	2.0	14.5	210.25
M	36	4.5	24	12.0	−7.5	56.25
N	30	18.0	21	17.0	1.00	1.00
O	37	2.5	18	19.0	−16.5	272.25
P	37	2.5	27	8.5	−6.0	36.00
Q	33	10.0	22	15.5	−5.5	30.25
R	28	19.5	17	20.0	−0.5	0.25
S	32	13.5	28	6.5	7.0	49.00
T	33	10.0	23	13.5	−3.5	12.25

$$\Sigma D^2 = 803.00$$

$N = 20$

$$\rho = 1.00 - \frac{6(\Sigma D^2)}{N(N^2 - 1)}$$

$$= 1.00 - \frac{6(803)}{20(400 - 1)}$$

$$= 1.00 - \frac{4818}{7980}$$

$$= 1.00 - .60$$

$$\rho = .40$$

1. Label columns for name, X, X², Y, Y², and XY.
2. Designate one set of scores as X, designate the other set as Y, and place the appropriate paired scores by the individual's name.
3. Find the sums of the X and Y columns (ΣX and ΣY).
4. Square each X score, place squared scores in the X² column, and find the sum of the column (ΣX^2).

5. Square each Y score, place squared scores in the Y² column, and find the sum of the column (ΣY^2).
6. Multiply each X score by the Y score, place the product in the XY column, and find the sum of the column (ΣXY).
7. Substitute the values in the formula

TABLE 3.2 Product-Moment Correlation Coefficient for Isometric and Isotonic Strength Scores

Name	Isometric Score X	X²	Isotonic Score Y	Y²	XY
A	63	3969	76	5776	4788
B	78	6084	80	6400	6240
C	46	2116	70	4900	3220
D	103	10609	102	10404	10506
E	74	5476	73	5329	5402
F	82	6724	87	7569	7134
G	95	9025	92	8464	8740
H	103	10609	93	8649	9579
I	87	7569	83	6889	7221
J	73	5329	79	6241	5767
K	78	6084	82	6724	6396
L	89	7921	90	8100	8010
M	82	6724	85	7225	6970
N	73	5329	81	6561	5913
O	92	8464	85	7225	7820
	1218	102032	1258	106456	103706

$N = 15$

$$r = \frac{N(\Sigma XY) - (\Sigma X)(\Sigma Y)}{\sqrt{N(\Sigma X^2) - (\Sigma X)^2}\sqrt{N(\Sigma Y^2) - (\Sigma Y)^2}}$$

$$= \frac{15(103706) - (1218)(1258)}{\sqrt{15(102032) - (1218)^2}\sqrt{15(106456) - (1258)^2}}$$

$$= \frac{1555590 - 1532244}{\sqrt{1530480 - 1483524}\sqrt{1596840 - 1582564}}$$

$$= \frac{23346}{\sqrt{46956}\sqrt{14276}}$$

$$= \frac{23346}{(216.69)(119.48)}$$

$$= \frac{23346}{25890.12}$$

$r = .90$

$$r = \frac{N(\Sigma XY) - (\Sigma X)(\Sigma Y)}{\sqrt{N(\Sigma X^2) - (\Sigma X)^2}\sqrt{N(\Sigma Y^2) - (\Sigma Y)^2}}$$

Table 3.2 illustrates the calculation of the Pearson product-moment correlation coefficient for isometric and isotonic strength scores.

Interpretation of the Correlation Coefficient

After calculating the correlation coefficient, you must interpret it. This interpretation should be done with caution. For example, a correlation of .70 may be considered quite high in one analysis, but low in another. Also, in your interpretation of the coefficient, you must remember that a high correlation does not indicate that one variable causes something to happen to another variable. Correlation is about the *relationship* of variables. The purpose for which the correlation coefficient is computed must be considered when making a decision about how high or low a coefficient is. Keeping the purpose of the correlation study in mind, use the following ranges as general guidelines for interpretation of the correlation coefficient. Note that negative values are considered in the same manner.

r = below .20 (extremely low relationship)

r = .20 to .39 (low relationship)

r = .40 to .59 (moderate relationship)

r = .60 to .79 (high relationship)

r = .80 to 1.00 (very high relationship)

Significance of the Correlation Coefficient

Your interpretation of a correlation coefficient should not be limited to the general interpretation described above. The **statistical significance,** or reliability, of the correlation coefficient should be considered also. In determining the coefficient significance, you are answering the following question: If the study were repeated, what is the probability of obtaining a similar relationship? You want to be sure that the relationship is real and did not result from a chance occurrence.

When r is calculated, the number of pairs of scores is important. With a small number of paired scores, it is possible that a high r value can occur by chance. For this reason, when a small number of paired scores is recorded, the r value must be large to be significant. On the other hand, if the number of scores is large, it is less likely that a high r value will occur by chance. Thus, a small r can be significant with a large number of paired scores.

A table of values is used to determine the statistical significance of a correlation coefficient. (In this discussion, .05 and .01 levels of significance and degrees of freedom are used. These terms will be explained in greater detail in the discussion of t-tests later in this chapter.) Before using the values table, you must first calculate the degrees of freedom (df) for the paired scores. The degrees of freedom equal N – 2 (N is the number of paired scores). In the calculation of r for isometric and isotonic strength scores in table 3.2, the degrees of free-

dom equal N – 2 = 15 – 2 = 13. To determine the statistical significance of r = .90, we will use the values in appendix B. Find the number 13 in the degrees of freedom column in appendix B. You see that a correlation of .514 is required for significance at the .05 level and .641 at the .01 level. These numbers indicate that, for 13 degrees of freedom, a correlation as high as .514 occurs only 5 in 100 times by chance, and a correlation as high as .641 occurs only 1 in 100 times by chance. Because the r value of .90 in table 3.2 is greater than both of these values, we conclude that the correlation is significant at the .01 level.

In summary, the obtained r is compared with the appropriate table values. If the obtained r is larger than the values found at the .05 and .01 level, r is significant at the .01 level. If the obtained r falls between these two table values, r is significant at the .05 level. If the obtained r is smaller than both table values, it is not significant. Significant correlation coefficients lower than .50 can be useful for indicating nonchance relationships among variables, but they probably are not large enough to be useful in predicting individual scores.

You should notice that the correlation needed for significance decreases with the increased number of paired scores. Remember the earlier statement that a large number of scores decreases the likelihood that a high r will occur by chance. The table values reflect the influence of chance. You also should notice that a higher correlation is needed for significance at the .01 level than at the .05 level. The reason is that we are reducing the odds that the correlation is due to chance (1 in 100 vs. 5 in 100).

Coefficient of Determination

The statistical significance of correlation is important, but to better determine the relationship of two variables, the **coefficient of determination** should be utilized. The coefficient of determination is the square of the correlation coefficient (r^2). It represents the common variance between two variables, or the proportion of variance in one variable that can be accounted for by the other variable. For example, imagine we administered a standing long jump test and a leg strength test to a group of male high school students, and we calculated a correlation coefficient of .85 between the two tests. We calculate that r^2 equals .72. We interpret this value to mean that 72% of the variability in the standing long jump scores is associated with leg strength. Or, we might say that 72% of both standing long jump ability and leg strength comes from common factors. We also can say that the two tests have common factors that influence the individuals' scores.

Using the coefficient of determination shows that a high correlation coefficient is needed to indicate a substantial to high relationship between two variables. In addition, coefficients of determination can be compared as ratios, whereas correlation coefficients cannot. For example, an r of .80 is not twice as large as an r of .40. By using the coefficient of determination, we see that an r of .80 is four times stronger than an r of .40 (r = .80, r^2 = .64; r = .40, r^2 = .16).

Negative Correlation Coefficients

There are occasions when a negative correlation coefficient is to be expected. When a smaller score that is considered to be a better score is correlated with a larger score that also is considered to be a better score, the correlation coefficient usually will be negative. The relationship between maximum oxygen consumption and the time required to run 2 miles is an example. In general, individuals with high values for maximum oxygen consumption will have lower times for the 2-mile run than individuals with low values for maximum oxygen consumption. In addition, a negative correlation will probably occur with performance that requires support of the body (weight correlated with pull-ups or dips).

Other Correlation Techniques

Although the Spearman rank-difference and Pearson product-moment correlation coefficients are widely used, there are occasions when they are not the appropriate techniques to use. To keep you informed, we will briefly describe additional techniques. The procedures for these techniques can be found in most statistical textbooks.

Phi Coefficient

The **phi coefficient** is used when the two variables are true dichotomies. A dichotomous variable is one that can have only one of two possible values. The following are examples of studies employing the phi coefficient:

- the relationship of the gender of an individual and success or failure on a particular task

- the relationship of the gender of an individual and response to the question, "Do you enjoy physical education?"

Point Biserial Coefficient

The **point biserial coefficient** is appropriate when one variable is continuous and one variable is dichotomous. It is based on the assumption that the discrete variable is a true dichotomy. Such classifications as male-female, participant-nonparticipant, and undergraduate student–graduate student are true dichotomies. This assumption is not appropriate for artificial dichotomies, such as skilled-nonskilled or enthusiastic-nonenthusiastic. The following are examples of studies that would employ the point biserial coefficient:

- the relationship of the gender of an individual and performance on a standardized test
- the relationship of the graduate/nongraduate (college) student and performance on a fitness test

Biserial Correlation Coefficient

The **biserial correlation coefficient** is appropriate when one of the variables is continuous and the other is an artificial dichotomy. A study of the relationship between the number of miles run per week and the time for running 5,000 meters would require the use of the biserial correlation coefficient. The miles run per week is the artificial dichotomous variable and might be divided into less than 50 miles per week and more than 50 miles per week.

Tetrachoric Correlation Coefficient

When both variables are forced into dichotomies, the **tetrachoric correlation coefficient** is required. This technique would be appropriate for a study of the relationship of success as a high school coach and college grade point average. It would be necessary to define successful and unsuccessful and to force the grade point average into a dichotomy (e.g., below 3.0 and above 3.0) to perform this study.

? ARE YOU ABLE TO DO THE FOLLOWING:

- define correlation, correlation coefficient, and coefficient of determination?
- interpret the correlation coefficient?

- construct a scattergram and interpret it?
- determine the Spearman rank-difference correlation coefficient and interpret it?
- determine the Pearson product-moment correlation coefficient and interpret it?

---

1. Using the rank-difference correlation coefficient method, determine the relationship between the height (inches) and weight (pounds) measurements of twenty individuals. After you have determined r, calculate the coefficient of determination, interpret the obtained value, and use appendix B to interpret the significance of r.

Student	Height	Weight	Student	Height	Weight
A	68	170	K	68	165
B	68	160	L	67	160
C	66	140	M	71	195
D	67	150	N	71	190
E	69	155	O	70	195
F	65	145	P	66	150
G	70	168	Q	69	170
H	71	182	R	66	148
I	74	208	S	65	140
J	65	144	T	76	210

2. Using the product-moment correlation coefficient method, determine the relationship between a 2-minute sit-up test and physical-fitness test scores. After you have determined r, calculate the coefficient of determination, interpret the obtained value, and use appendix B to interpret the significance of the correlation coefficient.

Student	Sit-Up Score	PF Score	Student	Sit-Up Score	PF Score
A	45	81	K	38	93
B	51	94	L	37	51
C	30	91	M	41	65
D	55	75	N	42	73
E	32	65	O	42	74
F	42	82	P	43	79
G	41	85	Q	38	42
H	52	65	R	39	65
I	61	73	S	45	54
J	39	85	T	43	63

3. Using the product-moment correlation coefficient method, determine the relationship between the daily sodium intake and the systolic blood pressure of twenty-five individuals. After you have determined r, calculate the coefficient of determination, interpret the obtained value, and use appendix B to interpret the significance of r.

Individual	Sodium Intake	Blood Pressure
A	7.2	189
B	6.9	175
C	7.1	160
D	7.0	163
E	6.6	147
F	7.2	188
G	6.5	140
H	7.1	178
I	6.9	164
J	7.0	182
K	6.6	150
L	7.3	188
M	7.0	170
N	6.7	154
O	6.9	165
P	7.1	157
Q	7.4	193
R	6.5	139
S	7.1	176
T	7.0	180
U	6.8	164
V	6.9	159
W	6.7	151
X	6.8	163
Y	6.5	137

Testing for Significant Difference Between Two Means

As a physical educator you may have occasions when you would like to compare different methods of instruction or programs. You may want to determine if a group has improved in skill, fitness, or knowledge after participation in a particular program.

To illustrate, imagine you are the instructor at a fitness center, and you have forty individuals of similar age in a cardiorespiratory fitness class. Rather than have all forty individuals participate in the same program, you decide to randomly assign each person to one of two groups. One group will participate in aerobic dance, three times per week, for 8 weeks. The other group will participate in a running program, three times per week, for 8 weeks. There are other factors about the two programs that you would have to consider (e.g., intensity and duration of each session), but you want to know if one program will develop fitness better than the other.

At the conclusion of the eight weeks, you administer the same cardiorespiratory fitness test to the two groups and notice that the group means are different. Can you say that one program developed cardiorespiratory fitness better than the other? You cannot reach such a conclusion by merely observing the means. It is not unusual for the means to be different. In fact, if one thousand random samples were drawn from a population and administered the same test, the sample means would approximate a normal curve. The question you must answer is, "Are the sample means significantly different?" To answer this question you must statistically analyze the scores.

The Null Hypothesis

In statistics, a hypothesis is a prediction about the relationship between two or more variables. The hypothesis that predicts there will be no statistical difference between the means of groups is the **null hypothesis.** The hypothesis that predicts there will be a difference is the **alternative hypothesis.** The hypotheses are written as

Null hypothesis $\quad\quad H_0 : \overline{X}_1 = \overline{X}_2$
Alternative hypothesis $\quad H_1 : \overline{X}_1 \neq \overline{X}_2$

This type of alternative hypothesis is used for a **two-tailed test,** meaning that the difference in means can be in either direction. If a statistical test of the null hypothesis presents no evidence that the hypothesis is false, you accept it and reject the alternative hypothesis. If the statistical test presents evidence that the null hypothesis is false (the mean for group I is larger or smaller than the mean for group II), you reject it and accept the alternative hypothesis.

It is acceptable to use an alternative hypothesis that is directional. This type of hypothesis is used for a **one-tailed test** and requires that the t distribution be used differently. The directional alternative hypothesis is written as

$$H_1 : \overline{X}_1 < \overline{X}_2 \text{ or } H_1 : \overline{X}_1 > \overline{X}_2$$

For most studies, the nondirectional alternative hypothesis (two-tailed) is sufficient.

Degrees of Freedom

The **degrees of freedom** (df) concept is used in all statistical tests. For the statistical procedures used in this chapter, the degrees of freedom are calculated by subtracting 1 from N (N − 1) for any set of scores. (The degrees of freedom are determined by the sample size.) The degrees of freedom indicate the number of scores in a distribution that are free to vary. For example, assume that you have determined the group mean for twenty scores. For this given mean, nineteen scores could vary. Once the nineteen scores are obtained, however, the twentieth score must assume a fixed value if the mean is to remain the same. To convince yourself of this concept, work with five scores that have a mean of 10 (the sum of the five numbers is 50). Assign four scores any value from 5 to 12. If the mean is to remain 10, you will see that the fifth score cannot be just any value. Its value is determined by the values that you assigned to the first four scores. In the case of a t-test where there are two groups, the degrees of freedom equal $(N_1 − 1) + (N_2 − 1) = N_1 + N_2 − 2$.

Level of Significance

The **level of significance** is the probability of rejecting a null hypothesis when it is true. The two most common levels of significance are .01 and .05. If you reject the null hypothesis at the .01 level of significance, there is 1 chance in 100 that you are rejecting the null hypothesis when it is actually true. At the .05 level, there are 5 chances in 100 that you are in error.

Two types of error, **Type I** and **Type II,** can be committed when accepting and rejecting hypotheses. If you reject a hypothesis when it is true, you commit a Type I error. The Type II error occurs when the hypotheses is false and should be rejected, but the test results appear to make the hypothesis true; that is, you accept the hypothesis when it is not true. Using the .01 level of significance, rather than the .05 level, reduces the risk of making a Type I error but increases the probability of making a Type II error. Owing to the probability of making a Type I error, only in unusual studies is a level of significance below .05 used. In general, the best way for a researcher to decrease the probability of making a Type II error is to increase the sample size (the number of subjects in the groups). As the sample size increases, the probability of making a Type II error decreases.

The level of significance and the degrees of freedom are used together to determine the value that a statistical test must yield for you to reject the null hypothesis. Appendix C shows the values used to determine significance. To use the table in appendix C, go down the df column to the degrees of freedom that you have determined and then go across to the values (critical values) under the .05 and .01 columns. These values will determine whether you reject or accept the null hypothesis. Notice that the greater the degrees of freedom, the smaller the value needed to reject the null hypothesis. Because the degrees of freedom are a result of the sample number, a large sample number is beneficial in terms of finding significant difference.

Standard Error of the Mean

If a large number of equal-size samples were randomly drawn from the same population and formed into a distribution, we would have a sampling distribution of means. From the sampling distribution of means, we can compute the standard deviation of the sampling distribution, called the **standard error of the mean** (SEM). When the means are in close agreement, the value of the standard error of the mean is small. Also, we are more confident that any one mean is near the value of the population mean.

Because it is not practical to calculate the standard error of the mean from a sampling distribution of means, a formula has been derived to provide an estimate of the standard error. The formula is

$$\text{SEM} = \frac{s}{\sqrt{N}} \quad (s = \text{standard deviation of sample scores})$$

Table 3.3 shows that, for the group running three days per week, the $\overline{X} = 80.9$ and the SEM = 0.38. The SEM value is added to and subtracted from the $\overline{X}$ (80.9 ± 0.38) to demonstrate the distribution of the means. The resulting values indicate that if this study were repeated a large number of times, 68.26% of the time the means for the group running 3 days per week would be in the range of 80.52 to 81.28. For the group running 5 days per week, 68.26% of the time the means would be in the range of 90.51 to 92.09 (91.3 ± 0.79).

Standard Error of the Difference Between Means

After calculating the standard error of the mean for each of the means, we can estimate the size difference to be expected between two sample means randomly drawn from the same population. To determine this value, called the **standard error of the difference,** we have to square the standard error of the mean of each group, add the results, and then find the square root of the sum. The standard error of the difference represents the standard deviation of all the observed differences between pairs of sample means. The formula is

$$s_{\overline{x}-\overline{x}} = \sqrt{\text{SEM}_1{}^2 + \text{SEM}_2{}^2}$$

In table 3.3, the difference between the means is 10.4 and $s_{\overline{x}-\overline{x}} = 0.87$. These values indicate that 68.26% of the time, the differences between the means would be in the range of 9.53 to 11.27 (10.4 ± 0.87).

t-Test for Independent Groups

The **t-test for independent groups** may be used to determine the significance of the difference between two independent sample means. In a comparison of the means of two independent samples, the following assumptions are made:

1. Initially the two sample groups come from the same population.
2. The population is normally distributed.
3. The two groups are representative samples; that is, they have approximately equal variances.

To illustrate the steps involved in the use of the t-test for independent groups, suppose you wanted to determine

TABLE 3.3 t-Test for Independent Groups: Harvard Step Test

Group Running 3 Days/Week		Group Running 5 Days/Week	
X_1	X_1^2	X_2	X_2^2
80	6400	88	7744
79	6241	92	8464
81	6561	93	8649
80	6400	95	9025
82	6724	91	8281
81	6561	89	7921
80	6400	88	7744
82	6724	90	8100
81	6561	94	8836
83	6889	93	8649
$\Sigma X_1 = 809$	$\Sigma X_1^2 = 65461$	$\Sigma X_2 = 913$	$\Sigma X_2^2 = 83413$

$\overline{X}_1 = 80.9$

$$s_1 = \sqrt{\frac{N\Sigma X^2 - (\Sigma X)^2}{N(N-1)}}$$

$$= \sqrt{\frac{10(65461) - (809)^2}{10(9)}}$$

$$= \sqrt{\frac{654610 - 654481}{90}}$$

$$= \sqrt{\frac{129}{90}}$$

$s_1 = \sqrt{1.43} = 1.20$

$$SEM_1 = \frac{s_1}{\sqrt{N_1}} = \frac{1.20}{\sqrt{10}} = \frac{1.20}{3.16} = 0.38$$

$$s_{\bar{x}-\bar{x}} = \sqrt{SEM_1^2 + SEM_2^2}$$

$$= \sqrt{(0.38)^2 + (0.79)^2}$$

$$= \sqrt{0.1444 + 0.6241}$$

$$= \sqrt{0.7685}$$

$s_{\bar{x}-\bar{x}} = 0.87$

$\overline{X}_2 = 91.3$

$s_2 = 2.50$

$SEM_2 = .79$

$$t = \frac{\overline{X}_1 - \overline{X}_2}{s_{\bar{x}-\bar{x}}}$$

$$= \frac{80.9 - 91.3}{.87}$$

$t = -11.95$ (compare with t-values in appendix C)

if running 5 days a week would develop cardiorespiratory endurance better than running 3 days a week. Your null hypothesis is that there will be no difference in the means of the two programs ($\overline{X}_1 = \overline{X}_2$). After randomly selecting the individuals for each group, you prescribe the same running program (intensity and duration for each day) for both groups. After 12 weeks, you administer the Harvard Step Test to both groups in the running program. Table 3.3

shows the test scores and the necessary calculations for the t-test. (For convenience, only ten individuals will be in each group.) The steps for the calculations are as follows:

1. Calculate the mean and standard deviations for each group.
2. Calculate the standard error of the mean (SEM) for each group.
3. Calculate the standard error of the difference between means $(s_{\bar{x}-\bar{x}})$.
4. Calculate the t-ratio by substituting the values in the formula

$$t = \frac{\overline{X}_1 - \overline{X}_2}{s_{\bar{x}-\bar{x}}}$$

5. Determine the degrees of freedom (df). For this comparison, the degrees of freedom = 10 + 10 − 2 = 18.
6. Refer to the t-values in appendix C. If the computed t-ratio is equal to or greater than the critical value in appendix C, reject the null hypothesis. If the t-ratio is less than the critical value, accept the null hypothesis. With 18 degrees of freedom, the t-ratio of 11.95 is greater than the t of 2.101 needed for significance at the .05 level and greater than the 2.878 needed for significance at the .01 level.

   Note: The negative sign is ignored because it is the result of subtracting $\overline{X}_2$ from $\overline{X}_1$. If the group running 5 days a week had been designated as group 1, the result would have been positive. The important consideration is the size of t, not its sign.
7. Reject the null hypothesis: you may conclude that running 5 days a week develops cardiorespiratory endurance better than running 3 days a week.

t-Test for Dependent Groups

If two groups are not independent but are related to each other, the **t-test for dependent groups** should be used. This test is also called the t-test for paired, related, or correlated samples. The only changes in the assumptions for the t-test for dependent groups, as compared with those for the t-test for independent groups, are the following:

1. The paired differences are a random sample from a normal population.
2. The equal variances assumption is unnecessary, since you will be working with one group.

To illustrate the steps involved in the use of the t-test for dependent groups, imagine that you wish to determine if participation in a basketball class will improve the scores of ninth-grade girls on a speed spot shooting test. Your null hypothesis is that there will be no difference in the means of the speed spot shooting pretest and posttest ($\overline{X}_1 = \overline{X}_2$). You administer the test the first day of the class and again at the conclusion of the basketball unit. Table 3.4 shows the pairs of scores and the necessary calculations for the t-test. (Again, for convenience, only ten pairs of scores will be used.) The steps for the calculations are as follows:

1. List the pairs of scores so that you can subtract one from the other.
2. Label a column D and determine the difference for each pair of scores.

TABLE 3.4 Test for Dependent Groups: Speed Spot Shooting Test

Pretest Scores	Posttest Scores	D	D²
10	12	2	4
12	15	3	9
9	10	1	1
11	10	−1	1
8	12	4	16
9	11	2	4
13	14	1	1
8	11	3	9
7	9	2	4
9	10	1	1
		ΣD = 18	ΣD² = 50

$\overline{D} = 1.8$

$$s_D = \sqrt{\frac{\Sigma D^2 - N(\overline{D}^2)}{N}} \qquad s_{\overline{D}} = \frac{s_D}{\sqrt{N}}$$

$$= \sqrt{\frac{50 - 10(1.8^2)}{10}} \qquad = \frac{1.33}{\sqrt{10}}$$

$$= \sqrt{\frac{50 - 10(3.24)}{10}} \qquad s_{\overline{D}} = \frac{1.33}{3.16} = .42$$

$$= \sqrt{\frac{17.6}{10}} \qquad t = \frac{\overline{D}}{s_{\overline{D}}}$$

$$s_D = \sqrt{1.76} = 1.33 \qquad t = \frac{1.8}{.42} = 4.29 \quad \text{(compare with t-values in appendix C)}$$

3. Label a column D², square each D, and sum D² (ΣD^2).

4. Calculate the mean difference ($\overline{D}$).

5. Calculate the standard deviation of the difference. The formula is

$$s_D = \sqrt{\frac{\Sigma D^2 - N(\overline{D}^2)}{N}}$$

6. Calculate the standard error of the difference ($s_{\overline{D}}$). The $s_{\overline{D}}$ is equivalent to the SEM and is obtained in a similar manner. The formula is

$$s_{\overline{D}} = \frac{s_D}{\sqrt{N}}$$

7. Calculate the t-ratio by substituting the values in the formula

$$t = \frac{\overline{D}}{s_{\overline{D}}}$$

8. Determine the degrees of freedom. For this comparison the degrees of freedom = 10 − 1 = 9.

9. Refer to the t-values in appendix C. With 9 degrees of freedom, the t-ratio of 4.29 is greater than the t-value of 2.262 needed for significance at the .05 level of significance and greater than the t-value of 3.250 needed at the .01 level.

10. Reject the null hypothesis. You may conclude that participation in the basketball class improved performance on the speed spot shooting test.

❓ARE YOU ABLE TO DO THE FOLLOWING:

- define and give examples of null hypothesis, degrees of freedom, level of significance, standard error of the mean, and standard error of the difference between means?
- define Type I and Type II errors?
- determine if there is a significant difference between two means through use of the appropriate t-test?

▶ REVIEW PROBLEMS ◀

1. An instructor used different methods to teach a health unit to two classes. Use the appropriate t-test to determine if the performances of the two classes on the knowledge test were significantly different.

Class 1					Class 2				
88	93	91	82	85	82	86	89	88	91
87	90	86	92	89	92	89	85	89	92
94	88	87	87	90	92	93	94	89	94

2. Use the appropriate t-test to determine if a group of twelve individuals experienced a significant change in percent body fat after participation in a 15-week exercise program.

Subject	Percent Body Fat Before Exercise Program	Percent Body Fat After Exercise Program
A	26	21
B	17	15
C	18	16
D	20	16
E	21	18
F	25	21
G	19	16
H	21	18
I	27	23
J	21	17
K	20	18
L	24	22

3. After participation in an adult fitness program, the resting heart rates of twelve smokers and twelve nonsmokers were measured. Use the appropriate t-test to determine if there is a significant difference in the heart rates of the two groups.

Smokers	Nonsmokers
74	69
75	68
76	70
70	68
68	73
71	70
77	73
75	71
70	70
76	69
74	70
75	71

4. Fifteen males participated in a diet and exercise program for 6 months. Use the appropriate t-test to determine if the participants experienced a significant change in their serum cholesterol after the diet and exercise program.

Participant	Preprogram Cholesterol	Postprogram Cholesterol
A	230	210
B	205	200
C	195	190
D	210	195
E	233	212
F	240	202
G	195	190
H	220	200
I	225	198
J	211	200
K	221	199
L	225	220
M	203	195
N	240	220
O	207	198

Testing for Significant Difference Among Three or More Means

The t-test is a method for testing hypotheses about two sample means, but there may be occasions that require the testing of hypotheses about more than two means. For example, you may elect to compare the effects of three or more methods of teaching, cardiorespiratory fitness programs, weight-training programs, or weight-reduction programs. **Analysis of variance** (ANOVA) is a method used to compare three or more means or even, at times, to compare two means. For these reasons, ANOVA is used in research more than any other statistical technique.

Special Terms and Symbols

Before attempting to perform the steps of the new techniques, you should have an understanding of these terms:

- N = number of scores
- n = the number of scores in a group (numbers in groups may be different)
- k = the number of independent groups or the number of trials (measures) performed on the same subjects (repeated measures)
- r = number of rows or subjects (repeated measures)
- grand ΣX = sum of all scores in all groups
- grand ΣX^2 = sum of the square of all scores in all groups
- total sum of squares (SS_T) = the sum of the squared deviations of every score from the grand $\overline{X}$; represents the variability of each score in all groups from the grand $\overline{X}$
- sum of squares within groups (SS_W) = the sum of the squared deviations of each score from its group $\overline{X}$; also referred to as sum of squares for error
- sum of squares between groups (SS_B) = the sum of the squared deviations of each group $\overline{X}$ from the grand $\overline{X}$; also referred to as treatment sum of squares
- mean square for the sum of squares within groups (MS_W) = variance within the groups
- mean square for the sum of squares between groups (MS_B) = variance between groups
- F-distribution = table values required to reject null hypothesis
- degrees of freedom within groups = (N – k); total number of measures or scores (N) minus number of groups (k); degrees of freedom for denominator in F-distribution
- degrees of freedom between groups = (k – 1); number of groups (k) minus 1; degrees of freedom for numerator in F-distribution
- $\dfrac{\text{degrees of freedom between groups}}{\text{degrees of freedom within groups}} = \dfrac{k-1}{N-k}$

Analysis of Variance for Independent Groups

The **analysis of variance for independent groups** is used when the sample groups are not related to each other. There are several assumptions for this ANOVA, but the basic assumptions are as follows:

1. The samples are randomly drawn from a normally distributed population.
2. The variances of the samples are approximately equal.

To illustrate the steps involved in the analysis of variance for independent groups, suppose that a fitness instructor wishes to determine if there is a difference in three programs designed to improve trunk extension. The null hypothesis is that there will be no difference in the means of the three programs ($\overline{X}_1 = \overline{X}_2 = \overline{X}_3$). The instructor randomly assigns the members of a fitness class to one of three groups, and each group participates for 10 weeks in a different program to improve trunk extension. At the conclusion of the training period, the groups are given the same trunk extension test. Table 3.5 shows the scores and the necessary calculations for the analysis of variance. As with previous illustrations, the total number of scores is intentionally small. The steps for the calculations are as follows:

1. Sum each group of scores to get ΣX_1, ΣX_2, and ΣX_3. Add the group sums to get a grand ΣX ($\Sigma X_1 + \Sigma X_2 + \Sigma X_3 = $ grand ΣX).
2. Square each score and sum the squared scores of each group (ΣX^2). Add the ΣX^2 for each group to get a grand ΣX^2 ($\Sigma X_1^2 + \Sigma X_2^2 + \Sigma X_3^2 = $ grand ΣX^2).
3. Calculate the correction factor (C). C is necessary because raw scores are used rather than deviations of the scores from the mean.

$$C = \frac{(\text{grand } \Sigma X)^2}{\text{total N}}$$

4. Calculate the total sum of squares (SS_T).

$$SS_T = \text{grand } \Sigma X^2 - C$$

5. Calculate the sum of squares between groups (SS_B).

$$SS_B = \frac{(\Sigma X_1)^2}{n_1} + \frac{(\Sigma X_2)^2}{n_2} + \frac{(\Sigma X_3)^2}{n_3} - C$$

6. Calculate the sum of squares within groups (SS_W).

$$S_W = SS_T - SS_B$$

7. Calculate the mean square for the sum of squares between groups.

$$MS_B = \frac{SS_B}{k-1}$$

8. Calculate the mean square for the sum of squares within groups.

$$MS_W = \frac{SS_W}{N-k}$$

9. Calculate the F-ratio.

$$F = \frac{MS_B}{MS_W}$$

10. Refer to the F-distribution in appendix D to determine if F is significant. To use the table in appendix D, locate the appropriate column for the numerator degrees of freedom (degrees of freedom between groups, $k - 1$). For the trunk extension study, there are 2 degrees of freedom between groups ($3 - 1 = 2$). We next find the row that corresponds to the degrees of freedom for the denominator (degrees of freedom within groups, $N - k$). We have $21(24 - 3)$ degrees of freedom within groups. The F-ratio of 8.57 is greater than the 3.47 table value at the .05 level and the 5.78 value at the .01 level, so we reject the null hypothesis at both levels of significance. The F-ratio permits us to conclude that there is a significant difference in the three means, but it does not indicate which mean is significantly superior or if two means are significantly superior to one mean. A follow-up test must be performed to identify the means that are significantly different from one another. Table 3.6 shows a summary of the ANOVA as it is usually reported in research publications.

Post Hoc Test

When the F-ratio indicates that there are significant differences between means, several tests may be used to identify which means are significantly different from each other. A test used for this purpose is referred to as a **post hoc test.** Only **Tukey's honestly significant difference test** (HSD) will be presented here.

The HSD calculates the minimum raw-score mean difference that must occur to declare a significant difference between any two means. The formula for computing the HSD value when the numbers of scores in the groups are equal is

$$HSD = q(\alpha, \ k, \ N - k) \sqrt{\frac{MS_W}{n}}$$

where q = value obtained from the table in appendix E, α = significance level, k = number of groups, N = total number of observations, $N - k$ = the degrees of freedom for the denominator in appendix E, MS_W = mean square for within-groups variance, and n = the number of scores in each group.

TABLE 3.5 ANOVA for Independent Groups: Trunk Extension Test

Group I		Group II		Group III	
X_1	X_1^2	X_2	X_2^2	X_3	X_3^2
22	484	20	400	18	324
23	529	19	361	19	361
21	441	18	324	17	289
22	484	19	361	22	484
19	361	18	324	18	324
21	441	21	441	19	361
22	484	20	400	20	400
21	441	19	361	19	361
$\Sigma X_1 = 171$	$\Sigma X_1^2 = 3665$	$\Sigma X_2 = 154$	$\Sigma X_2^2 = 2972$	$\Sigma X_3 = 152$	$\Sigma X_3^2 = 2904$
$\overline{X}_1 = 21.38$		$\overline{X}_2 = 19.25$		$\overline{X}_3 = 19.00$	

- $\Sigma X_1 = 171$, $\Sigma X_2 = 154$, $\Sigma X_3 = 152$

$\Sigma X_1^2 = 3665$, $\Sigma X_2^2 = 2972$, $\Sigma X_3^2 = 2904$

- grand $\Sigma X = 171 + 154 + 152 = 477$ (sum of all scores in all groups)

- grand $\Sigma X^2 = 3665 + 2972 + 2904 = 9541$ (sum of the square of all scores in all groups)

- correction factor $C = \dfrac{(\text{grand } \Sigma X)^2}{\text{total } N}$ (necessary because raw scores are used rather than deviations of the scores from the mean)

$$C = \frac{(477)^2}{24} = \frac{227{,}529}{24} = 9480.38$$

- $SS_T = \text{grand } \Sigma X^2 - C$ (sum of the squared deviations of every score from the grand $\overline{X}$)

$SS_T = 9541 - 9480.38 = 60.62$

- $SS_B = \dfrac{(\Sigma X_1)^2}{n_1} + \dfrac{(\Sigma X_2)^2}{n_2} + \dfrac{(\Sigma X_3)^2}{n_3} - C$ (sum of the squared deviations of each group $\overline{X}$ from the grand $\overline{X}$)

$$= \frac{(171)^2}{8} + \frac{(154)^2}{8} + \frac{(152)^2}{8} - 9480.38$$

$SS_B = 3655.13 + 2964.50 + 2888 - 9480.38 = 27.25$

- $SS_W = SS_T - SS_B$ (sum of the squared deviations of each score from its group $\overline{X}$)

$SS_W = 60.62 - 27.25 = 33.37$

- $MS_B = \dfrac{SS_B}{k-1} = \dfrac{27.25}{3-1} = 13.63$ (mean square for the sum of squares between groups; variance between groups)

- $MS_W = \dfrac{SS_W}{N-k} = \dfrac{33.37}{24-3} = 1.59$ (mean square for the sum of squares within groups; variance within groups)

- $F = \dfrac{MS_B}{MS_W} = \dfrac{13.63}{1.59} = 8.57$ (value required to reject null hypothesis; refer to appendix D)

TABLE 3.6 Summary for ANOVA for Trunk Extension Test

Source of Variation	Sum of Squares	df	Mean Square	F
Between groups	27.25	2	13.63	8.57*
Within groups	33.37	21	1.59	
Total	60.62	23		

*Significant at the .01 level.

When the n's in any two groups are unequal the formula is

$$\text{HSD} = q(\alpha,\ k,\ N-k)\sqrt{\frac{\text{MS}_W}{2}\left(\frac{1}{n_1}+\frac{1}{n_2}\right)}$$

Since the n's are equal in the example in table 3.5, the first equation will be used for our post hoc test. For the .01 level in the table in appendix E, we find that q is about 4.64 (k = 3 and N − k = 21, but since the table jumps from 20 to 24 for the denominator, we will use 3, 20). In table 3.6, MSW is 1.59 and n = 8. Our equation is

$$\text{HSD} = 4.64\sqrt{\frac{1.59}{8}}$$
$$= 4.64\sqrt{0.19875}$$
$$= 4.64(0.446)$$
$$\text{HSD} = 2.069$$

This value (2.069) represents the minimum raw-score difference between any two means that may be declared significant. In table 3.5,

$$\overline{X}_1 - \overline{X}_2 = 21.38 - 19.25 = 2.13$$
$$\overline{X}_2 - \overline{X}_3 = 19.25 - 19.00 = 0.25$$
$$\overline{X}_1 - \overline{X}_3 = 21.38 - 19.00 = 2.38$$

If minus signs had occurred in our example, we would ignore them. We are interested only in absolute differences. We see that $\overline{X}_1 - \overline{X}_2$ and $\overline{X}_1 - \overline{X}_3$ are greater than 2.069. We thus conclude that there is a significant difference between these groups at the .01 level but not between groups 2 and 3.

Analysis of Variance for Repeated Measures

The **analysis of variance for repeated measures** is used when repeated measures are made on the same subjects. Basic assumptions are as follows:

1. The samples are randomly selected from a normal population.
2. The variances for all measurements are approximately equal.

To illustrate this technique, we will assume that a basketball coach wishes to determine if loudness of sound is a factor in the making of foul shots. He arranges for the ten members of the basketball team to shoot fifteen foul shots under three different sound conditions (no sound, medium sound, and loud sound). The null hypothesis is that the means of the three trials will be no different ($\overline{X}_1 = \overline{X}_2 = \overline{X}_3$). Table 3.7 shows the scores and the necessary calculations for the analysis of variance. (Note that in this technique, N refers to the total number of measurements.) Ten subjects were measured three times, so N = 30. Also, k refers to the number of times that the group is measured. The steps for the calculations are as follows:

1. Calculate the grand ΣX and grand ΣX^2 as in the ANOVA for independent groups.
$$\Sigma X_1 + \Sigma X_2 + \Sigma X_3 = \text{grand } \Sigma X$$
$$\Sigma X_1^2 + \Sigma X_2^2 + \Sigma X_3^2 = \text{grand } \Sigma X^2$$

2. Calculate the correction factor as before.
$$C = \frac{(\text{grand } \Sigma X)^2}{N}$$

3. Calculate the total sum of squares (SS$_T$) as before.
$$\text{SS}_T = \text{grand } \Sigma X^2 - C$$

4. Calculate the sum of squares between groups (SS$_B$) as before (actually, this is the sum of squares between trials).
$$\text{SS}_B = \frac{(\Sigma X_1)^2}{n_1} + \frac{(\Sigma X_2)^2}{n_2} + \frac{(\Sigma X_3)^2}{n_3} - C$$

5. Calculate the sum of squares to determine the effects of the test-retest (SS$_{\text{subjects}}$): Add the scores of the three trials for each subject, square the sum, and then add the squared sums for each subject.

TABLE 3.7 ANOVA for Repeated Measures: Foul Shooting While Exposed to Different Sound Levels

No Sound		Medium Sound		Loud Sound			
X_1	X_1^2	X_2	X_2^2	X_3	X_3^2	ΣRows	$(\Sigma$Rows$)^2$
11	121	12	144	10	100	33	1089
9	81	10	100	9	81	28	784
10	100	12	144	9	81	31	961
8	64	10	100	9	81	27	729
12	144	12	144	10	100	34	1156
10	100	11	121	9	81	30	900
12	144	13	169	11	121	36	1296
9	81	9	81	9	81	27	729
10	100	11	121	8	64	29	841
9	81	10	100	10	100	29	841
$\Sigma X_1 = 100$	$\Sigma X_1^2 = 1016$	$\Sigma X_2 = 110$	$\Sigma X_2^2 = 1224$	$\Sigma X_3 = 94$	$\Sigma X_3^2 = 890$	grand $\Sigma X = 304$	$(\Sigma$rows$)^2 = 9326$
$\overline{X}_1 = 10$		$\overline{X}_2 = 11$		$\overline{X}_3 = 9.4$			

- grand $\Sigma X = 304$; grand $\Sigma X^2 = 3130$

- correction factor $C = \dfrac{(\text{grand } \Sigma X)^2}{\text{total } N} = \dfrac{(304)^2}{30} = \dfrac{92416}{30} = 3080.53$

- $SS_T = \text{grand } \Sigma X^2 - C = 3130 - 3080.53 = 49.47$

  (sum of the squared deviations of every score from the grand $\overline{X}$)

- $SS_B = \dfrac{(\Sigma X_1)^2}{n_1} + \dfrac{(\Sigma X_2)^2}{n_2} + \dfrac{(\Sigma X_3)^2}{n_3} - C$

  (sum of squares between trials; sum of squared deviations of each group $\overline{X}$ from grand $\overline{X}$)

  $= \dfrac{(100)^2}{10} + \dfrac{(110)^2}{10} + \dfrac{(94)^2}{10} - 3080.53$

  $SS_B = 3093.60 - 3080.53 = 13.07$

- $SS_{\text{subjects}} = \dfrac{(\Sigma \text{ rows})^2}{k} - C$

  (sum of squares to determine the effects of test-retest)

  $= \dfrac{(11+12+10)^2 + (9+10+9)^2 + \ldots (9+10+10)^2}{3} - 3080.53$

  $SS_{\text{subjects}} = 3108.67 - 3080.53 = 28.14$

- $SS_E = SS_T - SS_B - SS_{\text{subjects}}$

  (sum of squares for error; sum of squared deviations of each score from its group $\overline{X}$)

  $SS_E = 49.47 - 13.07 - 28.14 = 8.26$

- $MS_B = \dfrac{SS_B}{k-1} = \dfrac{13.07}{2} = 6.54$

  (mean square for the sum of squares between groups)

- $MS_{\text{subjects}} = \dfrac{SS_{\text{subjects}}}{r-1} = \dfrac{28.14}{10-1} = 3.13$

  (mean square for the sum of squares between subjects)

- $MS_E = \dfrac{SS_E}{(k-1)(r-1)} = \dfrac{8.26}{(2)(9)} = 0.46$

  (mean square for the sum of squares for error)

- F-ratio $= \dfrac{MS_B}{MS_E} = \dfrac{6.54}{0.46} = 14.22$

  (value required to reject null hypothesis; refer to appendix D)

The sum of the squared sums for each subject is divided by k (the number of trials), and C is subtracted from the resulting value.

$$SS_{subjects} = \frac{(\Sigma\ rows)^2}{k} - C$$

6. Compute the sum of squares for error (also referred to as within-group sum of squares); this calculation represents the sum of the squared deviations of each score from its group $\overline{X}$. Since this sum of squares remains after SS_B and $SS_{subjects}$, it is easy to calculate.

$$SS_E = SS_T - SS_B - SS_{subjects}$$

7. Calculate the mean square for the sum of squares between groups (trials). k = number of independent groups.

$$MS_B = \frac{SS_B}{k-1}$$

8. Calculate the mean square for the sum of squares between subjects. r = number of subjects.

$$MS_{subjects} = \frac{SS_{subjects}}{r-1}$$

9. Calculate the mean square for the sum of squares for error.

$$MS_E = \frac{SS_E}{(k-1)(r-1)}$$

10. Calculate the F-ratio.

$$F = \frac{MS_B}{MS_E}$$

11. Refer to the F-distribution in appendix D. The degrees of freedom for the numerator are $(k-1) = (3-1) = 2$. For the denominator, the degrees of freedom are $(k-1)(r-1) = (3-1)(10-1) = 18$. The F-ratio of 14.22 (6.54/0.46) is greater than the 6.01 value needed for significance at the .01 level, so we reject the null hypothesis. Tukey's honestly significant difference test (HSD) now should be

used to determine which means are significantly different. Table 3.8 shows the analysis summary.

Post Hoc Test

For ANOVA for repeated measures, the formula for computing the HSD value is

$$HSD = q(\alpha,\ k,\ [k-1][r-1])\sqrt{\frac{MS_E}{r}}$$

where q = value obtained from the table in appendix E, α = significance level, k = number of trials or measures performed on the same subjects, r = number of rows or number of subjects, $(k-1)(r-1)$ = degrees of freedom for denominator in appendix E, and MS_E = mean square for the sum of squares for error.

At the .01 level, we find q is 4.70 (k = 3 and $[3-1]$ $[10-1] = 18$). In table 3.8, $MS_E = 0.46$, so our equation is

$$HSD = 4.70\sqrt{\frac{0.46}{10}}$$
$$= 4.70\sqrt{0.046}$$
$$= 4.70(0.2145)$$
$$HSD = 1.008$$
$$\overline{X}_1 - \overline{X}_2 = 10 - 11 = -1$$
$$\overline{X}_2 - \overline{X}_3 = 11 - 9.4 = 1.6$$
$$\overline{X}_1 - \overline{X}_3 = 10 - 9.4 = 0.6$$

We see that $\overline{X}_2 - \overline{X}_3$ is greater than 1.008. There is a significant difference between medium sound and loud sound when shooting foul shouts. There is no significant difference between $\overline{X}_1$ (no sound) and $\overline{X}_2$ (medium

TABLE 3.8 Summary of ANOVA for Foul Shooting While Exposed to Different Sound Levels

Source of Variation	Sum of Squares	df	Mean Square	F
Subjects (rows)	28.14	9	3.13	14.22*
Between groups	13.07	2	6.54	
Error	8.26	18	0.46	
Total	49.47	29		

*Significant at the .01 level

sound) and between $\overline{X}_1$ (no sound) and $\overline{X}_3$ (loud sound). If we had tested at the .05 level, q would have been 3.61 and our HSD value would have been 0.774. We then would have found a significant difference between $\overline{X}_1$ (no sound) and $\overline{X}_2$ (medium sound) and between $\overline{X}_2$ (medium sound) and $\overline{X}_3$ (loud sound), but no significant difference between no sound and loud sound.

Intraclass Correlation Coefficient

The reliability, or consistency, of a test may be estimated through ANOVA. Test reliability will be discussed in chapter 4. Through ANOVA, the intraclass correlation coefficient (R) is computed. The Pearson product-moment correlation coefficient also can be used to estimate test reliability, but the intraclass correlation coefficient may be more accurate, for two reasons. First, product-moment correlation is limited to two trials. If more than two trials of a test are administered, it is necessary to reduce the scores to two sets, usually by averaging. Second, the Pearson product-moment correlation coefficient does not consider the variation of trial scores. It is possible that trial scores for the test performers may systematically increase or decrease, but the changes will not be detected if the product-moment correlation coefficient is used. Test reliability may be estimated as high, even though the scores systematically changed. Procedures for calculation of the intraclass correlation coefficient will not be described but can be found in other statistical sources.

☟ARE YOU ABLE TO DO THE FOLLOWING:

- define total sum of squares, sum of squares within groups, sum of squares between groups, mean square for the sum of squares within groups, and mean square for the sum of squares between groups?
- determine if there is a significant difference between two or more means through the appropriate one-way analysis of variance procedure?
- use Tukey's honestly significant difference test (HSD) to determine which means are significantly different from each other?

1. An elementary physical education teacher typically used two different methods to improve the agility of the students in her classes. Trying to determine if one program developed agility better than the other, she randomly assigned the students to one of two groups. After the students had been in the programs for 12 weeks, she administered the same agility test to the two groups. Use the appropriate t-test to determine if the group means are significantly different.

Scores for Group I		Scores for Group II	
13	12	14	13
13	11	12	15
10	8	10	12
11	14	11	10
12	10	13	14

2. A high school teacher was interested in determining if mental practice would improve badminton serving ability. He randomly selected ten subjects from a population of students who had never played badminton, taught the correct way to serve, and administered a short-serve test to them. He gave the students instructions about mental practice and asked them to mentally practice the badminton short-serve 10 minutes/day for 7 days. They were instructed not to practice badminton in any other way. He then tested the group again. Use the appropriate t-test to determine if the group mean for the short-serve test improved after mental practice.

Subject	Pretest Short-Serve Test Scores	Posttest Short-Serve Test Scores
A	37	43
B	42	46
C	36	38
D	50	55
E	34	32
F	44	51
G	51	53
H	42	48
I	45	43
J	52	55

3. A physical fitness instructor was interested in comparing three cardiovascular fitness programs. After three groups participated in the programs, she measured the oxygen uptake (ml/kg/min) of all the subjects. Use the appropriate ANOVA technique to determine if the group means are significantly different. If you find that there are significant differences in the group means, use the HSD to identify which means are significantly different.

Group I	Group II	Group III
46	47	49
46	50	51
48	50	50
47	48	49
50	49	52
48	47	53
47	51	49
51	50	52

4. A weight-training instructor was interested in determining the effects of external motivation on muscular strength. After a group of ten individuals had participated in a weight-training class for 15 weeks, the instructor tested the group for maximum strength on three different occasions. During one test, no external motivation was provided. During the second test, only the instructor shouted encouragement, and during the third test, he arranged for several spectators to shout encouragement. Use the appropriate ANOVA technique to determine if there is a significant difference in the group means of the tests. If you find that there are significant differences in the group means, use the HSD to identify which means are significantly different.

Subject	No External Motivation	Instructor Motivation	Spectator Motivation
A	81	84	88
B	88	89	93
C	92	94	97
D	83	85	88
E	81	83	85
F	79	80	85

G	84	84	87
H	87	86	93
I	88	90	94
J	84	86	88

5. A golf instructor used different instructional methods with three groups of females who were similar in age and golf experience. She then tested their ability to hit a golf ball for distance and accuracy with a 7-iron. Use the appropriate ANOVA technique to determine if there is a significant difference in the mean scores of the three groups. If you find there are significant differences in the group means, use the HSD to identify which means are significantly different.

Method I	Method II	Method III
110	105	115
115	112	120
112	105	118
98	100	110
120	118	126
90	93	110
119	115	124
125	120	130
111	112	118
102	113	115
116	113	125
118	108	130

6. The heart rate of twelve male college golfers was monitored during a golf match. Use the appropriate ANOVA technique to determine if their heart rates were significantly different when preparing to hit the drive, to hit approach shots to the green, and to putt. If you find that there are significant differences in the group means, use the HSD to identify which means are significantly different.

Player	Drive	Approach to Green	Putt
A	85	76	85
B	88	80	88
C	84	79	87
D	90	80	89
E	87	79	87
F	80	71	82

Player	Drive	Approach to Green	Putt
G	78	70	80
H	88	80	89
I	90	81	89
J	82	75	83
K	80	72	83
L	84	73	84

4 What Is a Good Test?

Upon completion of this chapter, you should be able to

1. Describe criterion-referenced and norm-referenced measurement and state when it is appropriate to use each;

2. Define validity and the types of validity for norm-referenced tests, give examples of each type, and describe how each may be estimated;

3. Describe how the criterion-referenced validity of a test can be determined through the use of behavioral objectives or testing before and after instruction;

4. Describe how domain-referenced validity and decision validity are used to determine criterion-referenced validity;

5. Define reliability and describe the four methods for estimating the reliability of norm-referenced tests;

6. Define objectivity and describe how it may be estimated; and

7. Describe the features of administrative feasibility that should be considered when selecting or constructing a test.

Note: Many of the testing examples in this chapter refer to the school environment, but the criteria for a good test also should be considered when testing in the nonschool environment.

As a physical educator you will often measure performances and attributes of individuals with a test, but it is irresponsible to randomly select a test. Before you select a test, or possibly construct your own test, consider (1) whether criterion-referenced measurement or norm-referenced measurement should be used and (2) the criteria for determining a good test—validity, reliability, objectivity, and administrative feasibility.

Criterion-Referenced Measurement

Criterion-referenced measurement is used when individuals are expected to perform at a specific level of achievement. In this type of measurement, one individual's performance is not compared with the performance of others;

a minimum level of acceptable performance (referred to as **criterion behavior**) is described. Most health-related physical fitness tests use criterion-related measurement. In the teaching environment, criterion-referenced measurement involves the use of behavioral objectives that describe the expected level of performance of the individual. The following are examples of criterion-referenced standards:

- For successful completion of the running fitness class, the student must be able to run 2 miles in 14 minutes or less and correctly answer 80% or more of the fitness knowledge test questions.
- For successful completion of the badminton class, the student must correctly answer a minimum of thirty-five questions on the knowledge test.

- To meet the YMCA Physical Fitness Test "good" standard for the bench press, the 18- to 20-year-old female must perform twenty-eight to thirty-two repetitions.
- To meet the ACSM Fitness Test "average" standard for the sit-and-reach test, the 40- to 49-year-old male must score 11–16 inches.

Again, with this type of measurement the individual's performance is not compared with the performances of other individuals.

Criterion-referenced measurement also can be used to determine grades. For example, in a running fitness class the grading standards for males might be as follows:

A: Run 2 miles in 13 minutes or less. Correctly answer 90% or more of the fitness knowledge test questions.

B: Run 2 miles in 13:01 to 13:30. Correctly answer 80% to 89% of the fitness knowledge test questions.

C: Run 2 miles in 13:31 to 14:00. Correctly answer 70% to 79% of the fitness knowledge test questions.

Determining what performance earns an A or any other grade may be a problem. If you choose to use criterion-referenced measurement for grading purposes, the standards should be well planned.

Criterion-referenced measurement has some limitations. When a pass/fail standard is used, it does not show how good or how poor an individual's level of ability is. In addition, when criterion-referenced measurement is used by teachers, too often the standard for success is arbitrary. Remember, we know that measurement may be used for several reasons, so there will be occasions when criterion-referenced measurement is appropriate. For example, criterion-referenced measurement is used with the health-related physical fitness tests described in chapter 15.

Norm-Referenced Measurement

Norm-referenced measurement is used when you wish to interpret each individual's performance on a test in comparison with other individuals' performances. This comparison is done using norms that enable the test administrator to interpret an individual's score in relation to the scores of other individuals in the same population. Examples of norms are percentiles, z-scores, and T-scores. Very often norm-referenced measurement is used by teachers to determine grades, but it may be used for other reasons, such as to establish appropriate levels of achievement for criterion-referenced standards. Norms for tests in physical education are usually reported by gender, weight, height, age, or grade level. In selecting a test with norms, the following factors should be considered:

1. The sample size used to determine the norms—in general, more confidence can be placed in a large sample.
2. The population used to determine the norms—for example, if a basketball skills test has norms for tenth-grade students, only tenth-grade students should have been used to develop the norms. Varsity basketball players or students in other grades should not have been used.
3. The time the norms were established—norms should be updated periodically.

Both criterion-referenced measurement and norm-referenced measurement may be used in the measurement of skills and knowledge. You should recognize when it is appropriate to use each.

❓ARE YOU ABLE TO DO THE FOLLOWING:

- define criterion-referenced and norm-referenced measurement?

Validity

Validity, the most important criterion to consider when evaluating a test, refers to the degree to which a test actually measures what it claims to measure. If a test is designed to measure accuracy of placement in the badminton low short-serve, it should accomplish that objective. In addition, validity is specific to a particular use. For example, although cardiorespiratory fitness may be a factor in a long tennis match, a fitness test should not be used to determine tennis ability. A valid tennis test should measure tennis skill.

Because the validity of tests varies, the selection of one test over another may depend on which test will best measure the desired trait. The validity coefficient indicates how well a test measures what it claims to measure, and, as discussed in chapter 3, the coefficient is determined through correlation techniques. The coefficient may range from -1.00 to $+1.00$, and the closer the coefficient is to $+1.00$, the more valid the test. A test being used as a substitute for another validated test should have a validity coefficient of about 0.80 or more. A test being used for predictive purposes may have a lower validity coefficient. Traditionally, predictive tests with validity coefficients of 0.50 have been accepted.

Validity of Norm-Referenced Tests

There are five types of validity for norm-referenced tests: face, content, predictive, concurrent, and construct validity. The type of validity used depends on the nature of the test and how the test scores are to be used. A test that has a high degree of content validity may not be a valid test to predict future performance. It is important that you understand the validity coefficient and the method used to find it when you select a standardized test or construct your own test.

Face Validity. A test has face validity, or logical validity, when it obviously measures the desired skill or ability. For example, if an individual is asked to run 40 yards as fast as possible, it is clear to the individual that the purpose of the test is to measure running speed. A written test has face validity if the questions are based on the unit or course objectives. Face validity is used often to test components of physical fitness.

When possible, it is best to establish the validity of a test through one of the other described procedures. A written test may be based on unit objectives, but it may contain too few or too many questions related to one or two objectives. Also, an item may appear to measure a physical component but actually not do so. For example, the sit-and-reach test appears to measure hamstring and lower back flexibility, but some studies have not supported this assumption.

Content Validity. Content validity is related to how well a test measures all skills and subject matter that have been presented to the test takers. To have content validity,

a test must measure the objectives for which the test takers are held responsible. As the test administrator you should administer knowledge tests that sample the subject matter covered. This means that regardless of how long or short the test is, it should measure how well the test takers have mastered the objectives. More than likely you would have no problem constructing a test of 150 items that measures the individuals' knowledge of all the subject matter that has been presented, but such a test may be too long for them to complete. To have content validity, the test must be reduced to a realistic number of items *(sample test)* and still represent the total content of the longer test.

Content validity is expected of skills test also. The test should measure the skills emphasized to a group. Content validity for most teacher-made tests is a subjective judgment, but by asking yourself, "Does the test measure what the test takers have been taught?" you will be provided with a good estimate of content validity. It may help to ask your fellow instructors to assist you in answering this question. Content validity also may be found by administering the sample test to a group and administering the total test (referred to as *universal content*) a short time later. The two tests are then correlated (product-moment correlation) to determine the content validity of the sample test.

Predictive Validity. When you wish to estimate future performance, you are concerned with predictive validity. In general, predictive validity is measured by giving a predictor test and correlating it with a criterion measure (obtained at a later date). In physical education, the later time is often after an instructional unit; in athletics, the later time could be after years of development.

The predictor test is the instrument used to measure the trait or ability of individuals. A sports skills test is an example. The criterion measure is the variable that has been defined as indicating successful performance of a skill, but the definition of successful performance is sometimes difficult to determine. One method of determining successful performance is through a panel of experts. For example, a volleyball coach could administer a volleyball skills test to all team members. A panel of experts may be asked to observe the team during games throughout the season and rate the players' performances. At the completion of the season, the coach would correlate (product-moment) the average of the experts' ratings (the criterion measurement) with the skills test administered at the beginning of the season to estimate the predictive validity of the test. College entrance examinations are used as predictor tests, with the criterion measure being success in college. Tests with predictive validity can be of value to you for the grouping of individuals when you know little about their level of skill and you expect improvement in their performance during the instructional unit.

Concurrent Validity. Concurrent validity might be called immediate predictive validity. It indicates how well the individual currently performs a skill. Concurrent validity is determined by correlating test results with a current criterion measurement rather than future information; a test and the criterion measurement are administered at approximately the same time. This procedure is often used to estimate the validity (how well a test measures what it claims to measure) of a test. Concurrent validity can be established in several ways. A new test could be correlated (product-moment) with expert ratings, tournament play, or a previous validity test. These procedures are described in chapter 7.

Concurrent validity is important if you want to administer a test requiring less equipment or time than other tests. To illustrate, consider the following. Maximum oxygen consumption is best measured through direct gas analysis and performance on a treadmill (equipment and time). However, the 12-minute running test is highly correlated with the treadmill test, so the run could be used to estimate the maximum oxygen consumption of an individual.

Construct Validity. Construct validity refers to the degree that the individual possesses a trait (construct), presumed to be reflected in the test performance. Anxiety, intelligence, and motivation are constructs. These qualities cannot be seen with the human eye, yet an individual who possesses one of these characteristics is expected to behave in a certain way. Construct validity applies to testing by the physical educator. The term *cardiorespiratory fitness* may be classified as a construct. Cardiorespiratory fitness tests are often based on the assumption that certain constructs, such as differences in pulse rates or the ability to run a distance in a specified time, reflect cardiorespiratory fitness. That is, the individual with good cardiorespiratory fitness will have a lower pulse rate after physical exertion and will perform better on a running test than the individual with poor cardiorespiratory fitness. Construct validity also applies to the measurement of sports skills. A tennis instructor assumes that when the individual learns the skills of the serve, the forehand and backhand, the overhead smash, and the volley, he or she will be able to put all the skills together and play tennis. These skills are constructs when referring to the total ability to play tennis. If a test includes items that measure these skills (constructs), it has construct validity.

Construct validity can be demonstrated by comparing higher-skilled individuals with lesser-skilled individuals. Again, consider a tennis skills test that is administered to both a tennis class and a varsity tennis team. With a test that has construct validity, the varsity players will most likely score higher than the members of the class.

Validity of Criterion-Referenced Tests

Criterion-referenced validity is related directly to predetermined behavioral objectives. The objectives should be stated in a clear, exact manner and be limited to small segments of the unit of instruction. To estimate the validity of a knowledge test, you should construct the items to parallel the behavioral objectives, and there should be several items for each objective. The validity of each group of items is subjectively estimated by how well they measure the behavioral objective.

A second method requires testing before and after instruction. Validity is accepted if there is significant improvement after instruction or if the behavioral objectives are mastered by an acceptable number of individuals. This method may be used for knowledge and physical performance tests.

The success of criterion-referenced testing depends on the predetermined standard for success. The standard for success should be realistic but high enough that the individuals are ready for the next level of instruction. If the individuals perform successfully at the next level, you can feel confident about the validity of a test.

Domain-referenced validity and **decision validity** are two techniques frequently used to validate criterion-referenced tests. The word *domain* is used to represent the criterion behavior. If the items, or tasks, on a test represent the criterion behavior, the test has logical validity. This logical validity is referred to as domain-referenced validity. This technique is similar to the face (logical) validity used to validate norm-referenced tests (i.e., validity is established through logic rather than through a statistical procedure). A criterion-referenced test usually measures only one skill objective, however.

The following example shows how domain-referenced validity could be determined for a topspin tennis serve test:

1. The topspin tennis serve form (technique) is analyzed (see table 6.1).
2. The most important components of the serve form are selected to be included in the criterion behavior.
3. Successful performance is defined—for example, form, number of successful serves out of attempted serves, and placement and speed of serves.

If this procedure were followed for the tennis forehand or backhand strokes, court position would need to be determined as well as how the ball would be presented to the test taker. (Will someone throw the ball, or will someone hit it?) A similar procedure could be followed for the establishment of domain-referenced validity of any skill test.

Decision validity is used when a test's purpose is to classify individuals as proficient (masters) or nonproficient (nonmasters) of the criterion behavior. With mastery testing, a cutoff score is identified, and individuals scoring above the cutoff score are classified as proficient. Individuals scoring below the score are classified as nonproficient.

Safrit (1986) and Safrit and Wood (1989) describe procedures for estimating domain-referenced and decision validity. You may wish to refer to these references for these descriptions.

Factors Affecting Validity

The validity of a test may be affected by several factors. Four of these factors are as follows:

1. The characteristics of the test takers—A test is valid only for individuals of age, gender, and experience similar to those on whom the test was validated.
2. The criterion measure selected—Several measures have been presented for estimating the validity of a

test. If all measures are correlated with the same set of scores, different correlation coefficients will be found.
3. Reliability—A test must be reliable to be valid. This concept is illustrated in the discussion of reliability later in this chapter.
4. Administrative procedures—If unclear directions are given, or if the test takers do not all perform the test in the same way, the validity will be affected. Environmental factors (e.g., heat and humidity) also may affect validity.

? ARE YOU ABLE TO DO THE FOLLOWING:

- define validity and the types of validity for norm-referenced tests, and give examples of each?
- describe the procedures for determining each type of norm-referenced validity?
- describe the procedures for determining criterion-referenced validity?
- list four factors that affect validity?

Reliability

Reliability refers to the consistency of a test. A reliable test should obtain approximately the same results regardless of the number of times it is given. A test given to a group of individuals on one day should yield the same results if it is given to the same group on another day. Of course, some individuals may not obtain the same score on the second administration of a test because fatigue, motivation, environmental conditions, and measurement error may affect the scores. However, the order of the scores will be approximately the same if the test has reliability.

For a test to have a high degree of validity, it must have a high degree of reliability. If test scores are not reliable, the validity of a test is limited. Imagine administering a test that measures the ability to hit the golf ball for distance to a beginning golf class. Many individuals will have a good score on one attempt but a poor score on another attempt. This lack of consistency influences the validity of the test, though high reliability does not necessarily mean high validity. A test may be consistent, but it may not measure what it claims to measure.

There are several methods to determine reliability, and all are reported in terms of a correlation coefficient that ranges from –1.00 to +1.00. The closer the coefficient value is to +1.00, the greater the reliability of a test. Some tests will have a greater reliability than others. Physical performance tests of running, jumping, and throwing generally have high reliability coefficients, whereas tests such as the tennis serve, badminton serve, and chip shot (in golf) usually have lower reliability coefficients. The lower coefficients are due to subjective judgment when declaring if an object landed within the marked boundaries.

Reliability of Norm-Referenced Tests

Four methods of estimating the reliability of norm-referenced tests are presented here: test-retest, parallel forms, split-half, and Kuder-Richardson Formula 21.

Test-Retest Method. The test-retest method requires two administrations of the same test to the same group of individuals, with the calculation of the correlation coefficient between the two sets of scores. The product-moment correlation method or analysis of variance (intraclass correlation coefficient) may be used to calculate the coefficient. In the school environment the greatest source of error in the test-retest reliability estimate is caused by changes in the students themselves. If knowledge tests are being administered, they are aware of the questions that will be asked on the retest and the answers they provided on the first test. The students also may have discussed the test. When a long interval of time elapses between the test and retest, maturational factors may influence the results of the retest, especially on physical performance tests. The appropriate time interval between administration of tests is sometimes difficult to determine. It could be as short as one day, or as long as several months, but if the test-retest method is used to estimate the reliability coefficient, the time interval must be considered.

Parallel Forms Method. The parallel forms method requires the administration of parallel or equivalent forms of a test to the same group and the calculation of the cor-

relation coefficient (product-moment or intraclass correlation coefficient) between the two sets of scores. Often, both forms are administered during the same test period or in two sessions separated by a short time period. The primary problem associated with this method of estimating reliability is the difficulty of constructing two tests that are parallel in content and item characteristics.

If the two tests are administered within a short time of each other, learning, motivation, and testing conditions do not influence the correlation coefficient. The reliability of most standardized tests in education is estimated through this method.

Split-Half Method. When the split-half method is used, a test is split into halves and the scores of the two halves are correlated. This method requires only one administration of the test and does not require construction of a second test. A common practice is to correlate the odd-numbered items with the even-numbered items. (This method assumes that all individuals being tested will have time to complete the test, so it is not appropriate when speed of completion is a factor in the test.)

The reliability coefficient calculated by this method is for a test of only half the length of the original test. Because reliability usually increases as a test increases in length, the reliability for the full test needs to be estimated. The Spearman-Brown formula is often used for this purpose. The formula is

$$\text{Reliability of full test} = \frac{2 \times \text{reliability on half test}}{1 + \text{reliability on half test}}$$

If the reliability between the two halves is found to be +.80, the reliability of the full test will be found as follows:

$$\text{Reliability of full test} = \frac{2 \times .80}{1 + .80} = \frac{1.60}{1.80} = .89$$

Though the split-half method may produce an inflated correlation coefficient, it is frequently used to estimate reliability coefficients for knowledge tests. It also can be used for some skills tests in which the odd and even trials are correlated.

Kuder-Richardson Formula 21. There are many ways to split a test to compute "half-test" scores for correlational purposes. For each split, however, a different reliability coefficient probably would be obtained. Kuder and Richardson developed a formula, K-R 20, that estimates the average correlation that might be obtained if all possible split-half combinations of a group of items were correlated. Two basic assumptions of the Kuder-Richardson formula are (1) the test items can be scored 1 for correct and 0 for wrong; and (2) the total score is the sum of the item scores. As was indicated with the split-half method, the Kuder-Richardson formula should not be used with a test in which speed of completion is a factor. Since K-R 20 requires much computation, the simpler formula, K-R 21, is often used to provide a rough approximation of K-R 20. The K-R 21 formula is

$$r_{KR} = \frac{n}{n-1}\left(1 - \frac{\overline{X}(n - \overline{X})}{n(s^2)}\right)$$

n = number of items

$\overline{X}$ = test mean (average number of items correct)

s^2 = test variance (variance of items answered correctly)

To illustrate the use of this formula, assume that

$$n = 50, \overline{X} = 40, \text{ and } s^2 = 25$$
$$r_{KR} = \frac{50}{49}\left(1 - \frac{40(50 - 40)}{50(25)}\right)$$
$$= \frac{50}{49}\left(1 - \frac{40(10)}{1000}\right)$$
$$= 1.02(1 - .40)$$
$$r_{KR} = 1.02(.60) = .61$$

Though K-R 21 is widely used, it gives a conservative estimate of reliability when the test items vary in difficulty, as they often do.

Reliability of Criterion-Referenced Tests

The reliability of criterion-referenced tests is defined as consistency of classification, or how consistently the test classifies individuals as masters or nonmasters. Ebel (1979) states that the reliability of criterion-referenced tests can be determined in much the same way as the reliability of norm-referenced tests; that is, test-retest, parallel forms, split-half, or Kuder-Richardson formulas. One important difference, however, is that whereas norm-referenced reliability applies to the total test score, criterion-referenced reliability applies to a single cluster of items (each cluster is intended to measure the attainment of a different objective). In other words, several reliability coefficients, one for each cluster, will be estimated for a criterion-referenced test.

The reliability of criterion-referenced tests may also be estimated through the proportion of agreement coefficient. With this procedure, a test is administered to a group; on the basis of the results of the test scores, each individual is classified as a master or a nonmaster. On another day, the group is administered the same test, and again each individual is classified as master or nonmaster. The proportion of agreement is determined by how many group members are classified as masters on both test days and how many group members are classified as nonmasters on both test days. Some classifications during the two test days may occur because of chance. The coefficient kappa technique may be used to correct for chance agreement. Refer to Safrit (1986) and Safrit and Wood (1989) for a description of this procedure.

Factors Affecting Reliability

The reliability of a test may be affected by many factors, including the following:

1. The method of scoring—The more objective the test, the higher the reliability. A discussion of objectivity follows.
2. The heterogeneity of the group—Coefficients based on scores from 15-year-olds will probably be smaller than those based on a similar-sized group that includes 14-, 15-, and 16-year-olds. Therefore, when the reliability coefficient of a test is based on test scores from a group ranging in abilities, it will be overestimated. If you wish a test to measure a particular skill of 15-year-olds, the reliability coefficient of the test should be based on 15-year-old individuals. When you read background information about a standardized test, note the heterogeneity of the group on which the reliability was estimated.
3. The length of the test—The longer the test, the greater the reliability. This relation is true of physical performance and knowledge tests. Remember, we used the Spearman-Brown formula to demonstrate that the reliability coefficient for a

whole test was larger than the reliability coefficient for one-half of the test.

4. Administrative procedures—The directions must be clear; all test takers should be ready to be tested, motivated to do well, and perform the test in the same way; and the testing environment should be favorable to good performance.

? ARE YOU ABLE TO DO THE FOLLOWING:

- define reliability?
- determine reliability of a test through the test-retest, parallel forms, split-half, and Kuder-Richardson Formula 21 methods?
- list four factors that affect the reliability of a test?

Objectivity

A test has high objectivity when two or more persons can administer the same test to the same group and obtain approximately the same results. Objectivity is a specific form of reliability and can be determined by the test-retest (with different individuals administering the test) correlational procedure. Certain forms of measurement are more objective than others. True-false, multiple-choice, and matching tests have high objectivity when scoring keys are available, whereas essay tests have very low objectivity. Measurements of jumping ability, free-throw shooting, throwing for distance, and success in archery are objective, but judgments of the quality of performance in gymnastics, diving, and figure skating are not.

Objectivity is more likely to take place when the following factors are present:

1. Complete and clear instructions for administration and scoring of the test are given.
2. Trained testers administer the test. All testers must administer the test in the same way.
3. Simple measurement procedures are followed. If the measurements are complicated, mistakes are more likely to occur.
4. Appropriate mechanical tools of measurement are used. Use of appropriate measurement tools decreases the chances for measurement errors.

5. Results are expressed as numerical scores. Scores expressed in phrases or terms are less likely to reflect objectivity.

? ARE YOU ABLE TO DO THE FOLLOWING:

- define objectivity?
- determine the objectivity of a test?
- list the factors that provide for objectivity?

Administrative Feasibility

Administrative feasibility, along with validity, reliability, and objectivity, must be considered when selecting or constructing a test. In fact, if two tests are fairly equal in validity, reliability, and objectivity, the following administrative considerations may determine which test you should choose:

1. Cost—Does the test require expensive equipment that you do not have or cannot afford to purchase?
2. Time—Does the test take too much instructional time? Many authorities recommend that testing use no more than 10% of total instructional time. A test that requires several class or group meetings to administer may not be feasible to administer.
3. Ease of administration—(a) Do you need assistance to administer the test? If so, do you train assistants or ask other instructors to assist you? The training of student testers usually requires much time, but it is essential that whoever administers the test be qualified to do so. (b) Are the instructions easy to follow? The test takers should be able to understand the directions and, regardless of who administers the test, the results should be the same. (c) Is the test reasonable in the demands that are placed on the test takers? They should not be ill or sore after taking the test.
4. Scoring—Will the services of another individual affect the objectivity of the scoring? In an effort to duplicate the actual activity, some tests require the services of another individual (e.g., in some tennis tests, the ball is hit to the person being tested; in softball hitting, the ball is pitched to the hitter). Tests such as these have a place in the measurement of skill, but the helper should be qualified to perform

the services. The scoring of the test should not hinder the differentiation among the levels of ability.

5. Norms—Are norms available to compare your test takers with others? If your test takers score well below published norms, you should attempt to determine the reason. When published test norms are used, the factors described in the discussion of norm-referenced measurement should be considered. As a teacher, you may wish to establish local norms to reflect the progress your students have made in a particular program.

One final comment about a good test: When selecting a sports skills test, try to find a test that is similar to game performance. Individuals enjoy taking this type of test more than taking one that has no resemblance to the game skill for which they are being tested. The use of this type of test is an important component of authentic assessment, which is described in chapter 6.

?ARE YOU ABLE TO DO THE FOLLOWING:

- describe the administrative criteria that should be considered in the selection and construction of tests?

You should now feel capable of selecting good physical performance and knowledge tests. Complete the review problems, and then we'll begin to prepare you to construct knowledge tests.

►REVIEW PROBLEMS◄

1. Describe how you might use criterion-referenced measurement in a seventh-grade soccer class.
2. Select three sports skills tests and three other physical performance tests (e.g., agility, physical fitness, balance) described in this book and determine how well they meet test selection criteria.

5 Construction of Knowledge Tests

Upon completion of this chapter, you should be able to

1. List and describe the steps for knowledge test construction;

2. Construct a table of specifications and explain its use;

3. State the purposes of item analysis;

4. Define item difficulty, index of discrimination, and response quality;

5. Conduct item analysis;

6. Contrast the advantages and disadvantages of various test items; and

7. Construct true-false, multiple-choice, short answer, completion, matching, and essay test items.

Because many good standardized psychomotor tests are available, you may construct only a few of these tests while performing your responsibilities as a physical educator. The same cannot be said of knowledge tests. (The term *knowledge test* refers to tests that measure thought processes.) If you enter the teaching profession, it is likely that you will construct many types of knowledge tests throughout your career. If your responsibilities are in a fitness or wellness club, there probably will be occasions when you will wish to determine the club members' knowledge of health-related matters. The information that you gather from the tests can help you determine the needs of the members and plan appropriate programs.

As you gain experience in constructing knowledge tests, it will be less difficult to complete the task. However, at no time should you feel that a test can be constructed within a few minutes or the night before it is to be administered. It takes time and planning to construct a good knowledge test. You can expect only problems from a haphazard test. In addition, a poorly constructed test will not adequately fulfill the reasons for measurement, as described in chapter 1.

Steps in Construction of a Test

There is more to test construction than writing the items. To construct a good test, you should follow these five steps: test planning, test item construction, test administration, item analysis, and item revision. Guidelines for these five steps, as well as construction of various types of objective items and essay items, are covered in this chapter.

Test Planning

The first step in planning test items is to consider content validity. The test should be representative of the instructional objectives and the content presented in the unit of on. The test should measure how well the student... have fulfilled the objectives of the instructional t.

With the unit objectives in mind, you should next develop a table of test specifications, which serves as an outline for construction of the test. Planning and adhering to a table of test specifications ensure that all material is covered and that the correct weight is given to each area. The table of test specifications indicates the following:

- kinds and number of test items
- kinds of tasks (thought processes) the items will present and number of each kind of task
- content area and number of items in each area

(Some teachers also include an estimate of item difficulty.) Table 5.1 is an example of specifications for a volleyball test.

The most commonly used kinds of objective items are multiple-choice, true-false, matching, and completion. The total number of test items is usually determined by the length of the class period, the length of the items, the difficulty of the items, the conditions under which the test is to be administered, and the age of the students. Students should have time to attempt to answer all of the items when working at a normal rate. You might estimate that the slowest student will be able to answer multiple-choice items at the rate of one per minute and true-false items at the rate of two per minute. As you administer similar tests to similar groups, your ability to estimate the time needed to complete a test will improve.

Several tasks, or thought processes, may be included on a test. In addition to knowledge (factual information), the test may require the students to demonstrate the ability to comprehend, synthesize, evaluate, apply, and analyze. You must decide if you only want a factual information test. Certainly it is easier to construct factual information items. If you attempt to construct the test items in a short period of time, you probably will put together this type of test. Though there is a need for items that measure knowledge, a good test will include various kinds of tasks. With adequate planning and practice, you can develop the skill to write a test with such variety. When you plan the test specifications, plan for different kinds of tasks and the number of items for each task.

The content area deals with the areas covered during instruction. In a physical activity class, content might include such things as history, terminology, rules, equipment, technique or mechanical analysis, strategy, and physiological benefits of participation. Before you begin construction of a test, plan the content areas and the number of items for each area. Too often physical education instructors spend only part of one class period describing the history of an activity and later administer a test that includes many historical questions. A good physical activity class test will include items dealing with rules, equipment, technique, and strategy.

Item difficulty, which is determined by the proportion of students who pass the item, should be related to the purpose of the test. It can be determined only after a test has been administered, and the ability to estimate it improves with experience. (Item difficulty will be discussed later in the section on item analysis.)

Observe table 5.1 again. Notice that fifteen items are related to the rules of volleyball, but only five of the fif-

TABLE 5.1 Specifications for a 50-Item Multiple-Choice Volleyball Test

Content Area	Task (Number of Questions and Percentages of Total)			
	Knowledge	Comprehension	Analysis	Application
History	2 (4%)			
Rules	5 (10%)	5 (10%)		5 (10%)
Technique	2 (4%)	5 (10%)	8 (16%)	
Offensive strategy	4 (8%)			5 (10%)
Defensive strategy	4 (8%)			5 (10%)

teen items are concerned directly with knowledge. The other ten items cover comprehension and application of the rules. Development of test specifications makes you aware of each item's purpose.

Test Item Construction

Regardless of the type of test items you construct, observe the following general guidelines:

1. Allow enough time to complete the test construction. Put it aside after a few hours and work with it again a day or two later. It is rare that anyone is able to construct a good test without time to revise the items.
2. No item should be included on a test unless it covers an important fact, concept, principle, or skill. Ask yourself three questions before you write the item: Why is the student responsible for this? What is the value of this point? What future benefit will it have?
3. Items should be independent of each other. This means that you should avoid items that provide answers to other items; correctly answering one item should not depend on correctly answering a previous item.
4. Write simply and clearly. Using correct grammar is essential, but try using terms and examples that the students understand. Avoid obvious, meaningless, and ambiguous terms. Textbook wording should be used rarely. The item should test the students' ability as related to the subject matter, not their ability to interpret the item.
5. Be flexible. As a general rule the test should include more than one type of item. No one item is best for all situations or all types of material. Also, some students can better demonstrate their ability on certain types of items. (When using more than one type of item, place all items of a particular type together.)
6. If easy items are to be part of the test, place them at the beginning. When students have difficulty with the first few questions, they often are unable to concentrate on the remainder of the test. Easier items will build the confidence of the students.
7. As you construct the items, record the test number of each item in the table of test specifications. (For example, the numbers of the items that cover knowledge of history, application of rules, analysis of technique, and other content areas and tasks are recorded in the appropriate row and column of the table.) You may find that you want to change some of the specifications, but remember to monitor the content area and task of each item.
8. Prepare clear, concise, and complete directions. Leave no doubt as to how the items are to be answered.
9. Ask other instructors to review the test. If they have problems with the wording of an item, it is likely the students will have problems also.

Test Administration

If you have correctly followed the preceding guidelines and also observe the following ones, you likely will have few problems during test administration.

1. Provide a typed copy of the test. It is annoying to have to interpret handwriting when taking a test.
2. Start the test on time. If you have constructed a test that requires approximately 50 minutes to complete, make sure the students have 50 minutes.
3. Be sure the test is administered under normal conditions. Whether you consider the test easy or difficult, it is not fair to the students to have to take the test under abnormal conditions.
4. Read the directions to the students. In their haste to begin the test, many students will begin before reading the directions.

Item Analysis

After you have administered and scored the test, you are ready to determine the quality of the items through a statistical procedure called **item analysis.** Item analysis serves the following purposes:

- indicates which items may be too easy or too difficult
- indicates which items may fail to discriminate clearly between the better and poorer students for reasons other than item difficulty
- indicates why an item has not functioned effectively and how it might be improved
- improves your skills in test construction

The exact procedures used in item analysis depend on the type of items and test, the number of test takers, the computational facilities available, and the purpose of analysis. More confidence can be placed in item analysis when 100 or more tests are analyzed, but you can obtain an indication of the quality of the items through analysis of a smaller number of tests. Most item analyses are concerned with **item difficulty, discrimination power,** and **response quality.** The first three steps in item analysis are as follows:

1. Arrange the scored tests in order from high score to low score.
2. Determine the upper 27% of the test scores and place them in one group. Do the same for the bottom 27% of the test scores. These groups are referred to as upper group (UG) and lower group (LG). Although upper and lower groups of 27% are considered the best for maximizing the difference between the two groups, any percentage between 25% and 33% may be used.
3. Tally the number of times the correct response to each item was chosen on the tests of each group.

Item Difficulty.   Item difficulty is defined as the proportion of test takers who answer an item correctly. If upper and lower groups are not formed, the **difficulty index** (p) may be found by dividing the number of test takers correctly answering each item by the total number taking the test.

$$p = \frac{\text{number answering correctly}}{\text{total number in group}}$$

If fifty students completed a test and thirty-one correctly answered an item, the item difficulty would be .62.

$$p = \frac{31}{50} = .62$$

Another acceptable method for determining the difficulty index requires the use of upper and lower groups.

$$p = \frac{\text{number correct in UG} + \text{number correct in LG}}{\text{number in UG} + \text{number in LG}}$$

If the number of test takers who answered correctly in the upper group is 16, the number who answered correctly in

the lower group is 7, and the total number of test takers in each group is 20, the item difficulty is

$$p = \frac{16 + 7}{20 + 20} = \frac{23}{40} = .58$$

Since it is necessary to separate the test scores into upper and lower groups to determine the index of discrimination, you may prefer to use the second method to determine item difficulty. You should note that an easy item has a high index and a difficult item has a low index.

The typical norm-referenced test includes items with a range of difficulty, but the average test item difficulty should be around 50%. The difficulty for criterion-referenced tests is established at the minimum proficiency level, and, ideally, every student should pass every item at the end of the instructional unit. Because this is an unrealistic goal, however, items on criterion-referenced tests are usually constructed so that at least 80% to 85% of the students are expected to pass.

Interpretation of item difficulty is not always an easy task. The item may be easy either because its construction makes the answer obvious or because the students have learned the material in the item. On the other hand, it may be difficult either because it is constructed poorly or because the students have not learned the material. You should consider all of these things if the item difficulty indicates the item is unacceptable as it has been presented to the students. Table 5.2 shows the indices that may be used to evaluate item difficulty.

TABLE 5.2   Evaluation of Item Difficulty

Difficulty Index	Item Evaluation
.80 and higher	reject item
.71–.79	accept if index of discrimination is acceptable, but revise if discrimination is marginal
.30–.70	accept item
.20–.29	accept if index of discrimination is acceptable, but revise if discrimination is marginal
.19 and below	reject item

Item Discrimination. Item discrimination determines how well the item differentiates between the good student and the poor student. If the item discriminates, more students with high scores will answer the item correctly than will students with low scores. The index of discrimination (D) is found by subtracting the number of correct responses of the lower group from the number of correct responses of the upper group and dividing the difference by the number of scores in each group. The formula is

$$D = \frac{\text{number correct in UG} - \text{number correct in LG}}{\text{number in each group}}$$

With the same values that were used previously to determine an item difficulty of .58, the index of discrimination is

$$D = \frac{16 - 7}{20} = \frac{9}{20} = .45$$

The index of discrimination can range from +1.00 to −1.00, but rarely do these extremes occur. A negative index indicates that more students in the lower group answered the item correctly than did students in the upper group. An item with a negative index has no place in a test. Generally, an index of .40 or above on a norm-referenced test indicates that the item discriminates well.

TABLE 5.3 lists the rules for evaluating the index of discrimination for norm-referenced tests.

The usual item discrimination indices will not work for criterion-referenced tests. One possible way to identify discriminating items for such tests is to administer the same item before instruction (pretest) and after instruction (posttest). Before instruction, few students should answer the item correctly, but after instruction most students should answer it correctly. If there is a large difference in the proportion of correct answers from pretest to posttest, the item discriminates.

A test item with a difficulty index between .30 and .70 has a good chance of being a discriminating item, but you should not assume this always to be true. Before you judge the quality of an item, consider both the difficulty index and the index of discrimination.

Response Quality. The choices of answers for each item in a multiple-choice test are called *responses*. The incorrect responses are referred to as *distractors* or *foils*.

Ideally, in a multiple-choice test, each response should be selected by some of the students. If a response is not selected by any student, it has contributed nothing to the test. As a rule of thumb, a response should be selected by at least 2% to 3% of the test takers.

Another consideration is the pattern of incorrect responses by the upper and lower groups. For example, if an incorrect response is selected by many students in the upper group but few in the lower group, the item might need revision. The item analysis of a multiple-choice test should include a record of the number of students who selected each response as well as the item difficulty and index of discrimination. Table 5.4 shows the analysis of five multiple-choice items.

Item Revision

After completing the item analysis, you are ready to perform any necessary revision. Revision usually involves discarding or rewording some items, changing responses, and changing items to different types (for example, changing multiple-choice items to true-false items). If you perform the preceding steps the first time you administer a test, and analyze and revise the test after at least one additional administration of the test to a similar group, you will have a good test.

TABLE 5.3 Evaluation of Index of Discrimination

Index of Discrimination	Item Evaluation
.40 and above	item discriminates; accept item
.30–.39	item provides reasonably good discrimination; may need improvement, particularly if item difficulty is marginal
.20–.29	item provides marginal discrimination; consider revision
below .20	item does not discriminate; reject item

Source: R. L. Ebel, *Essentials of educational measurement,* 3d ed., Englewood Cliffs, N.J.: Prentice Hall, 1979.

TABLE 5.4 Example of Item Analysis for Multiple-Choice Test

60 students completed the test
Groups of 27% (16 test scores in each group); correct responses in bold print

Item			Responses				p	D
		A	B	C	D		.50	.63
1	Upper Group	1	**13**	2	0			
	Lower Group	4	**3**	5	4			
		A	B	C	D			
2	Upper Group	0	1	**12**	3		.53	.44
	Lower Group	3	4	**5**	4			
		A	B	C	D			
3	Upper Group	0	**8**	0	8		.50	.00
	Lower Group	1	**8**	0	7			
		A	B	C	D			
4	Upper Group	**11**	3	2	0			
	Lower Group	**4**	10	2	0		.47	.44
		A	B	C	D			
5	Upper Group	2	4	3	**7**		.25	.38
	Lower Group	7	4	4	**1**			

Item 1. All responses considered; difficulty and discrimination good. Retain item.
Item 2. All responses considered; difficulty and discrimination good. Retain item.
Item 3. Response C not considered and A considered only once; no discrimination. Reject item.
Item 4. Response D not considered; difficulty and discrimination acceptable. Retain item but replace D.
Item 5. All responses considered; difficulty and discrimination marginal. Revise item.

?ARE YOU ABLE TO DO THE FOLLOWING:

- describe the five steps in constructing knowledge tests?
- construct a table of test specifications and explain its use?
- define item analysis, item difficulty, and index of discrimination and conduct item analysis on test items?

Objective Test Items

Many individuals claim that objective test items permit correct responses through simple recognition, rote memory, or association and do not measure the thought processes of comprehension, analysis, and application. These same individuals also believe that only essay tests can truly measure these thought processes. Objective items can measure different kinds of thought processes, but it takes time and effort to construct the items. [*In the discussion of objective test items, examples of items are provided. The thought process measured by each of the items is indicated in brackets for illustrative purposes. You should not indicate these thought processes on tests that you construct.*]

True-False Items

The true-false item is a declarative statement, and the test taker must decide if the statement is correct or incorrect. The true-false item is widely used in teacher-made tests because items can be written rapidly and scored with ease.

Many teachers limit true-false items to factual content, but they can be used to test applications and principles. In addition, knowledge in the form of propositions can be measured. The following tennis items are examples of propositions:

If the score is 15–30, the server is ahead in points.

If the score is 15–30, the serve should be to the receiver's left service court.

Another excellent way to use the true-false item is to describe a situation and then to ask the students to respond to items about the situation. Game situations and strategies are very appropriate for this approach.

The following are advantages of true-false items:

1. A wide range of material may be covered in a single testing period. The response time required by a true-false item is less than that required by multiple-choice or completion items, so more items can be included on a test.
2. The scoring is easy.
3. In general, items are easy to construct. However, if true-false items are to measure thought processes other than simple knowledge, they will require some time to construct.

The following are disadvantages of true-false items:

1. Because there are only two possible answers, guessing could produce a score of 50% correct. Realizing this, many students do not study as they should.
2. Because the students have a 50% chance of guessing the correct answers, the reliability of the test items tends to be lower than that of other types of items.
3. The correct answer often depends on one word.

Guidelines for Constructing True-False Items. True-false items can be used effectively if you adhere to the following guidelines:

1. Avoid the use of absolute and relative modifiers. Words such as *all, always, never, no,* and *none* are clues that the item is probably false. Words such as *sometimes, usually,* and *typically* suggest that the item is probably true.

2. Include an equal number of true and false items, or include more false items than true ones. False items tend to discriminate more than true items.
3. Avoid the exact language of the textbook.
4. Avoid trick items. For example, using the wrong first name of an individual to make an item false is not a good practice.
5. Avoid negative and double negative terms. The inclusion of double negatives may confuse the students and does not test their ability in terms of the subject matter. If you feel that negative statements should be used, *underline* the negative term or terms.
6. Avoid ambiguous statements. There should be no doubt the statement is completely true or completely false.
7. All items should be of the same approximate length. Some teachers have a tendency to make true statements longer than false statements.
8. Limit each item to a single concept. Items that include more than one concept are often confusing to the students.

One final comment about true-false items: An alternative format for the true-false items is to require the students to correct false statements. The major disadvantage of this technique is that often the item can be corrected in several ways. A better technique is to have the students identify only the false element in the item.

Examples of True-False Items. For each of the following statements, print a *T* in the blank in front of the statement if you believe it to be true and an *F* if you believe it to be false. Each item has a value of 3 points.

_____ 1. If the standard deviation of a group of scores increases, the variability increases. [*comprehension*]

_____ 2. A T-score of 60 is located one standard deviation above the mean. [*knowledge*]

_____ 3. A correlation coefficient of +.60 is twice as significant as a correlation coefficient of +.30. [*analysis*]

_____ 4. If the tail of a distribution curve is to the right, the skew is negative. [*comprehension*]

Read the described tennis situation and the statements that follow. If you believe the statement to be true, print a *T* in the blank in front of the statement. If you believe the statement to be false, print an *F*. Each item has a value of 3 points.

Player A makes a good serve and player B successfully returns it. Either player will now lose a point if

_____ 1. the ball bounces twice on his or her side of the court.

_____ 2. the player hits the ball and it touches the net before it lands in the opponent's court.

_____ 3. after hitting the ball, the racket slips out of the player's hand.

_____ 4. the player hits the ball before it crosses the net. [*application*]

Multiple-Choice Items

The multiple-choice item consists of two main components: the stem and three to five responses (one correct response and two to four incorrect responses, referred to as distractors or foils). The stem may be more than one sentence long, but it is usually a direct question or an incomplete statement. It should present the problem in enough detail so that there is no ambiguity about what is being asked. Multiple-choice items have several advantages:

1. They can measure almost any understanding or ability. However, as do other test items, they measure different abilities only if they are designed to do so. Too often multiple-choice items are constructed to measure only rote memory.
2. They can be used to test most types of material.
3. The chances of guessing the correct answer are much less than they are for true-false items.
4. They can be scored easily.

Multiple-choice items also have several disadvantages:

1. They are more difficult to construct than other objective tests. Considerable time is required to develop good items that each include at least four responses.
2. They sometimes encourage memorization of facts rather than understanding of concepts. As noted earlier, this deficiency can be corrected if the items are well planned.
3. Because fewer items can be asked than with true-false items (owing to the time element), less material can be covered.

Guidelines for Constructing Multiple-Choice Items. Multiple-choice items are not easy to construct, but the following guidelines will aid you in the task:

Stem Construction

1. The stem should be concise, be easy to read and understand, and contain the central issue of the item. It should not be necessary to repeat words in the responses. Avoid the use of irrelevant material in the stem. A properly constructed item has meaning by itself so that the good student knows the correct answer before reading all the responses. If the stem is an incomplete sentence or question, make the responses complete the stem.
2. Avoid absolute modifiers such as *always, never, all, none,* and so on.
3. Avoid negative wording; state the stem positively. If it is necessary to use negative words, capitalize each letter of the words or *underline* them.
4. Although not mandatory, it sometimes helps the student if the stem begins with a *w* word such as *which, why, where, what, when,* or *who.* This introduces the stem with the main point of the item.
5. Do not word the stem so that you are asking the student's opinion. If you use a stem that calls for an opinion, you may have difficulty defending one correct answer.
6. If the item is testing the definition, or meaning, of a word, the word to be defined should be in the stem and the responses should consist of alternative definitions or meanings.

Response Construction

1. All responses should be plausible, but there should be only one correct response. Ridiculous or obvious responses have no place in the test. The student who does not immediately know the correct response after reading the stem should have to consider all responses. If distractors are not chosen by some of the students, they should be eliminated from the test.
2. Use at least four responses for each item. If you can think of five good responses, use them. The use of five responses keeps the guessing factor at .20. However, if you can think of only three acceptable responses for an item, use just three.
3. All responses should be grammatically consistent, homogeneous in content, and approximately the

same length. If some responses begin with a vowel but other responses in the same item do not, use "a(n)" in the stem to introduce the responses. Avoid the tendency to include more information in the correct response than in the incorrect responses (such as wording the stem so that the correct response needs to be qualified).

4. If the items are numbered, use *A, B, C, D,* and *E* to designate the responses. Also, unless limited by the number of pages, place the responses in vertical order rather than horizontal order for ease in reading.

5. Avoid patterns in the positions of the correct responses. Make it a point to place the correct response in each position approximately an equal number of times; that is, use *A, B, C, D,* and *E* equally.

6. Use the response "none of the above" or "all of the above" with care. If you use "none of the above," all options must be clearly wrong, or one must be clearly correct. If the student has only four responses to consider, the use of "all of the above" reduces the student's discrimination task to three responses. It would probably be best to include a plausible fourth response rather than use "all of the above."

7. When possible, list the responses in logical or sequential order. When variables or dates are arranged in sequence, the correct response occasionally should be first or last in the sequence. This arrangement helps the student to overcome the tendency to disregard the extremes of the sequence as probably not correct.

Examples of Multiple-Choice Items.   Print the letter of the one correct answer on the blank line to the left of the item number. Each item has a value of 2 points.

_____ 1. For a knowledge test, a score of 55 has a percentile rank of 40. What do these values indicate?
  A. 40 students answered 55% of the test correctly.
  B. 40% of the students had a score of 55 or less.
  C. 55% of the students had a score of 40 or less.

  D. 40% of the students had a score of 55 or more. [*analysis*]

_____ 2. If the correlation coefficient between two variables is −.80,
  A. the relationship is quite small.
  B. the relationship does not always exist.
  C. the two variables are significantly unrelated.
  D. the value of one variable decreases as the value of the other variable decreases.
  E. the value of one variable increases as the value of the other variable decreases. [*comprehension*]

_____ 3. Which muscle extends the lower leg and flexes the upper leg?
  A. quadriceps femoris
  B. biceps femoris
  C. gluteus maximus
  D. gastrocnemius [*knowledge*]

_____ 4. What is the approximate maximum heart rate (beats per minute) of a 20-year-old individual?
  A. 180
  B. 190
  C. 200
  D. 210 [*application*]

Short-Answer and Completion Items

The differences between a short-answer item and a completion item are primarily the length and the format of the response. A short-answer item requires the student to respond to a question in a word, a phrase, or a sentence or two. In a completion item, the simplest short-answer form, one to several words are omitted from a sentence, and the student is asked to provide the missing information. Both items are suited to measure factual knowledge, comprehension of principles, and ability to identify and define concepts. Identification items also are a form of short-answer items.

The advantages of short-answer and completion items are the following:

1. They are affected much less by guessing than are true-false or multiple-choice items.
2. They come closer to assessing recall, as contrasted with recognition, than does any other type of

objective test item. Recall usually requires intensive study on the part of the student.

3. They are valuable when steps or procedures are to be learned.
4. They are easy to construct.

The disadvantages of these items are the following:

1. Scoring takes longer than for choice-type items, especially when only correct spelling is accepted.
2. Often, unless extreme care is taken in the construction of each item, a number of answers might be wholly or partially correct. The scorer has to decide which responses are acceptable and how much credit to give for each variation. This feature usually means that only the test constructor is able to score the tests.
3. They encourage rote learning; however, there are occasions when recall and memorization are appropriate (first aid and cardiopulmonary resuscitation [CPR], for example).

Guidelines for Constructing Short-Answer and Completion Items.
Though short-answer and completion items are easier to construct than other objective test items, these guidelines should be observed when constructing the items:

1. Be sure that the item can be answered with a unique word, phrase, or number and that only one answer is correct.
2. Be sure the students know what type of response is required. Indicate also how precise the response should be. (Specifying the level of precision is especially important when computation of fractions or decimals is involved.)
3. Think of the answer first. Then try to write an item to which that answer is the only appropriate answer. By using this approach you can avoid constructing items that have multiple correct answers.
4. With completion items, try to place the blank near the end of the sentence. This placement usually makes the intent of the item clearer and avoids the possibility of multiple answers.
5. Use no more than two blanks in an item. Too many blanks make the item confusing to the student.
6. Avoid lifting items directly from the textbook. One sentence taken out of context from a paragraph may fail to adequately present the concept of the entire paragraph.
7. Make the actual blanks for the responses the same length. Varying the length of the blank according to the length of the expected answer provides clues for the students. (For ease of scoring, provide short blank lines in the item and blank lines of appropriate length in a column to the right or left of the items for the student to write the responses.)

Examples of Short-Answer Items.
Answer the following questions. They have a value of 3 points each.

1. What are the three measures of central tendency? [knowledge]
2. In a study of leg strength and hand grip, a correlation of −.90 was found. Interpret this correlation. [comprehension]
3. In a distribution of scores, the mean is 22 and the standard deviation is 2. What percent of the scores are between the scores of 16 and 28? [application]

Examples of Completion Items.
Complete the items by writing the correct answer on the blank line to the left of each item. Each item has a value of 2 points.

_____ 1. The _____ is usually the most reliable measure of variability. [knowledge]
_____ 2. A T-score of 75 is found _____ standard deviations above the mean. [application]
_____ 3. In a T-scale, the mean is assigned to a T-score of _____. [knowledge]

Matching Items

The matching test usually consists of a column of items (stimulus words or phrases) on the left-hand side of a page and a column of options (alternatives) on the right. The student's task is to select the option that is correctly associated with the item. Matching items are similar to multiple-choice items in that the options serve as alternatives for all the items. They also are similar to short-answer items because they usually are limited to specific factual information (names, dates, labels).

The following are advantages of matching items:

1. They are easy to construct and score.
2. They provide many scoreable responses on each test page or for each unit of testing time.

3. They motivate students to integrate their knowledge and to consider relations among the items.

4. The odds of guessing the correct answer are low.

The following are disadvantages of matching items:

1. They are time consuming for students to complete.

2. They usually test only factual information.

3. They are limited to association tasks.

Guidelines for Constructing Matching Items. To construct an effective and fair matching item test, use the following guidelines:

1. Include only homogeneous material in each matching exercise.

2. Make the basis for matching each item and option clear in the directions. The directions should inform the students if an option can be used more than once, if each item has only one correct answer, and how the marking is to be done.

3. Keep the sets of items relatively short (five or six in the lower grades and ten to fifteen in the upper grades). The shorter lists enable the students to respond more rapidly. If more matches are desired, arrange for several matching groups within a single test. Ideally, each group of matching items will involve a different topic.

4. Place all items and options for a matching exercise on one page. This arrangement enables the students to complete the exercise in less time and reduces the likelihood of errors caused by turning pages back and forth.

5. Use an appropriate format. Usually it is best to list the homogeneous items on the left and the options on the right. For ease of scoring, leave a blank space beside each numbered item for the letter of the matched option.

6. Arrange the responses in alphabetical or logical order. This arrangement reduces the time required for the student to find the correct answer.

7. Develop more options than items. Having two or three more options will reduce guessing.

Examples of Matching Items. Select the letter of one option from Column II that best associates with a term in Column I. Print your answer on the appropriate line. Each response has a value of 3 points. [*knowledge or association*]

Column I	Column II
_____ 1. Turnverein	A. Bloomer
_____ 2. Royal Central Institute of Gymnastics	B. Hitchcock
	C. Jahn
_____ 3. vertical jump	D. Ling
_____ 4. physical education costume for women	E. Naismith
	F. Sargent
_____ 5. basketball	G. Williams

Essay Test Items

All the test items we have covered are considered objective items. The final item to be discussed is the essay item, which is evaluated subjectively. Essay items are designed to measure the students' ability to use higher mental processes—identifying, interpreting, integrating, organizing, and synthesizing—and to express themselves by writing. [*In the provided examples of essay questions, the measured thought processes are indicated in brackets for illustrative purposes. You should not indicate the measured thought processes on your constructed tests.*]

The following are advantages of essay items:

1. They are easily and quickly constructed.

2. They can measure complex concepts, thinking ability, and problem-solving skills.

3. They encourage students to learn how to effectively organize and express their own ideas.

4. They minimize guessing.

The following are disadvantages of essay items:

1. They usually are very time consuming to score.

2. The scoring requires some decision making on the part of the scorer; thus, reliability may be decreased.

3. Because they take longer to answer, only a few items can be answered during one class period. This time constraint limits the field of knowledge that can be covered.

Guidelines for Constructing Essay Items

Though essay items seem the easiest test items to construct, the following guidelines should be observed when preparing them:

1. They should require the students to demonstrate a command of essential knowledge. Too often essay items call only for reproduction of materials presented in the textbook or class lectures.

2. Each item should be phrased so that only one answer is correct. When items have more than one correct answer, it is difficult to evaluate the student's level of achievement.

3. Indicate the scope and direction of the required answer. Vague phrasing leads to a wide variation of responses and makes the task of evaluating the items even more difficult.

4. Require all students to answer the same items. If students answer different items, the basis for comparing the scores is limited. When students choose the items they can answer best, the range of test scores will probably be smaller, decreasing the reliability of the scores.

5. Indicate the approximate amount of time for the students to devote to each item, and the point value of each item. Many students need guidelines in how to budget their working time. In addition, stating the amount of time that should be devoted to each item gives a clue as to the detail expected on a given item.

6. In general, it is better to use several short essay items rather than a few long ones. Short essay items are likely to be less ambiguous to the student and easier to score.

7. Write the ideal answer to the item. Writing the ideal answer gives you a clear idea of the item's reason and aids you in scoring the item.

Guidelines for Scoring Essay Items

Essay items can be difficult to evaluate. These guidelines may help.

1. Develop a method for scoring the tests. Some teachers identify essential points that should be included. Other teachers rank each item according to the quality of response.

2. Evaluate the same item on all the students' papers before going on to the next item. It is also wise to occasionally check your consistency by reviewing how you evaluated an item on the first few papers you scored.

3. Try to conceal the name of the student whose test you are evaluating. Not knowing whose paper is being evaluated prevents the influence of any biases you may have toward students.

Examples of Essay Items

Read each item carefully and answer each one as completely as possible. The approximate amount of time that you should spend on each item and the point value of each item are indicated in parentheses.

1. Define *correlation,* and contrast the Spearman rank-difference correlation coefficient and the Pearson product-moment correlation. (10 minutes, 20 points) [*analysis, interpretation, organization, application*]

2. Define *standard scores,* and contrast T-scores, z-scores, and percentiles. (10 minutes, 20 points) [*analysis, interpretation, organization, application*]

3. A teacher is interested in determining whether her new teaching method is effective. Describe how she can determine its effectiveness. Include in your discussion
   a. what testing procedures she should use;
   b. when she should test; and
   c. what statistical analysis she should use. (15 minutes, 30 points) [*synthesis, integration, comprehension, analysis, application*]

⁇ ARE YOU ABLE TO DO THE FOLLOWING:

- contrast the advantages and disadvantages of the objective and essay items described in the text?
- construct true-false, multiple-choice, short answer and completion, matching, and essay test items?

You have completed your study of knowledge test items. As you now know, much work is required for construction of a good test, and each type of test item has advantages and disadvantages. All test items, however, can serve to measure the cognitive achievement of the students if the items are well constructed.

1. Construct a knowledge test for a high school tennis class. The test should include a table of specifications, thirty multiple-choice items, and twenty true-false items. Ask a friend to take the test and provide comments about any items that might need to be rephrased or responses that are obviously incorrect or obviously correct.

2. A physical education teacher administered a fifty-item knowledge test to her 200 ninth-grade students. After scoring the tests, she determined the upper 27% and the lower 27% of the scores. She tabulated the following results for the first five items:

Item	Group	No. of Correct Answers
1.	Upper	44
	Lower	8
2.	Upper	45
	Lower	39
3.	Upper	35
	Lower	28
4.	Upper	14
	Lower	2
5.	Upper	37
	Lower	14

Calculate the item difficulty and index of discrimination for each item, and interpret your findings.

6

Assessing and Grading the Students

Upon completion of this chapter, you should be able to

1. Define assessment, formative assessment, and summative assessment;

2. List and describe the characteristics of authentic assessment;

3. Describe portfolio assessment;

4. List and describe the use of grades;

5. List the three behavior areas and the factors commonly graded in these areas, and state why some factors should not be graded;

6. List and describe the criteria for grades;

7. Define norm-referenced grading and the grading methods of natural breaks, standard deviation, percentage, and norm, then describe the advantages and disadvantages of these methods;

8. Define criterion-referenced grading and the grading methods of contract and percentage correct, then describe the advantages and disadvantages of these methods;

9. Define the weighting of factors and describe a method for performing this technique;

10. Describe four methods for reporting term grades; and

11. Describe your grading philosophy and develop a grading method that could be used in a teaching assignment.

Assessment and the assignment of grades are two important teaching responsibilities. These responsibilities are related, but they are also separate responsibilities. Occasionally, some individuals will use the words *assessment* and *evaluation* interchangeably. You should recall how these terms were defined in chapter 1. Evaluation is the interpretation of measurement; evaluation is an important part of assessment. Assessment is a process that includes measurement, evaluation, identification, and prescription.

Assessment should be performed continuously throughout the teaching of a skill. Through assessment the teacher can help the students perform at their maximum level and succeed in their class endeavors. Grading means that the teacher determines (through assessment) the achievement level of each student toward class objectives and assigns the appropriate grade at the conclusion of the teaching unit. Many U.S. citizens do not believe teachers are fulfilling these responsibilities in an acceptable manner. Because of demands for school improvement and accountability for student learning, individuals and professional groups are seeking better ways to assess student performance. As a result of these efforts, many school programs expect teachers to conduct **authentic assessment** of students. Authentic assessment provides ways for data or information to be gathered and organized so that accurate judgments can be made about each student. Once class goals have been stated, authentic assessment allows a teacher to do the following:

- monitor the students' performance and determine where they are experiencing difficulties
- prescribe a correction for learning problems
- keep track of students' progress toward class goals and objectives
- fairly assign grades

Characteristics of Authentic Assessment

Authentic assessment includes the characteristics described below. By including these characteristics, the teacher will experience greater success with authentic assessment.

Formal Record Keeping

Authentic assessment requires the maintenance of formal records. The completion of accurate records is time consuming, and, although the teacher is responsible for the records, students may assist in this function. The need for records and the role of the students in completing these records will be described in the context of other authentic assessment characteristics.

Natural Surroundings

Authentic assessment is conducted while students are performing in a game or under gamelike conditions. Skills tests may be used for authentic assessment, but the students should be able to connect the expected skills to real-life (game) situations. For this reason, skill test components should be as gamelike as possible. In addition, rating charts of the skills that have been taught may be used to assess the students during game participation or skill practice. The form or technique of the students can be documented with the appropriate chart (described later in this chapter). Records also may be kept of the students' successful completion of skills during game play. The number of tennis serves returned during a match, the number of rebounds during a basketball game, and the number of successful passes during a soccer match are examples of the types of skills that can be recorded.

Formative and Summative Assessment

When conducted throughout the teaching unit, authentic assessment enables the teacher to provide students with regular feedback about progress toward the class goals and objectives. This assessment, called **formative assessment,** allows teachers to diagnose learning problems and prescribe any necessary changes in the teaching unit. Regular assessment does not imply daily assessment, but it does mean that it is done routinely and is not limited to designated testing times or days. Further, when done as part of the regular teaching process, authentic assessment can serve to motivate students to achieve the learning goals. Authentic assessment also should determine students' achievements of class goals and objectives at the conclusion of the teaching unit (called **summative assessment**). Typically, summative assessment is used in the assigning of grades, but both types of assessment should be used.

Technique (Form) and End Result

Assessments of each student's technique or form in performing the skills are conducted in authentic assessment. This assessment may be more subjective than objective, but the use of checklists, rating charts, and criteria sheets will make the assessment more objective (an example of a checklist for the topspin tennis serve is provided in table 6.1). This assessment is especially useful when the end result of a performance is not good even though the student's form is mechanically sound. The golf swing, tennis stroke, archery form, and heading of a soccer ball are examples of such skills.

The end result also should be assessed. Does the golf ball land in the desired area? Does the tennis ball go over the net and land in the appropriate area of the court? Does the arrow hit the target? Is the soccer ball headed in the right direction with the appropriate height? This assessment usually can be objectively scored (counted, mea-

TABLE 6.1   Checklist for Topspin Tennis Serve (Right-Handed Player)

Yes	No	Preparation
____	____	Continental grip (racket is held 1/8 of a turn from Eastern grip)
____	____	Body sideways to net
____	____	Lower arm straight from elbow to fingers
____	____	Feet spread about shoulder-width apart
____	____	Court position correct in relation to center mark
____	____	Ball held in thumb and first three fingers
____	____	Hand with ball placed lightly against racket face
____	____	Racket held at waist height and pointed toward service court

Yes	No	Toss
____	____	Both hands drop simultaneously
____	____	Racket hand moves across and in front of body
____	____	Weight shifts to back foot as racket goes back
____	____	Both hands are lifted into a Y shape
____	____	Tossing arm extends completely before ball is released
____	____	As ball leaves hand, racket is lowered into back-scratching position with palm of racket hand near ear
____	____	Toss is slightly higher than server can reach
____	____	If ball were allowed to drop, it would hit court in front of baseline and in front of heel

Yes	No	Contact
____	____	Shoulders turn in throwing motion as ball rises
____	____	Weight shifts to front foot as racket is "thrown" at ball
____	____	Racket comes forward just as ball begins to drop; contact is made at the 1:00 position with slight outward roll of the forearm

Yes	No	Follow-Through
____	____	Racket continues through ball toward target and finishes across body
____	____	Palm of racket hand faces back leg
____	____	Right leg falls across the baseline into playing court

sured, or timed). Skills tests often are used to assess the end result.

Self-Assessment and Peer Assessment

Authentic assessment should include student self-assessment and peer assessment. The teacher should explain and demonstrate assessment techniques, but the students can be taught how to assess their own skill. The students must understand how the assessments will be used and the necessity of accuracy and consistency.

End-result assessment usually is easy for the students to conduct. Just as the teacher does, the students count, time, or measure their own or their peers' performance. Daily accomplishments can be recorded as well as the number of times a skill is practiced. Directions as to how the end result is to be recorded should be provided.

Technique assessment is more difficult for the students. Charts or forms that include clearly stated performance criteria must be provided. The same charts or forms used by the teacher can be used by the students (see table 6.1). Students may perform self-assessment if

Assessing and Grading the Students   **81**

their performance can be videotaped; otherwise, peer assessment of technique probably is best. The teacher should spot-check the records and regularly review performance expectations. In addition to assisting in the assessment process, watching and analyzing the performance of their peers will help the students learn more about a skill.

Portfolio Assessment

Portfolio assessment can be included in authentic assessment. With portfolio assessment, the students are responsible for the collection of the portfolio contents. The portfolio may include written assignments (e.g., analysis of a skill and historical report of a sport); a preassessment of skill level; performance goals; a planned program for improvement; a self-assessment of performance through a videotape; a technique or form assessment by a peer; a record of practice sessions; written tests; class notes; and other items on which the teacher and students have agreed. The purpose of the portfolio is to document and exhibit the students' progress, achievements, and effort. In addition, the teacher may use the students' portfolios to determine if class objectives were fulfilled, to communicate with parents, and to evaluate the program.

If portfolio assessment is used, the students must understand how the portfolio will be evaluated. In addition, guidelines and directions should be provided regarding organization and construction style. The following are a few important considerations: What is the date of completion? Is there a designated form for skill assessment? Are all items to be dated and placed in a notebook, or may some other method be used? When and where will the portfolios be collected? When and where will they be returned? Other considerations will become apparent as portfolio assessment is used. It is important to communicate these considerations to the students early in the process.

Grading

As we begin the discussion of grading in physical education, think back to your junior and senior high school days. Do you remember the grades you received in your physical education classes? Do you remember the factors that were used to determine your grades? Did you and the other students feel you were graded fairly? Your instruc-

tors may have explained the factors that would be used to determine the grades and that all students would be evaluated objectively, but many instructors do not choose objective factors for grade determination. Instead, they base grades merely on attendance, participation, and effort. Students who miss some classes, fail to always take part in class activities, and appear to be giving less than their best effort do not receive high grades. In other words, the instructor subjectively categorizes the students. There is nothing wrong with rewarding students for effort, but grades earned in physical education classes should involve more than attendance, participation, and effort.

Proponents of grades based on participation argue that if objective grading is used, some students earn low grades and lose interest in physical education. It is possible that a few students who do not earn high grades will be upset, but they will not lose interest in a class because of grades. They lose interest when effective teaching does not take place. Effective teaching includes fair and objective grading.

Grades are recognized as symbols that denote progress and achievement toward established criterion-referenced or norm-referenced course objectives. As the teacher, you will decide whether the course objectives will be criterion-referenced or norm-referenced, but grades should always be related to the objectives. Different acceptable grading methods are available, and formative and summative assessment can be used with most, if not all, of them. The choice is yours. It is essential, however, that you be consistent and fair.

Use of Grades

If you enter the teaching profession, you will have the responsibility of reporting grades for every one of your students each term. Grades may be reported differently, but they have important uses for four groups: students, parents, teachers, and administrators. You should be prepared to discuss with the four groups your grading policies and how you determine the students' grades.

Students

Grades inform the students of their achievement levels. When students know the course objectives, the evaluation methods, and the grade standards, they usually are not surprised by the grades they earn. However, most students like to be informed of their achievement levels by the teacher, and certain students will be challenged by this feedback to work for higher marks. This motivation is more likely to occur if you provide feedback to the students throughout the term and if the students feel that you have a sincere interest in them. Unfortunately, for some students a good grade, rather than the attainment of course objectives, becomes the primary goal. Though it is difficult to prevent, you should attempt to counsel the students about this type of attitude.

Parents

Grades inform the parents of the progress and achievement of their children. Displeased when their children do not get the grades hoped for, some parents will ask you why their son or daughter did not receive a better grade in physical education. You will have a difficult time with many of these parents if you explain that their children did not have a good attitude, did not work hard enough in the class, and therefore did not deserve a better grade. On the other hand, if you explain the objectives of the instructional unit and how you evaluate the students, and provide the scores their children earned, your task will be less difficult. Not all parents will agree with your methods of evaluation, but at least they will understand and probably appreciate the seriousness with which you consider grades. You may avoid such disagreements by sending the parents information about the purposes and objectives of physical education, and your grading philosophy, at the beginning of the school year.

Teachers

To determine the students' grades, you must do a comprehensive evaluation of all students. This evaluation will enable you to better know the strengths and weaknesses of the students. In addition, after evaluating the accomplishments of the students, you can evaluate the effectiveness of your teaching and the efficiency of the program. If many students are failing to complete the objectives of the program, you need to examine your teaching methodology and the expectations of the program. It may be necessary to make changes in both.

The students' grades from previous physical education classes may be beneficial to you at the beginning of each school year. If the grades indicate the students' level of skill, you can readily identify the higher-skilled students and, if necessary, group the students. However, since different factors often are used to determine grades in physical education, you should assume that the grades indicate the skill level of the students only if you are familiar with the grading philosophy of the previous teacher.

Administrators

School administrators use grades to make decisions related to promotion, graduation, academic honors, athletic eligibility, and guidance. They also use grades to determine if students have fulfilled educational objectives. Further, administrators place grades in every student's permanent record, which can have a positive or negative influence when the student applies for a job or admission to college.

?ARE YOU ABLE TO DO THE FOLLOWING:

- list and describe the uses of grades?

Factors Used in Grading

Many factors are used by physical educators to determine the grades of students. All factors can be grouped into three behavior areas: affective, cognitive, and psychomotor.

Affective Factors

Participation in a physical education program should influence the affective behavior (attitudes and feelings) of students. Let's examine the factors that are usually considered to reflect affective behavior. (Affective behavior measurement is covered in chapter 19.)

Sportsmanship. You always should insist that the students play fairly. They should exhibit good sportsmanship as winners or losers in a game or event. Those who do not should be disciplined. But, can you expect students who exhibit poor sportsmanship at the beginning of the term to change after participation in your class?

Usually, poor sportsmanship is due to emotional problems other than those that arise during a game situation, and more than grades is required to improve these behaviors. When sportsmanship is used in determining the grade, students are likely to interpret their grade as a penalty for misbehavior rather than as something that is earned.

Perhaps the best method for dealing with sportsmanship problems is to insist upon sportsmanship during class participation and to individually counsel students about their behavior. This method requires that you keep written records of incidents of poor sportsmanship. Try this approach, and your students may realize that you have a sincere interest in their personal development.

Attendance, Participation, and Showering. Skill development takes place through proper instruction, participation, and practice of fundamentals. Students who fail to attend class regularly and who have poor skills usually do not improve or fulfill other course objectives. If grades are related to the extent that the students fulfill course objectives, students who do not regularly attend class and who have poor skills will not earn good grades. A teacher may not have an attendance policy, but these students will be penalized for their poor attendance.

On the other hand, there may be highly skilled students who are able to complete the course objectives at a satisfactory level, or better, without regular attendance. Should you lower the grades of these students? Since most school programs have attendance policies, problems related to attendance should be handled by the principal, not by the teacher. Base your grades on completion of course objectives, not on attendance.

Perhaps more of a problem occurs when students attend class but, for some reason, do not come dressed to participate. Again, it is best not to use the grade as a threat but to attempt to make the class enjoyable and challenging for the students. If you are successful in developing this type of class atmosphere, the students will want to participate.

Similar to these two factors is the practice of grading the students on showering. Though the students should be instructed in the importance of showering after physical activity, there may be reasons that some students do not want to shower. For example, the showers may not permit privacy for the students who desire it. Or, the instructor may not allow enough time to cool down before showering. Even if these are not the reasons students avoid showering, grading for showering is not a good practice. Advise and encourage, but do not reward students for showering or penalize them for failing to shower.

Effort. Effort is difficult to evaluate objectively. A poorly skilled individual may appear to be putting forth much effort, whereas a highly skilled individual appears to be putting forth little effort. Should the highly skilled student be penalized? If effort is graded, it is possible that the poorly skilled individual will receive the same grade as the highly skilled individual. Is it fair to give these two students the same grade? Some teachers argue that when effort is graded the students are motivated to try harder. Perhaps this is true, but as a teacher you have the responsibility to promote inner motivation. Even though it sounds idealistic, the students' desire to excel should come from within, not from external rewards.

If you wish to include effort as a course requirement, seek to develop an objective method for evaluating it. The authentic assessment techniques described earlier can be used to document effort. You also should develop realistic grading standards so that anyone who puts forth the effort can at least meet the minimum standards for the class.

Cognitive Factors

General agreement exists that grading in physical education should include mental factors. Though many teachers limit the cognitive evaluation to knowledge of rules, history, and fundamentals, the student also should be required to demonstrate the ability to understand, apply, and analyze rules, strategy, and technique. As stated in chapter 5, it takes time to construct tests that properly measure these factors, but the teacher has the responsibility to do so.

Psychomotor Factors

Most physical educators grade the psychomotor skill of students. The degree of emphasis will vary, but teachers usually grade skill in terms of the activity, game performance, and fitness.

The Activity. Two aspects of skill are generally used when grading the skill in an activity: achievement and improvement. Grading for achievement consists of measuring the skill of the students at the conclusion of an instructional unit and assigning the appropriate grades. As they will for any cognitive or psychomotor skill, the levels of ability will vary; unless the standards for skill are very low, only a portion of the students are likely to earn high grades.

Perhaps the most important consideration when grading skill achievement is to establish realistic norm-referenced or criterion-referenced objectives. If a school system has a coordinated physical education program, it is easier to plan realistic objectives because teachers are aware of the students' movement experiences. Knowing the physical education objectives for the previous years and the skills the students were expected to develop enables a teacher to plan the appropriate objectives.

When a class has some students with limited movement experiences and other students with good movement experiences, it is difficult to establish fair objectives. The skill objective may be too low for the students with good movement backgrounds and too difficult for the other students. (The availability of beginning and advanced classes helps prevent this problem, but such classes are not always possible in many school programs.) When this dilemma does occur, the approach of some teachers is to homogeneously group the students in a class and use different grading standards for each group. However, if this method is used, problems can occur: (1) some students with better than average skill may deliberately seek to be placed in the lower-skilled group in an attempt to ensure a good grade; and (2) if the student's record does not indicate placement in a beginning or advanced class, what do the grades for the different groups mean? Does the grade of B earned by a student in the lower-skilled group mean the same as a B earned by a student in the higher-skilled group? For these reasons, many physical education teachers agree that the level of achievement should be evaluated in the same way for all students in a particular class.

Some physical educators believe that students should be graded on skill improvement. It is desirable that all students improve their skill through participation in a physical education instructional unit, but is it fair to all students to grade on improvement? In addition, can improvement be measured accurately? Usually, improvement is measured by administering one test at the beginning and another at the end of an instructional unit and subtracting the first score from the second score. The difference in the scores is interpreted as the improvement score. Several problems are associated with this technique:

1. When students know that improvement is a factor in grading, some may deliberately score low on the first test to show much improvement on the second.
2. Testing some skills before a minimum level of proficiency has been developed can be dangerous (in gymnastics and wrestling, for example). In addition, fitness testing should not be done on poorly conditioned individuals.
3. For some activities, the instructional term may not be long enough for students to practice and show improvement. Also, if the instructional term is too long, the improvement of some students may be due to physical maturity rather than ability.
4. If all students perform at their best on the test given at the beginning of the instructional unit, the low-skilled students may have an advantage in the earning of high grades because they have greater potential for improvement. The high-skilled students will probably improve very little. To correct for this inequity, the instructor must develop a scale for improvement for each skill level. Several hundred scores should be collected and analyzed to develop such a scale. The students with high skill should not be expected to improve as much as the students with low skill.
5. Subject areas such as math, English, science, and history do not grade on improvement. If physical education is to be viewed in the same way as other subjects, grades should not be based on improvement.

You can see that the disadvantages of grading on improvement appear to far outweigh the advantages. If you feel that it is important to report improvement, do so with a form separate from the grade report.

Game Performance.   Grading game performance for individual activities may be done through tournament play. Tournaments should be double elimination or round-robin play, however. Game performance also may be graded through the authentic assessment procedures previously described in this chapter.

Fitness. Though the educational objective of physical fitness is unique to physical education, many physical educators do not include it in the grading process of all activities. It may not be practical to provide class time in all instructional units for fitness activities, but after a fitness unit has been completed, the students should be expected to maintain a specified level of physical fitness throughout the school term. The specific level of fitness for each student may vary, however. In addition, it is probably best to avoid the use of fitness tests for grading purposes. If physical fitness is a factor in the grading process, perhaps it is best to permit the students to earn participation points in fitness activities. The reasons for measurement of physical fitness are discussed in chapter 15.

❓ARE YOU ABLE TO DO THE FOLLOWING:

- list the three behavior areas and the factors commonly graded in these areas, and state the reasons why some of these factors should not be graded?

Criteria for Grades

As you now are aware, many factors can be considered in the grading of students. Some factors can be accurately and fairly graded, but other factors should be reported directly to the students and parents (rather than included in the reported grade). Barrow and McGee (1979) provide the following criteria for grades. If you observe these criteria, you will have a grading process that is educationally sound and fair to the students.

1. Grades should be *related to the educational objectives*. If a factor has not been included as an instructional objective, it should not be graded.
2. The grades should have *validity, reliability,* and *objectivity*. Grades should indicate achievement of the factors that they purportedly represent. The validity of a grading method is low when the grades are not related to the instructional objectives.

    A grading system should be consistent. It should yield the same grade for the same performance, regardless of the number of times the grade is calculated. In addition, unless modifications are made, it should yield the same results for the same performance from year to year.

    Though it may be necessary to grade some factors subjectively (e.g., gymnastics), a grading system should be as objective as possible. A grading system has high objectivity if several teachers can perform the same measurements on students and arrive at the same final grade. If some factors can be measured only subjectively, checklists or rating scales should be used. Grades that are determined subjectively are usually unreliable and difficult to defend if challenged.

3. The **weight** (the percentage or portion of the total grade) of each graded factor should be related to the emphasis placed on the factor during the instructional unit. It is possible, but unlikely, that all graded factors will have equal weight. (Assigning weights to factors will be discussed later in this chapter.)
4. The weights of the factors and the method with which the final grade is determined should be *understandable* to the students and parents. Each student should be able to determine the earned grade before it is provided by the teacher. The technique for determining grades should neither be a secret to the students and parents nor so complicated that they do not understand it.
5. Whether grades are norm-referenced or criterion-referenced, they should *discriminate* the good student from the poor student. Students who perform at a high level should receive better grades than students who perform at a lower level. As in other subject areas, physical education grades should discriminate between the levels of attainment.
6. The grades should have *administrative economy*. An educationally sound grading system should be used, but the system should be feasible in terms of time, cost, and personnel. Remember, clerical help for the teacher is limited, and grades must be prepared in a short time period. If the grading system requires so much time that other teaching responsibilities suffer, it is not practical. Microcomputers are now being used to record and determine grades, giving teachers more time for class preparation.

- list and describe grading criteria?

Methods of Grading

Many grading methods are used by physical education teachers. Regrettably, not all are good. Grading systems are classified as either norm-referenced or criterion-referenced, and both include acceptable methods of grading.

Norm-Referenced Grading

The norm-referenced system of grading is based on the normal probability curve that was described in chapter 2. Norm-referenced standards compare the performance of the students with each other. Levels of performance that discriminate among ability groups are developed. The levels of ability may range from high to low; the appropriate grade is used to indicate the attained ability. There are many methods of norm-referenced grading, not all of which are acceptable. Several methods follow.

Natural Breaks Method. In general, when test scores are ranked, gaps occur in the distribution. These breaks may be used as cutoff points for letter grades. Though quick and convenient for the teacher, this method is not recommended. A student's grade depends only on where the gaps occur, and there certainly is no consistency from one term to another. A numerical grade may be a B one term but an A another term. Table 6.2 shows how this method may be used.

Standard Deviation Method. This method assumes that the scores are normally distributed and that the standard deviation can be used to determine the grades. So, the first thing you must do is to calculate the mean and the standard deviation of a distribution of scores. You then have several choices for arranging the distribution into sections for grading purposes. Table 6.3 shows three arrangements. For illustration purposes, look at the following calculations for a sample knowledge test that has a mean of 74 and a standard deviation of 6. The arrangement in example 3 of table 6.3 is used.

TABLE 6.2 Grades Assigned by Natural Breaks Method

95		79	
95		77	
93		77	
93		76	
92		76	
91		75	
91	A	73	
. . . . . .		73	
88		72	
87		72	C
87		. . . . . .	
86		69	
85		68	
85		66	
83		64	
82	B	63	D
. . . . . .		. . . . . .	
		57	
		55	F
		. . . . . .	

The C range is determined first, since its range affects the B and D ranges. The C range is found as follows:

$$C = \overline{X} \pm 0.5s$$
$$= 74 \pm (.5)6$$
$$= 74 \pm 3$$
$$C = 71 \text{ to } 77$$

The upper limit of the B range is found as follows:

$$B = \overline{X} + 1.5s$$
$$= 74 + (1.5)6$$
$$B = 83$$

The lower limit of the D range is found as follows:

$$D = \overline{X} - 1.5s$$
$$= 74 - (1.5)6$$
$$D = 65$$

TABLE 6.3   Grades Assigned by Standard Deviation Method

Example 1

Grade	Standard Deviation Range	Percent
A	2.0s or more above mean	2
B	Between +1.0s and +2.0s	14
C	Between +1.0s and –1.0s	68
D	Between –1.0s and –2.0s	14
F	2.0s or more below mean	2

Example 2

Grade	Standard Deviation Range	Percent
A	1.75s or more above mean	4
B	Between +0.75s and +1.75s	19
C	Between +0.75s and –0.75s	54
D	Between –0.75s and –1.75s	19
F	1.75s or more below mean	4

Example 3

Grade	Standard Deviation Range	Percent
A	1.5s or more above mean	7
B	Between +0.5s and +1.5s	24
C	Between +0.5s and –0.5s	38
D	Between –0.5s and –1.5s	24
F	1.5s or more below mean	7

The ranges for the grades are as follows:

A = above 83

B = 78 to 83

C = 71 to 77

D = 65 to 70

F = below 65

If this method is used with a small class, the percentage of scores for each grade is not likely to be exactly the same as presented in table 6.3. (A small number of scores does not usually result in a normal distribution.) The standard deviation method of grading is best when scores are collected for several classes and grouped into one distri-bution. It may be necessary to collect the scores over two or more years, but the larger set of scores will result in an approximately normal distribution. Once you have established a grade range based on a large distribution of test scores, you can convert subsequent scores for the test into letter grades. Used in this manner, the standard deviation method is an acceptable norm-referenced grading system.

Percentage Method.   Using the percentage method, the teacher decides what percentage of the class is to receive each letter grade, lists the scores in order, and assigns the grades. For example, suppose a teacher has a class of thirty students. Table 6.4 shows how many students would receive each letter grade with three different groups of percentages.

Examples 1 and 3 of table 6.4 also show one of the problems encountered with this method. The selected percentage may require the rounding of numbers, which results in a different total number of students than the actual number of students. Example 1 has a total of 29 students, and example 3 has 31 students. When the total is different from the actual number of students, the teacher must decide which letter grade is to be received by more or fewer students than indicated by the percentage.

There is another problem with this method. Suppose that in example 2, when the scores are listed in order, the highest five are the following:

94

92

91

91

91

Only the highest three scores should receive the grade of A, but scores 3, 4, and 5 are the same. The teacher must decide whether only the highest two scores will receive an A or the highest five. If only two scores receive the grade of A, more than six students will be given a B. If five scores are given the grade of A, fewer scores will be given a B. This problem could occur anywhere in the distribution and with any percentage group.

This method has other disadvantages. Average-ability students will receive higher grades in a class with low-ability students than in a class with high-ability students.

TABLE 6.4 Grades Assigned by Percentage Method (Class of 30 Students)

Grade	Example 1		Example 2		Example 3	
	% of Students	No. of Students*	% of Students	No. of Students	% of Students	No. of Students*
A	7	2	10	3	15	5
B	24	7	20	6	20	6
C	38	11	40	12	30	9
D	24	7	20	6	20	6
F	7	2	10	3	15	5

*Will not total 30 because of rounding of numbers.

Also, consider what occurs if the class is homogeneous in ability. Though all students are approximately equal in ability, some students will receive high grades and some will receive low grades. Finally, there is no consistency with this method. The grade assigned to a particular score may vary from term to term.

The disadvantages of the percentage method can be overcome if it is used in the same way as the standard deviation method. A large number of scores should be collected before the percentage groups are designated. Once the percentage groups (A, B, C, D, and F) have been determined with a large number of scores for a particular test, subsequent test scores can be assigned the appropriate letter grade. The problems of the percentage method still may occur, but only during the initial determination of the letter grades. Once the letter grades have been assigned to the scores, these problems are eliminated. Used specifically in this manner, the percentage method is acceptable for norm-referenced grading.

Norms Method. Norms are performance standards based on analysis of scores. They are developed by collecting scores for a large number of individuals of the same gender and similar age, experience, ability, and other such characteristics. Norms may be developed at the national, state, or local level. At any of these levels, several hundred scores should be collected and analyzed before the norms are accepted. Percentiles, T-scores, and z-scores are forms of norms.

The norms method is an excellent system for norm-referenced grading for several reasons. The norms may be used for several years before new norms need to be developed. Also, they are unaffected by the group being tested because all students in the group could excel in performance and earn a high grade. Finally, they have consistency in that the grade for a given performance will be the same for a group during any school term. (The procedures for developing norms are described in chapter 2.)

Criterion-Referenced Grading

Criterion-referenced standards are clearly defined; the students know exactly what is expected of them. Standards may be developed for each grade that can be earned, or the standards may be pass/fail. When standards are developed for each grade, the students choose to work for a particular grade, and they are not in competition with each other. If pass/fail, the standards represent the level of ability that most students should be able to achieve during the instructional unit.

Contract Method. The contract grading method can be used with a class or with each student. With the class contract, the quality, amount, and type of work to be performed to earn the various grades are the same for all members of the class. For example, in a tenth-grade softball class, the A grade standards for each girl might be the following:

- Score 19 or above on the overhand throw for accuracy
- Score 19 or above on the fielding test
- Score 90 or above on the written test

- Write a one-page report on the technique of bunting
- Write a one-page report on the technique of fielding a ground ball in the outfield and throwing to home plate

Other standards would be written for the remaining grades. The teacher may or may not permit the class to assist in developing the contract. With the individual contract, the teacher and student agree upon the type, amount, and quality of work the student must do to earn a particular grade. Each student could have a different contract, and every student could earn an A grade.

This method of grading allows for individual differences in ability and for successful performance, as defined by the student. Too often when this method is used, however, the emphasis is on the quantity of work rather than on the quality of work. If quality standards can be designed, this system is acceptable for criterion-referenced grading.

Percentage Correct Method. Teachers often use the percentage correct method for grading. With this method, the student is advised what percentage of attempts must be correct to earn the various grades. Table 6.5 shows four examples of this method. The percentage correct method also can be used with physical performance scores, but there will be no maximum score for performances such as throwing and jumping events. In these events the grade of A or A+ would be any score greater than a specified score. The standards for the grades should be based on previous test scores that have been analyzed, not on standards the teacher arbitrarily selects.

When the percentage correct method is used, it is sometimes difficult to compare different tests, because the level of difficulty for the tests will not always be the same. A grade of 85 on one knowledge test may be a better score than a grade of 85 on another test, depending on the test difficulty. (This problem could occur with psychomotor tests also.) When one test is considered more difficult than another, different weights may be assigned to the tests.

The percentage correct method is an acceptable criterion-referenced grading system if the grade standards are determined as objectively as possible. It is a better system when the instructor assigns weights to factors or tests with different degrees of difficulty. There are no limits on the number of students who may earn high

TABLE 6.5 Grades Assigned by Percentage Correct Method

Grade	Percentage Correct Score	
	Example 1	Example 2
A	90 to 100	93 to 100
B	80 to 89	85 to 92
C	70 to 79	77 to 84
D	60 to 69	70 to 76
F	below 60	below 70
	Example 3	Example 4
A+	98 to 100	98 to 100
A	94 to 97	95 to 97
A–	90 to 93	93 to 94
B+	87 to 89	91 to 92
B	83 to 86	87 to 90
B–	80 to 82	85 to 86
C+	77 to 79	83 to 84
C	73 to 76	79 to 82
C–	70 to 72	77 to 78
D+	67 to 69	75 to 76
D	63 to 66	72 to 74
D–	60 to 62	70 to 71
F	below 60	below 70

grades, and the students know exactly what they must do to earn a particular grade.

☝ ARE YOU ABLE TO DO THE FOLLOWING:

- define norm-referenced grading and the grading methods of natural breaks, standard deviation, percentage, and norms?
- describe the advantages and disadvantages of each?
- define criterion-referenced grading and the grading methods of contract and percentage correct?
- describe the advantages and disadvantages of each?

TABLE 6.6 Use of Weights in Determining Grades for Tennis

Area	Weighting of Area	Factor	Weighting of Factor	Grade	Points
Psychomotor	6	Skill test	1	C+	6
		Game performance	2	B+	18
		Tournament standing	2	A+	24
		Technique	1	A–	10
Cognitive	2	Knowledge test	2	A–	20
TOTALS	8		8		78
COMMENTS	Grade = 78/8 = 9.75 (A–)				

Which Method of Grading Is Best?

Only a few of the grading methods used in physical education have been presented in this chapter. These, and many others, are not without faults. As teachers gain experience, they develop a method that suits them best. However, all teachers, beginning and experienced, should use a grading system that fulfills the grading criteria previously described and that they agree with philosophically. If you teach, a major decision will be whether to use criterion-referenced grading or norm-referenced grading. Both have a place in the grading process, so you should be prepared to use either, depending on which best serves your needs and the needs of your students.

The Weighting of Factors

Usually a teacher emphasizes certain factors in a teaching unit; that is, the teacher gives these factors more value than other factors in determining the unit grade. The importance of these factors is reflected in the weight (percentage of the total grade) assigned to each. If evaluation scores for all factors are averaged without the assigning of weights, all scores will have equal value. As previously stated, the use of weights should be considered with knowledge and physical performance tests, as well as when one test is more difficult than another. Table 6.6 shows how weights might be used to determine grades in a tennis unit. Note that the psychomotor area has a weight three times greater than the cognitive area. Also note that game performance and tournament standing are important components in the

TABLE 6.7 Numerical Conversion Table for Letter Grades

A+ = 12	B– = 7	D+ = 3
A = 11	C+ = 6	D = 2
A– = 10	C = 5	D– = 1
B+ = 9	C– = 4	F = 0
B = 8		

psychomotor area. If you choose to include game performance, use authentic assessment procedures to determine the grade. In addition, technique rating may include self-assessment, peer assessment, or teacher assessment or some combination of the three. If letter grades are assigned for weighted factors, a numerical table for conversion of letter grades, as shown in table 6.7, should be available.

? ARE YOU ABLE TO DO THE FOLLOWING:

- define the weighting of factors and describe a method for performing this technique?

Reporting of Final Grades

Teachers may choose a grading method, but they usually do not choose how the grades are to be reported. All teachers within a school, or school system, are required to report grades in the same way.

Letter. The letter grades A, B, C, D, and F are most commonly used. Some school systems use + and – with the grades: A+, A, and A–. Often the use of letter grades requires the teachers to convert numerical grades into letter grades, so a system, as shown in table 6.5 is needed.

Numerical. The numerical average is reported rather than a letter grade. The grade may be the average of the actual scores or of the percentage correct. Though letter grades are not reported with this method, some schools equate the numerical ranges with letter grades: A = 93 to 100, B = 85 to 92, and so forth.

Pass/fail. The grade indicates only whether the student has been successful or unsuccessful in completing the course objectives.

Descriptors. Words, terms, and phrases are used to describe the student's performance. Examples are "excellent," "above average," "average," "below average," "working at near capacity," "making moderate use of ability," "working substantially below ability," "outstanding progress," "appropriate progress," "progress below capabilities," and "little or no progress."

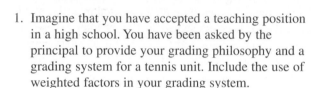

ARE YOU ABLE TO DO THE FOLLOWING:

- describe four methods for reporting grades?

Grading is not always an enjoyable task, but it is a necessary one. It is not a responsibility to be taken lightly. A grading system should be fair, consistent, related to the educational objectives, and as objective as possible. Teachers who arbitrarily devise grading systems fail in their responsibilities to the students, parents, and administrators.

REVIEW PROBLEM

1. Imagine that you have accepted a teaching position in a high school. You have been asked by the principal to provide your grading philosophy and a grading system for a tennis unit. Include the use of weighted factors in your grading system.

7

Construction and Administration of Psychomotor Tests

Upon completion of this chapter, you should be able to

1. Describe the four components of the psychomotor domain;

2. Select psychomotor tests that have been constructed properly;

3. Describe the steps for construction of a psychomotor skill rating scale;

4. Describe the procedures for construction of a psychomotor test;

5. Describe the pretest, testing, and posttest responsibilities for the administration of psychomotor tests;

6. Properly administer psychomotor tests; and

7. Define motor ability, motor capacity, and motor educability.

Test Construction Guidelines

Jansma (1988) describes four fundamental components of the psychomotor domain: physical, motor, fitness, and play. The physical component deals with the individual's anatomical or structural status. The motor component deals with the quality of movement patterns, or how well the individual moves. The fitness component refers to the quantity of movement, or how much movement can be sustained. The play component represents the culmination of development within the psychomotor domain. To be a good player, the individual needs physical, motor, and fitness competence.

Many published tests are available to measure these psychomotor domain components. There may be occasions, however, when no published test meets the particular needs of the group you wish to test, or you feel that you are capable of devising a better test. The following

guidelines will help you construct a good test. Because there is agreement on the techniques for estimating the validity and reliability of norm-referenced tests, it probably would be best if you first developed a norm-referenced test. The guidelines presented here, or ones similar to them, were followed in the development of most of the tests presented in the following chapters.

Know What Is Required of a Good Test

Before constructing a psychomotor test, you should be familiar with the criteria of a good test. Review the criteria in chapter 4.

Define the Performance to Be Measured

The new test might be designed to measure a sports skill, a game situation, fitness, strength, flexibility, or other related performances. You should define the exact performance you want to measure and state the objective of the new test. The test taker should be able to relate the test to real-life situations (e.g., the components of a skill test should be similar to gamelike conditions). Suppose you want to construct a new tennis serve test. Do you want to include measurement of power in the test or just measurement of the ability to serve the ball into the correct area? If it is to be a strength test, do you want to measure the strength of the leg, arm, or another body part? It may be wise to name the muscles to be tested. If it is to be a flexibility test, you should identify the joint or body part that will be involved in the measurement of flexibility. Also, include in your definition characteristics of the group that will take the test (e.g., gender and grade).

After you have identified and defined the performance to be measured, ask yourself the following questions:

1. Has the performance been included in the unit of instruction?
2. Can the performance be objectively measured?
3. Is there an existing test that will meet my needs?

Once you are satisfied with your answers to these questions, you are ready to analyze the performance that will be measured.

Analyze the Performance

To construct a good test, you must analyze the performance to be measured by identifying all the components needed for successful performance. (For example, performance in softball involves hitting, catching, throwing, and running.) After you have identified the components, select the ones you want to measure. It is important that you give careful thought to this guideline. The components that you identify will determine the items you include in your test.

Suppose you want to construct a test to measure hitting ability. The skill of hitting may be broken down into four parts: grip, stance, swing, and follow-through. Successful performance of the test should require the student to perform the fundamentals of these four parts in a mechanically sound way.

Review the Literature

You should review tests that measure the same performance or related performance and the research performed to develop the tests. This review will serve several purposes:

1. You will become familiar with developing physical performance tests. You may find useful ideas that will aid you in your project.
2. You may choose to include previously published test items in your test.
3. You may find a previously validated test to use in establishing the validity of your test.
4. You will become more familiar with the performance components.

Devise the Test Items

You now are ready to devise the item or items that will be included in your test. (You may also select published test items.) It is a good idea to develop more items than you actually plan to include in the test and to select the best ones after analyzing all the items. Keep the following principles in mind:

1. Make the items as realistic as possible. If a sports skill is being measured, the item should be similar to the game situation. This consideration (authentic assessment) is described in chapter 6. The items also must be appropriate for the gender and age of the individuals being tested.
2. Make the items simple to perform. You do not want to include an item the students have difficulty remembering. If they hesitate or forget during test performance, the validity and reliability of the test will be affected.
3. Make the items practical. They should be inexpensive and require a minimum amount of time to administer.
4. Determine the test layout—dimensions and administrative order of items.
5. Make the scoring simple. Simplicity of scoring will aid objectivity, lessen the time required to train any assistants needed to administer the test, and better enable the students to understand the scoring.

Prepare the Directions

The directions must be clear and precise, or the reliability and objectivity of the test will be affected. In addition, clear directions will prevent confusion among the students. When writing the directions, try to imagine questions that might be asked after the directions have been given to a group. Review the directions of tests found in this book and other textbooks to aid you in the wording.

Have the Test Reviewed by Your Peers

This is not the time to be hesitant in asking for assistance in your project. Ask other instructors to study your test and offer constructive criticism. What may be clear or obvious to you may not be to others. Asking for input now may prevent problems once you administer the test. Remember, when you ask for help, do not be oversensitive if the other instructors do not agree with everything you have written. You do not have to accept all their suggestions; however, open-mindedness is important in constructing successful tests.

Administer the Test to a Small Group of Students

At this point it would be wise to administer the test to a small group of students to determine if there are any problems with the directions, administration, and scoring. Though not essential, having another instructor administer the test to a class while you observe and make notes of any problems may be beneficial. The class must be representative of the group for which the test is designed. After the sample group has completed the test, make any necessary changes. If you administered more items than you plan to include in the final version of the test, you can remove the items that appear to be troublesome.

Determine the Validity, Reliability, and Objectivity

Having completed the previous guidelines, you are ready to determine the validity, reliability, and objectivity coefficients of your test by administering it to a large number of students. As was the small group, this large group must be representative of the group for which the test is designed.

For norm-referenced tests, concurrent validity is usually desired. Concurrent validity can be estimated through one of the following methods.

Tournament Play. If the test measures a sports skill, the scores can be correlated with tournament play. It is better to use a round-robin tournament because it provides the opportunity for the more skilled student to win. If the test

is valid, the students who score well on the test will also place high in the tournament, and those who do poorly on the test will place low in the tournament.

Previously Validated Test. The scores of your test can be correlated with the scores of a previously validated test. With this method it is necessary that you administer your test and the validated test; high correlation means that your test is valid. The obvious problem with this method is that you probably are devising your own test because the validated test is not acceptable (owing to expense, time, or some other reason). However, if a validated test is available, this is a good method.

Ratings of Experts. The test scores can be correlated with the ratings of experts (individuals with a high degree of skill or knowledge in the sport). If using this method, you must select or devise a rating scale. Hensley, Morrow, and East (1990) and Verducci (1980) offer the following steps for construction of a rating scale:

1. Determine the specific skills that are to be evaluated. The rating scale must reflect the objectives of the instructional program, and the objectives should be stated in terms of observable behavior.
2. Identify the traits that determine success. The expected traits for success at the beginner's level are different from the traits at the level of the experienced player. The rating scale should include the skills that are necessary for the level of play that is to be evaluated.
3. Determine the levels of success or ability for each skill. A five-point rating scale usually provides enough spread to differentiate the ability levels.
4. Define each category or ability level by observable behavior. Descriptive phrases should accompany each numerical value, and there must be no doubt as to the ability level that is expected for each numerical value.
5. The form should permit the immediate recording of the rating of the observed skill.

Hensley, Morrow, and East (1990) also offer guidelines for use of a rating scale:

1. Strive to minimize the sources of error associated with rating scales. The halo effect, the physical

appearance and personality of the individual being rated, and the previous ratings are examples of influences on the results of rating scales.

2. The individual being rated should be observed on more than one occasion, and the ratings should be averaged.

3. Ratings must be completed while the individual performs; no rating should be completed from memory.

4. When possible, several experts should be used and their ratings averaged.

5. Discuss the scale with the experts; be sure all experts agree with the scale.

6. Allow adequate time for the experts to complete their task.

An example of a rating scale for execution of the tennis forehand is found in table 7.1.

Reliability can be estimated through the methods of test-retest, parallel forms, split-half, and Kuder-Richardson formulas as described in chapter 4. Use of the test-retest method will enable you to estimate reliability and objectivity coefficients at the same time.

Develop the Norms

If you have constructed a norm-referenced test, a table of norms is needed. Review the calculations of z-scores, T-scores, and percentiles described in chapter 2; remember, norms are usually reported by age and gender. Because a large number of scores is required to develop the norms, it will be necessary to test several classes. If this

TABLE 7.2 Guidelines for Construction of Psychomotor Tests

Review criteria of a good test
   Consider validity, reliability, objectivity, and administrative feasibility
Define the performance to be measured
   Identify components for successful performance
Review the literature
   Research tests that measure the same performance or related performance
Devise the test items
   Make items realistic, simple, and practical; determine layout; make scoring simple
Prepare directions
   Be clear and precise
Have test reviewed by peers
   Be open-minded
Administer test to small group
   Make sure small group is representative of group for which test is designed
Determine validity, reliability, and objectivity
   Administer test to large group; make sure group is representative of group for which test is designed
Develop norms
   Base norms on large number of scores

is not possible, you can accumulate test scores over a period of two or three years. You must administer the test the same way each time, however. Table 7.2 summarizes the guidelines for construction of physical performance tests.

Determine Intercorrelations

Determining intercorrelations is necessary only if your test includes several items (referred to as a *test battery*). When a test includes more than one item, all items should have high correlation with the criterion and low correlation with each other. The correlation of the items with each other is determined through a multiple correlation procedure. This procedure has been used with other statistical procedures to develop many of the physical fitness, motor ability, and sports skills tests used in physical education programs. In the construction of a test

TABLE 7.1 Rating Scale for the Ability to Perform the Tennis Forehand

5	Exceptional ability; ball consistently stroked with power; ball consistently lands close to baseline
4	Above average ability; ball usually stroked with power; ball usually lands close to baseline
3	Average ability; occasional power; capable of hitting ball deep but inconsistent in doing so
2	Below average ability; no power; ball consistently hit into opponent's forecourt
1	Inferior ability; ball is rarely hit over net

battery, not all the items initially administered to the subjects are expected to be included in the final test battery. When two items are highly correlated with each other, the two items are considered to measure the same thing. The item that has the highest correlation with the criterion remains as part of the test; the other item is discarded. Since multiple correlation will not be discussed in this book, you should refer to a statistics book for the appropriate procedure.

❓ARE YOU ABLE TO DO THE FOLLOWING:

- describe the four components of the psychomotor domain?
- select psychomotor tests that have been constructed properly?
- describe the steps for construction of a psychomotor skill rating scale?
- describe the procedures for construction of a psychomotor test?

Test Administration Responsibilities

Do you remember taking psychomotor tests during your middle grades and senior high school physical education classes? When the students arrived for class, were the instructors prepared to administer the tests, or were they rushing to complete test preparations? Were they familiar with the test items, or did they appear to be unsure as to how the items should be administered? Did they require all students to perform the items correctly, or did they permit some students to perform the items incorrectly? Did they interpret the test results to the class, or were the students informed of the test results only through a grade? These questions illustrate the many responsibilities associated with the administration of psychomotor tests.

The administration of psychomotor tests requires pretest, testing, and posttest responsibilities. If a test is to be effective and the purposes of testing are to be fulfilled, the responsibilities in all three areas must be completed. The following testing responsibilities are (1) appropriate for a school or nonschool environment and (2) described

as if the test has more than one item. These responsibilities are basically the same, however, regardless of what type of group is tested or how many items are included in a test.

Pretest Responsibilities

Pretest responsibilities include everything that is to be done before the actual testing of the students. These responsibilities are as follows:

1. Develop a test schedule. Consider the days and minutes necessary for testing and the order in which the items will be administered.
2. If the entire class cannot be tested at the same time, plan an appropriate testing procedure. It may be necessary to have a class activity with which all students are familiar. While part of the group is tested, the other students can participate in the activity.
3. Provide opportunities for the students to practice the test items or activities similar to the items. Through practice, the students will know how to perform the items and know exactly what is expected during the testing. The purpose of the test also should be described.
4. Prepare the scorecards. The scorecards should be easy to follow and to use. If scorecards are not to be used, be prepared to score the results in another manner.
5. Train all test assistants, and make sure they are familiar with their responsibilities. They should know how to administer the test and be aware of all safety precautions. In addition, they should be prepared to deal with any unplanned developments that may occur during testing.
6. Know exactly how the test instructions are to be given to the group. Practice giving the instructions. If the instructions are rather involved, it may be wise to write them on paper.
7. If smaller groups are needed, plan how they are to be formed. If the absence of several students could affect your method for forming groups, plan more than one method.
8. Review all safety precautions. No one should be injured while performing the test as a result of your failure to take safety precautions.

9. Provide all necessary equipment and floor or court markings. Test the equipment for safety, and make sure that nothing on the field or court is unsafe.

Testing Responsibilities

When all pretest responsibilities are completed, the testing responsibilities are easier to perform. The essential responsibilities are as follows:

1. Organize the group for instructions. The purpose of the test should have been discussed during a previous class meeting, but if it has not been, do so at this time.
2. Give test instructions. Always face the group and speak clearly. Do not attempt to give the instructions or demonstrate the items with your back to the group.
3. Demonstrate test items. If more appropriate, items may be demonstrated after smaller groups are formed. Whenever possible, have someone demonstrate the items while you describe them.
4. If test assistants are available, form smaller groups. The number of groups formed may depend on the number of items on the test.
5. Administer the test items. Insist that all individuals perform the items correctly. Remember that the validity and reliability of the test are affected if not all students are required to perform the items in the same way.
6. If time allows, gather the group for reaction to the test and discussion.

Posttest Responsibilities

If the test is to have meaning to the students, the following posttest responsibilities should be completed:

1. Score all test items. Scoring the test may require the use of norms. If norms (standardized or local) are available, scoring is a simple task. If they are not available, develop your own. Whether the test is norm-referenced or criterion-referenced, you should calculate the mean, mode, median, deciles, and standard deviation of the test. These values will be useful in reporting the test results to the class and in comparing classes.

2. If you are testing for grading purposes, determine the grade for each student.
3. Interpret the test results to the students. This interpretation should be presented immediately after the test has been taken, and it should involve more than just reporting the students' grades. If some students did not perform well on the test, discuss the possible reasons with them. Discussion of a student's performance should not embarrass the student. If necessary, conduct the performance review in a private conference with the student. Also, if criterion-referenced standards are used, students will want to know how the class did as a group.
4. Evaluate the test. Did the test fulfill your reasons for testing? Was it a learning experience for the students? Did the pretest, testing, and posttest procedures go well? Make notes of any changes you should make in your next administration of the test.

These are the major responsibilities for the administration of psychomotor tests. Test administration becomes easier with experience, but you should never take test responsibilities lightly.

⸮ARE YOU ABLE TO DO THE FOLLOWING:

- describe the proper procedures for administration of psychomotor tests?

Types of Psychomotor Tests

Different types of psychomotor tests evolved during the twentieth century. During the first half of the century, there was much interest in measurement of an individual's **motor ability** (defined as the innate and acquired ability of an individual to perform motor skills of a general nature, exclusive of highly specialized sports or gymnastic skills). However, the measurement of motor ability is no longer popular, and its decline can be attributed to three reasons. First, many physical educators question the existence of a general motor ability; they feel that abilities are highly specific to the performance task. Second, the construct validity of motor ability test batteries has never been established. Last, a consensus does not exist on what the components of motor ability are.

During the time that motor ability testing was common, tests were designed to measure **motor capacity** (the individual's potential ability to perform motor skills) and **motor educability** (the individual's ability to learn new motor skills). These tests also are no longer popular. Rather, it appears that now many physical educators measure the physical performance components of agility, balance, cardiorespiratory endurance, flexibility, muscular strength, and muscular endurance. Though there is no common agreement on the basic components that underlie physical performance, it cannot be disputed that individuals with poor abilities in these areas are not likely to succeed in sports and other physical activities. Tests often are used to identify these individuals so that appropriate activities may be prescribed to improve their weak abilities. In addition, physical educators employed in schools and fitness centers are measuring the components of health fitness (cardiorespiratory fitness, flexibility, muscular strength, muscular endurance, and body composition) because of the current emphasis on well-being and health fitness.

Conducted since the early 1900s, **sports skills** measurement is very popular today. Most, if not all, middle grade and high school physical education programs include the development of sports skills as a major objective. It is important that valid, reliable, and objective tests be used to measure these skills. Very few new sports skills tests or norms have been developed in recent years. The American Alliance for Health, Physical Education, Recreation, and Dance, however, is revising existing tests and developing new tests in some sports.

ARE YOU ABLE TO DO THE FOLLOWING:

- define motor ability, motor capacity, and motor educability?

▶ REVIEW PROBLEMS ◀

1. Select three psychomotor tests (at least one of them should have several items) described in this book and refer to the provided references for descriptions of their construction procedures. Note whether the procedures are similar to the ones described for you. Also note how the validity and reliability of the tests were determined.
2. Construct a rating scale for performance of a sports skill.

8 Agility

Upon completion of this chapter, you should be able to

1. Define and measure agility;

2. State why agility should be measured; and

3. Prescribe activities to improve agility.

Agility, sometimes referred to as the maneuverability of the body, is the ability to rapidly change the position and direction of the body or body parts. Heredity is a major factor in an individual's level of agility, but agility also depends on strength, speed, coordination, and dynamic balance. Many individuals are able to improve agility by increasing their ability in these variables. Agility also can be improved through direct instruction, training, and practice of agility drills.

Agility is important in all activities and sports. Individual and team sports involve quick starts and stops, rapid change of direction, efficient footwork, and quick adjustments of the body or body parts. Individuals with good agility have a better chance of success in a physical activity than individuals with poor agility. Agility test items are usually of three types: (1) change in running direction, (2) change in body position, and (3) change in body part direction. Examples of the three types are the dodge or obstacle run (change in running direction), squat thrusts (change in body position), and a test that requires a change in the position of the hands or feet (change in body part direction). Agility tests that require only movement of the hands or feet are rarely used in physical education. Agility may be specific to an activity or sport; you should not expect, therefore, each individual to do equally well on all agility tests. Most valid agility tests serve to identify individuals with poor agility.

Why Measure Agility?

Improvement in agility is an acceptable objective for a physical education class. As an objective, agility improvement should be determined through measurement. It is doubtful, however, that the agility levels of the students should be used in determining grades. How much improvement in agility will occur in the amount of time spent on agility instruction in the school environment is questionable. But, if agility is an important factor in the performance of sports, and if you grade sports skills, agility is graded. Agility tests are sometimes used to classify students for a particular activity or sport, but a test that measures the skill within the activity or sport should be used for classification purposes.

Agility tests are best used for diagnostic purposes, to determine which individuals have poor agility. In testing for diagnostic purposes, criterion-referenced measurement is more appropriate than norm-referenced measurement. A predetermined score should be used to place students into acceptable and unacceptable agility groups, and activities designed to improve agility should be prescribed for the individuals placed in the unacceptable group. It is the instructor's responsibility to determine the appropriate activities. Individuals with unacceptable agility may need strength, speed, coordination, and dynamic balance development exercises; or simple agility drills may serve the purpose, depending on the individual. After completion of the prescribed activities or drills, improvement in agility can be determined by the administration of the same agility test.

? ARE YOU ABLE TO DO THE FOLLOWING:

- define agility and state why it should be measured?

Tests of Agility

The agility tests selected for review are practical, inexpensive to administer, and satisfactory for both sexes. Objectivity coefficients and norms are not reported for all the tests. Norms can be developed to meet your specific needs. You may want to develop local norms for the tests for which norms are reported. Your primary purpose in developing norms should be to establish a criterion-referenced standard for the tests that you choose to use.

Obtaining consistency and comparability of results requires that the agility tests be performed on a nonslip surface, and all students should wear shoes that provide good traction. In addition, the students should practice performing the agility tests and should be familiar with the performance requirements.

■ Right-Boomerang Run
(Gates and Sheffield 1940)

Test Objective. To measure running agility.
Age Level. Ten through college-age.
Equipment. Stopwatch, tape measure, a chair or similar object for center station, and four cone markers for outside points.
Validity. With the sum of T-scores for a fifteen-item agility battery as the test criterion, a validity coefficient of .72 has been reported for females. With a similar sixteen-item battery, coefficients ranging from .78 to .87 have been reported for junior high males.

TABLE 8.1 Norms in Seconds for Right-Boomerang Run for Seventh- and Eighth-Grade Males

Performance Level	Score
Above average	12.9 and below
Average (42% to 69%)	13.0 to 13.9
Below average	14.0 and above

Adapted from B. L. Johnson and J. K. Nelson, *Practical measurements for evaluation in physical education,* 4th ed., Edina, Minn.: Burgess Publishing, 1986.

Reliability. .93 for females and .92 for males.
Norms. Table 8.1 reports norms for boys in seventh and eighth grades.
Administration and Directions. A chair is placed 17 feet from the starting line, and a cone marker is placed 15 feet on each side of the center point. On the signal, "Go," the student runs to the center station, makes a quarter turn right, runs around the outside station and returns to the center, makes another quarter turn, and completes the course as shown in figure 8.1. The student should be instructed to run as fast as possible through the course and not to touch the chair or cones.
Scoring. The score is the time to the nearest one-tenth of a second to complete the course. A penalty of one-tenth second is deducted from the score for each time chairs or markers are touched.

■ Sidestepping
(North Carolina Motor Fitness Battery 1977)

Test Objective. To measure agility, endurance, and speed of lateral movement.
Age Level. Nine through seventeen.
Equipment. Stopwatch, measuring tape, and marking tape.
Validity. Face validity.
Reliability. Not reported.
Norms. Table 8.2 includes norms for males and females, ages nine through seventeen.
Administration and Directions. Two parallel lines are placed on the floor 12 feet apart as measured from the inside of the lines. The test performer assumes a starting position inside the lines, with one foot touching a line. On the signal, "Start," the test performer (1) moves sideward with a sidestep, leading with the foot nearest the line to be approached; (2) repeats the sidestep until the foot has touched or gone beyond

FIGURE 8.1 Right-boomerang run.

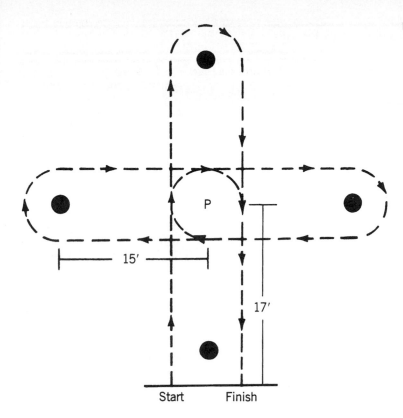

15'

17'

Start   Finish

the line; and (3) moves to the other line in the same manner. The test performer must face the same direction at all times, must not cross his or her feet, and must not leap.

Scoring. One point is scored each time a foot touches or goes beyond a sideline. The final score is the number of times a line is touched in 30 seconds.

■ **SEMO Agility Test**
(Kirby 1971)

Test Objective. To measure agility while moving the body forward, backward, and sideward.

Age Level. High school and college.

Equipment. Four cone markers and a stopwatch.

Validity. .63 when correlated with the AAHPERD shuttle run test.

Reliability. .88 for high school and college males.

Objectivity. .97.

Norms. Kirby provided norms for college males.

Administration and Directions. Cones are placed in each corner of the free-throw lane of a basketball court or in the corners of a 12-by-19-foot rectangle that is on a good running surface (see figure 8.2). Beginning at point A facing the free-throw line, on the signal, "Go," the test performer (1) sidesteps to outside of point B; (2) backpedals from B to D, passing inside D to be in a position facing A; (3) sprints to A, passing around the cone; (4) backpedals from A to C, passing inside C to be in a position facing B; (5) sprints to B, passing around the cone; and (6) sidesteps from B to finish line at A.

Scoring. Two trials are permitted, with the better time recorded to the nearest one-tenth of a second. Practice trials should be given before the test is administered. Do not permit crossover steps when the sidestep is performed. Also, require the student to keep the back perpendicular to an imaginary line connecting the corner cones when performing the backpedal. If the student performs any part of the test incorrectly, the test is invalid. The test should be administered until the student performs one trial correctly. With Kirby's norms, if a college male requires more than 13.02 seconds to complete the course, he is classified as an advanced beginner. Johnson and Nelson (1986) report that a college female who requires more than 14.50 seconds also is classified as an advanced beginner.

TABLE 8.2 Norms in Percentiles for Sidestep Test for Ages Nine Through Seventeen

Percentile	Age								
	9	10	11	12	13	14	15	16	17
	Males								
95	19	19	20	21	23	23	25	23	26
90	17	18	19	19	21	21	23	22	25
85	16	17	18		20		22	21	23
80	15		17	18	19	20	21		22
75		16					20	20	21
70			16	17	18	19			
65	14	15					19	19	20
60			15	16	17	18			
55	13	14						18	19
50				15			18		
45			14		16	17		17	18
40	12	13					17		
35			13	14	15	16			17
30	11	12					16	16	
25			12	13	14	15			16
20	10	11					15	15	15
15	9	10	11	12	13	14	14	14	14
10	8	9	10	11	11	13	13	13	12
5	7	8	8	9	10	11	11	10	10
	Females								
95	18	19	21	20	20	21	21	21	21
90	16	17	18	18	19	19	20	19	20
85	15	16	17		18		19	18	
80			16	17		18	18		19
75		15			17			17	18
70	14		15	16		17	17		
65					16			16	
60		14				16			16
55	13		14	15			16		
50		13						15	
45					15				15
40	12		13	14		15	15		
35		12						14	
30	11		12	13	14				
25		11				14	14	13	14
20	10		11	12	13			12	13
15	9	10	10		12	13	13	11	
10	8	9	9	11	11	12	11	10	11
5	7	7	7	8	10	11	10	9	10

Adapted from *North Carolina Motor Fitness Battery,* Raleigh, N.C.: North Carolina Department of Public Instruction, 1977.

FIGURE 8.2 SEMO agility test.

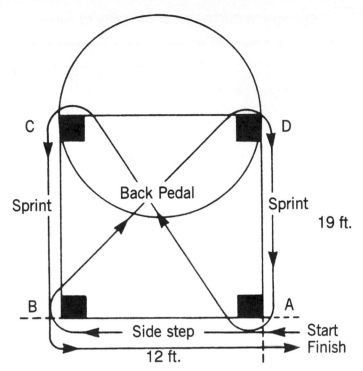

■ AAHPERD Shuttle Run
(AAHPERD 1976a)

Test Objective. To measure agility while running and changing direction.

Age Level. Nine through college-age.

Equipment. Stopwatch, measuring tape, marking tape, and two blocks of wood (2" × 2" × 4").

Validity. Not reported by AAHPERD.

Reliability. Not reported by AAHPERD.

Norms. Table 8.3 provides quartile norms for ages nine through seventeen and up. The President's Challenge, described in chapter 15, includes the shuttle run as a test component. To qualify for the National Physical Fitness Award, a student must score no less than the fiftieth percentile on all components of the President's Challenge. Comparing the shuttle run fiftieth percentile scores in tables 8.3 and 15.14, you will note that they differ. The percentile scores for the Challenge were established at a later date than the AAHPERD shuttle run percentiles.

Administration and Directions. Lines are placed 30 feet apart with marking tape. The two blocks are placed adjacent to and outside of the line not being used as the starting line. On the signal, "Go," the test performer (1) runs from the starting line to the blocks and picks one up; (2) returns to the starting line and places the block behind the line; (3) runs to pick up the second block; and (4) returns to the starting line and places the second block behind the line.

Scoring. Two trials are permitted. The better time to the nearest one-tenth second is accepted as the score. Rest should be allowed between trials. The student is not permitted to throw or drop the blocks. To eliminate this problem, test givers sometimes administer the test without the blocks; the student is instructed to touch behind the line.

■ Barrow Zigzag Run
(Barrow and McGee 1979)

Test Objective. To measure agility while running and changing direction.

Age Level. Junior high through college. (Though this test was originally designed for males, it may be satisfactorily used with junior high through college-age females.)

Equipment. Stopwatch and five standards that are used for high jump, volleyball, or badminton. Cones also may be used.

Validity. .74, with the total score for twenty-nine test items measuring eight factors.

Reliability. .80.

Agility   **105**

Objectivity. .99.

Norms. Table 8.4 reports norms for males in grades seven through eleven.

Administration and Directions. The course is designed as shown in figure 8.3. On the signal, "Go," the test performer runs, as fast as possible, the prescribed course in a figure eight fashion for three complete laps. The standards should not be touched in any manner. If a foul is committed or the course is run improperly, the student is required to run the course again. (The validity and reliability of the test would probably be affected minimally if you required the students to run only two laps.)

Scoring. The score is the time to the nearest one-tenth second required to complete the course three times.

Activities to Develop Agility

If you diagnose some students with poor agility, you should attempt to improve this agility. McClenaghan and Gallahue (1978) suggest the following activities for the development of agility in young children. These activities, or modifications of them, also may be used for junior and senior high students with poor agility.

Changes in the Height of the Body in Jumps

1. Alternate jumping maximum and minimum heights.
2. Alternate fast and slow jumping.
3. Jump while tossing an object to yourself.
4. Hop on one foot.
5. Hop two to four times on one foot, then the same number of times on the other foot.
6. Jump over a stationary rope.
7. Jump over a swinging rope.
8. Jump over a turning rope.
9. Jump over a rope you are turning.
10. Jump rope with a partner.

Changes in Distance

1. Jump as far as you can.
2. Jump as near as you can.
3. Jump and land with your feet in different positions.
4. Jump backward.
5. Walk backward.
6. Run backward or sideward.
7. Leap over objects.

TABLE 8.3 Norms in Seconds for AAHPERD Shuttle Run for Ages Nine Through Seventeen+

	Age							
Percentile	9–10	11	12	13	14	15	16	17+
	Males							
95	10.0	9.7	9.6	9.3	8.9	8.9	8.6	8.6
75	10.6	10.4	10.2	10.0	9.6	9.4	9.3	9.2
50	11.2	10.9	10.7	10.4	10.1	9.9	9.9	9.8
25	12.0	11.5	11.4	11.0	10.7	10.4	10.5	10.4
0	17.0	20.0	22.0	16.0	18.6	14.7	15.0	15.7
	Females							
95	10.2	10.0	9.9	9.9	9.7	9.9	10.0	9.6
75	11.1	10.8	10.8	10.5	10.3	10.4	10.6	10.4
50	11.8	11.5	11.4	11.2	11.0	11.0	11.2	11.1
25	12.5	12.1	12.0	12.0	12.0	11.8	12.0	12.0
0	18.0	20.0	15.3	16.5	19.2	18.5	24.9	17.0

Adapted from AAHPERD, *AAHPERD youth fitness test manual,* Reston, Va.: American Alliance for Health, Physical Education, Recreation and Dance, 1976.

Performance Level	Grade				
	7	8	9	10	11
Above average	25.2 and below	24.5 and below	24.6 and below	25.8 and below	25.8 and below
Average (T-score 45 to 55)	29.0 to 25.3	29.5 to 24.6	27.9 to 24.7	28.9 to 25.9	28.9 to 25.9
Below average	29.1 and above	29.6 and above	28.0 and above	29.0 and above	29.0 and above

Adapted from H. M. Barrow and R. McGee, *A practical approach to measurement in physical education,* 3d ed., Philadelphia: Lea & Febiger, 1979.

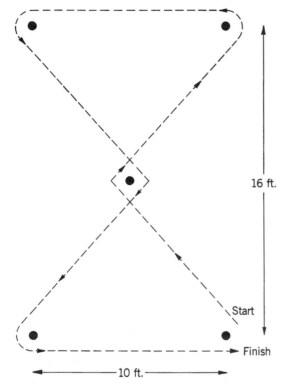

FIGURE 8.3 Barrow zigzag run.

8. Jump different heights.
9. Jump and land lightly.
10. Jump and land on different surfaces.

Changes in Direction

1. Jump and turn (quarter, half, three-quarter, and full turn).
2. Jump forward, then sideward, then backward.

3. Jump in a circle, square, triangle, and so forth.
4. Run between chairs.
5. Run forward and change direction quickly, on command.
6. Slide sideways and change direction quickly, on command.
7. Jump over a turning rope and change your body position.
8. Move forward, sideward, or backward while jumping over a rope you are turning.
9. Run through a series of tires (laid flat on the ground).
10. Do tumbling tricks requiring your body to roll in various ways (log rolls, forward rolls, backward rolls, and so on).

Other Agility Activities

Side-Straddle Hop (Jumping Jacks). Stand erect with arms at sides and feet together; jump, spreading the legs to the side and at the same time bring the arms overhead; jump and return to starting position; attempt to perform in a smooth and continuous action. One side-straddle hop is counted each time you return to the starting position.

Heel Touch. Stand erect with hands at the sides; jump and touch both heels with the fingers. Each jump is counted as one.

Treadmill. Assume push-up position with right leg forward; keep hands in place while alternately bringing one leg forward and extending the other leg in a running position. One treadmill is counted each time the right leg is forward.

Zigzag Run. Arrange chairs in a position to provide a zigzag course; run as fast as possible in a zigzag course around the chairs.

Student	10-Second Squat Thrust (Number)	AAHPERD Shuttle Run (Seconds)
A	7.00	9.8
B	6.50	10.8
C	5.50	11.4
D	7.50	9.6
E	5.25	12.0
F	6.50	10.4
G	6.75	10.5
H	6.00	11.0
I	5.75	11.4
J	5.00	12.5
K	6.00	11.3
L	6.75	10.3
M	5.75	11.2
N	6.50	10.7
O	5.75	11.5

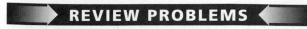

REVIEW PROBLEMS

1. Review additional agility tests found in other textbooks. Note the groups for whom the tests are intended and the validity, reliability, and objectivity coefficients.
2. Administer one of the tests described in this chapter to several of your fellow students. Ask them to provide constructive criticism of your test administration.
3. An elementary physical education teacher administered the 10-second squat thrust and the AAHPERD shuttle run tests to fifteen 10-year-old boys. Determine the relationship of the two groups of scores. Interpret the correlation coefficient.

9 Balance

Upon completion of this chapter, you should be able to

1. Define and measure static and dynamic balance;

2. State why balance should be measured; and

3. Prescribe activities to improve balance.

Balance is the ability to maintain equilibrium against the force of gravity. The balance center (semicircular canal) in the inner ear, the kinesthetic sense in the muscles and joints ("feel" of an activity), and visual perception contribute to balance. In certain positions, balance also is affected by strength. If the supporting muscles cannot hold the body weight, body parts, or an external weight firmly in position, balance is limited. For some individuals, increased strength results in improved balance.

Basically, there are two types of balance: **static** and **dynamic.** The recovery of balance, after the body's balance has been disturbed, may also be considered a type of balance. Static balance, the ability to maintain equilibrium while stationary, is often thought of as steadiness. Maintaining static balance requires that the person's center of gravity be over the base of support. Assuming a position to shoot a rifle, looking through a microscope, and posing for a photographer are examples of static balance.

Dynamic balance is the ability to maintain equilibrium while in motion or to move the body or parts of the body from one point to another and maintain equilibrium. Dancing, walking, driving a golf ball, and bowling are examples of dynamic balance. Static and dynamic balance are necessary for successful performance in physi-

cal activity, but the ability to recover balance is also essential in many activities. Running, kicking, hopping, dismounting from gymnastics apparatus, performing gymnastic floor exercises, and wrestling are examples of such activities. In fact, all human motion occurs as a result of the disturbance of the body's balance.

Why Measure Balance?

Balance is necessary not only in sports and related physical activities but also in our usual, everyday activities. Individuals with poor balance are at a disadvantage in efficiently performing most physical activities. Though heredity may be a factor, an individual's ability to maintain balance can be improved through appropriate physical activities. Thus, since performance of any physical skill requires some degree of balance and since balance can be improved, balance tests should be used to identify those individuals with poor balance. Activities then should be prescribed to improve their balance. However, as balance is specific to a body part or parts and may be specific to a sport or physical activity, different types of balance tests should be used for diagnostic purposes. Also, different types of activities designed to improve balance should be prescribed.

As was recommended for agility, specific improvement in balance should not be used to determine grades. If balance is an important component of a physical activity, the student's performance in that activity will be affected by the degree of balance. Through the assigning of grades for performance in an activity, balance has been graded.

?ARE YOU ABLE TO DO THE FOLLOWING:

- define balance and state why it should be measured by the physical educator?

Tests of Balance

Balance tests are classified as static or dynamic. The tests reviewed are practical, inexpensive to administer, and satisfactory for both sexes. Reliability and objectivity coefficients are not available for all the tests, and, regrettably, the published norms are primarily for college-age individuals. It will be necessary to develop local elementary, middle grades, or high school norms for your use. It is recommended that balance test norms be used in the same manner as agility norms to develop criterion-referenced standards. Though not a factor in all balance tests, fatigue may influence the performance of some students. For this reason, it is best not to administer balance tests after any strenuous activity. So that the test performers will be familiar with the test, permit them to practice the test. Practice enables many students to score better.

Static Balance Tests

■ Stork Stand
(Johnson and Nelson 1986)

Test Objective. To measure stationary balance while the body weight is supported on the ball of the foot of the dominant leg.
Age Level. Ten through college-age.
Equipment. Stopwatch.
Validity. Face validity.
Reliability. Coefficients of .85 and .87 have been reported using the test-retest method.
Objectivity. Johnson and Nelson (1986) report a study that found an objective coefficient of .99.
Norms. Table 9.1 reports norms for college students.
Administration and Directions. Individuals may be tested in pairs. The test performer stands on the foot of the dominant leg, places the other foot against the inside of the supporting knee, and places the hands on the hips as shown in figure 9.1. On the signal, "Go," the performer raises the heel of the dominant foot from the floor and attempts to maintain balance as long as possible. The test administrator counts aloud the seconds. The partner of the test performer records the number

TABLE 9.1 Norms in Seconds for Stork Stand, Bass Stick Test (Lengthwise), and Bass Stick Test (Crosswise) for College Students

Performance Level	Stork Stand	Bass Stick (LW)	Bass Stick (CW)
	Males		
Above average	37 and above	306 and above	165 and above
Average	15 to 36	221 to 305	65 to 164
Below average	14 and below	220 and below	64 and below
	Females		
Above average	23 and above	301 and above	140 and above
Average	8 to 22	206 to 300	60 to 139
Below average	7 and below	205 and below	59 and below

Adapted from B. L. Johnson and J. K. Nelson, *Practical measurements for evaluation in physical education,* 4th ed., Edina, Minn.: Burgess Publishing, 1986.

FIGURE 9.1 Stork stand.

FIGURE 9.2
Bass lengthwise stick test.

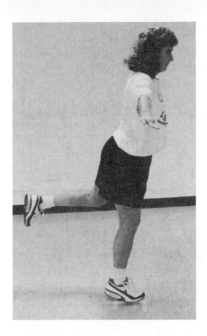

of seconds the performer is able to maintain balance. The trial is ended when the hands are moved from the hips, when the ball of the dominant foot moves from its original position, or when the heel touches the floor. Three trials are administered.

Scoring. The best time, in seconds, of the three trials is the score. Since there is no time limit, and some individuals may be able to maintain their balance for some time, you may choose to halt the performance of those individuals who exceed the norm for above average.

▪ Bass Stick Test (Lengthwise)
(Bass 1939)

Test Objective. To measure stationary balance while the weight of the body is supported on a small base of support on the ball of the foot.

Age Level. Ten through college-age.

Equipment. Sticks 1" × 1" × 12" (you may test one-half of the class at the same time if you have enough sticks), stopwatch, and adhesive tape.

Validity. Face validity is accepted.

Reliability. .90.

Norms. Table 9.1 reports norms for college students.

Administration and Directions. All sticks should be taped to the floor. Individuals may be tested in pairs. The test performer places a foot lengthwise on the stick (ball of the foot and heel should be in contact with the stick). On the signal, "Go," the performer lifts the opposite foot from the floor, raises the heel of the dominant foot from the stick, and attempts to hold this position for a maximum of 60 seconds (see figure 9.2). The test administrator counts aloud the seconds while the partner of the performer records the number of seconds the performer is able to maintain balance. The trial is ended when any part of either foot touches the floor. Three trials are taken on each foot. If any performers lose their balance within the first 3 seconds of a trial, the trial is not considered an attempt.

Scoring. The score is the total time in seconds for all six trials, three on each foot.

▪ Bass Stick Test (Crosswise)
(Bass 1939)

The crosswise stick test is the same as the lengthwise test except that the ball of the foot is placed crosswise on the stick. Table 9.1 includes norms for college students.

You will find additional static balance tests directly related to gymnastics performance in other measurement textbooks. Head balance, head and forearm balance, and handstands are examples of such tests.

Dynamic Balance Tests

■ Johnson Modification of the Bass Test of Dynamic Balance
(Johnson and Nelson 1986)

Test Objective. To measure the ability to maintain balance during movement and upon landing from a leap.

Age Level. High school through college.

Equipment. Stopwatch, tape measure, and floor tape.

Validity. Face validity; .46 when correlated with Bass test of dynamic balance.

Reliability. .75 using test-retest.

Objectivity. .97.

Norms. Johnson and Nelson (1986) provide norms for college women.

Administration and Directions. Eleven pieces of tape (1" × ¾") are placed in the pattern shown in figure 9.3. The test performer (1) stands with the right foot placed on the starting mark; (2) leaps to the first tape mark, lands on the ball of the left foot, and attempts to hold for 5 seconds; (3) leaps to the second tape mark, lands on the ball of the right foot, and attempts to hold for 5 seconds; and (4) continues to the other tape marks, alternating feet and attempting to hold a steady position for 5 seconds. The ball of the foot must completely cover the tape. The test administrator should count aloud the seconds of each balance.

Scoring. The test scoring is as follows:

5 points for landing successfully on the tape mark (tape completely covered)

1 point (up to 5 seconds) for each second the steady position is held on the tape marks

A maximum of 10 points per tape mark and 100 points for the test may be earned. The test performer is penalized 5 points for any of the following landing errors:

- failing to stop upon landing
- touching the floor with any part of the body other than the ball of the landing foot
- failing to completely cover the tape mark with the ball of the foot

If the test performer makes a landing error, the correct balance position may be assumed and held for a maximum of 5 seconds.

If the test performer lands successfully on the tape mark but commits any of the following errors before completing the 5-second count, a penalty of 1 point is taken away:

- touching the floor with any part of the body other than the ball of the landing foot

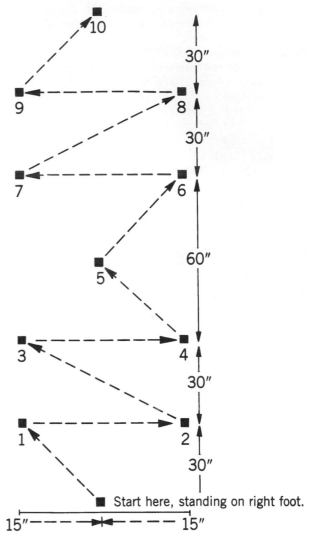

FIGURE 9.3 Floor pattern for modified Bass dynamic balance test.

- failing to hold the landing foot steady while in the steady position

If balance is lost, the test performer must return to the proper mark and leap to the next mark.

■ Balance Beam Walk
(Jensen and Hirst 1980)

Test Objective. To measure balance while walking on a balance beam.

Age Level. Nine through college-age.

Equipment. Regulation balance beam and stopwatch.

Validity. Face validity.

Norms. No norms reported.

Administration and Directions. Standing on one end of the beam, the test performer slowly walks the full length of the beam, pauses for 5 seconds, turns around, and walks back to the starting point. Three trials are allowed.

Scoring. Pass/fail. There is no time limit for this beam walk (the test performer walks until he or she falls), so the test could require much class time to administer. You may want to shorten the time for test administration or to increase the difficulty of the test by limiting the amount of time permitted to complete the test. The test difficulty may also be increased through the use of a 2-inch balance beam.

■ Modified Sideward Leap

(Scott and French 1959; Safrit 1986)

Test Objective. To measure the ability to maintain balance during movement and upon landing from a leap.

Age Level. Junior high through college.

Equipment. Stopwatch, tape measure, and floor tape.

Validity. Face validity.

Reliability. .66 to .88 at differing age levels.

Norms. No norms reported.

Administration and Directions. Place three 1-inch square spots in a straight line, 18 inches apart as shown in figure 9.4. Place additional spots at right angles to the line. These spots should be 3 inches apart and range in distance from spot A (24 to 40 inches) according to the height of the test performers. Three or four spots properly placed will usually cover the range in height. Place a small cork (may be the bottom of an old badminton bird) or other light object on spot B.

The test performer (1) places the left foot on mark X with the right side toward spot A (the correct spot for each individual may be determined through practice); (2) leaps sideward and lands on the ball of the right foot on spot A (the leap should require both feet to be off the floor at the same time, but it should not require extensive effort); (3) immediately leans forward and, using only one hand, pushes the cork off spot B (the floor should not be touched with either hand); and (4) holds a balanced position for 5 seconds (the position may be either forward or erect). Four trials are administered: two as above, and two with the student placing the right foot on mark X, landing on the ball of the left foot, and leaning forward to spot C.

Scoring. The maximum number of points for each trial is 15:

1. 5 points for landing correctly on spot A
2. 5 points for leaning and pushing object off spot B or C
3. 1 point for each second that balance is held on spot A, up to 5 seconds

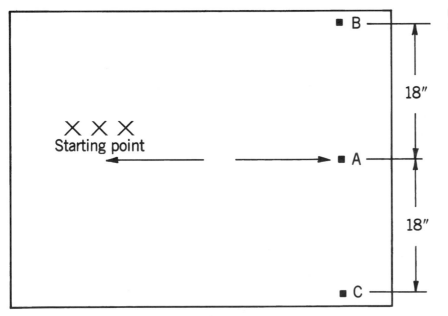

FIGURE 9.4 Floor marking for the modified sideward leap test.

Activities to Develop Balance

Balance can be improved through extensive practice of activities that place individuals (1) in balanced positions that they attempt to maintain and (2) in balanced positions that help them develop a "feel" (kinesthetic sense) for such positions. Balance also can be improved through activities that place individuals in a state of imbalance, forcing them to attempt to recover balance. Nichols, Arsenault, and Giuffre (1980) recommend the following activities for the teaching of balance to elementary students, but the activities, or modifications of them, may be practiced at any level of instruction.

Static Balance Activities

Knee Balance. In a kneeling position, attempt to balance on one knee while the arms are to the side. The position is held for 10 to 15 seconds, then the other knee is used.

Stork Stand. While in the same position as the stork stand test, attempt to hold the position for 10 to 20 seconds.

Swan Stand. Lean forward at the hips and lift the right foot off the floor. While balancing on the left foot, lift the right leg behind as high as possible. Hold for 10 to 15 seconds. Repeat on the other foot.

V-Sit. Sit on the floor and lift the arms and legs into the air while balancing on the buttocks. Hold for 10 to 20 seconds.

Dynamic Balance Activities

Tape Line. Tape a line on the floor, then (1) walk forward, backward, and sideways; (2) walk while balancing a book or a beanbag on the head; and (3) run, hop, or skip in different directions.

Hopping. Try to (1) hop over objects using the left foot and then the right; (2) hop with the eyes closed; (3) hop while holding on to different objects; or (4) hop in and out of tires.

Rug Twister. Place a rug sample so that the rubber backing faces upward. Stand on the rug and twist back and forth to move around the floor.

Hop Leap. Place tape marks on the floor approximately 1 yard apart. Leap from mark to mark, alternating the landing foot. Maintain a one-foot static balance on each mark for 5 seconds.

Recapturing Balance Activities

1. Jump off a low bench, landing with both feet inside a hoop.
2. Jump forward off a chair and clap the hands above the head while in midair.
3. Jump forward off a chair with one foot going forward and the other backward, and land with the legs back together.
4. Jump forward off a low bench, make a half turn in midair, and land facing the bench.
5. Jump sideways off a low bench. Jump backward.
6. Jump forward off a chair and catch a ball in midair.

The balance beam and walking boards can be used for many types of balance activities. The boards should be different widths, heights, and inclines to provide challenges that increase in difficulty. When the students are first using the balance beam, it may be best to have it at a low height. As the students gain confidence, the height can be increased.

▶ REVIEW PROBLEMS ◀

1. Review additional balance tests found in other textbooks. Note the groups for whom the tests are intended and the validity, reliability, and objectivity coefficients.
2. Administer one static balance test and one dynamic balance test described in this chapter to several of your classmates. Ask them to provide constructive criticism of your test administration.

10 Cardiorespiratory Fitness

Upon completion of this chapter, you should be able to

1. Define and measure cardiorespiratory fitness;

2. State why cardiorespiratory fitness should be measured; and

3. Prescribe activities and exercises to develop cardiorespiratory fitness.

Cardiorespiratory fitness is the ability to perform large muscle, whole body physical activity of moderate to high intensity for relatively long periods of time. It is the ability of the circulatory and respiratory systems to adjust to vigorous exercise and to recover from the effect of such exercise. It involves the functioning of the heart and lungs, the blood and its capacity to carry oxygen, the blood vessels and capillaries supplying blood to all parts of the body, and the muscle cells, which use the oxygen to provide the energy necessary for endurance exercise. Activities such as aerobic dance, distance running, brisk walking, swimming, bicycling, and cross-country skiing are associated with cardiorespiratory fitness. Terms such as aerobic power, aerobic fitness, cardiovascular endurance, and cardiorespiratory endurance essentially mean cardiorespiratory fitness.

Cardiorespiratory fitness indicates a high state of efficiency of the circulatory and respiratory systems in supplying oxygen to the working muscles. The more oxygen you are able to take in and utilize, the longer you are able to work (exercise) before fatigue or exhaustion occurs. Generally, the more intense the work or performance of an activity, the greater the amount of oxygen processed by the body (oxygen uptake). The greatest rate at which oxygen can be taken in and utilized during exercise is referred to as *maximum oxygen consumption* (VO_2 max). Maximum VO_2 is also termed maximum oxygen intake, maximum oxygen uptake, or aerobic capacity. Because oxygen consumption is related to body weight, VO_2 max is usually reported as the volume of oxygen consumed per kilogram of body weight per minute of work (ml/kg/min). The maximum VO_2 an individual can attain measures the effectiveness of the heart, lungs, and vascular system in the delivery of oxygen during heavy work and the ability of the working cells to extract it. The higher the VO_2 max attained, the more effective the circulatory and respiratory systems. VO_2 max in untrained college males generally ranges from 42 to 45 ml/kg/min of work, whereas values for females are 3 to 4 milliliters lower at the same level of fitness. Many endurance athletes have been able to achieve values as high as 65 to 80 ml/kg/min.

Why Measure Cardiorespiratory Fitness?

Because flexibility, muscular strength, and muscular endurance exercises may reduce the frequency of musculoskeletal problems and other health problems, they should be included in an exercise program. However, the most important aspect of an exercise program is cardiorespiratory

115

conditioning. Performed with the correct intensity, duration, and frequency, cardiorespiratory conditioning activities serve the following purposes:

1. increase physical working capacity at all ages
2. decrease the risk of developing obesity and problems associated with obesity
3. decrease the risk of coronary heart disease
4. aid in the management of both stress and depression
5. enable most people to feel better, physically and mentally

These health benefits are very important. As a physical educator, you should be prepared to help individuals attain them. Through measurement you can identify individuals who have poor cardiorespiratory fitness and then prescribe the appropriate activities for them. Some individuals are motivated when taking the test to adopt or to continue an active and healthful lifestyle. In addition, cardiorespiratory tests may be used to screen individuals for other activities. However, the screening test should not take the place of a medical examination, and maximal effort should not be required unless the test is conducted under proper conditions (emergency care equipment available with qualified personnel to use the equipment).

Cardiorespiratory fitness testing is often performed before and after participation in physical conditioning activities to measure changes in fitness. Sometimes, in the school environment, the cardiorespiratory test results may be included in the determination of a unit grade. Unless prohibited because of medical problems, all individuals can experience change in cardiorespiratory fitness through proper conditioning activities. However, if a score on a cardiorespiratory fitness test is to be used in the grading process, reasonable objectives should be stated at the beginning of the unit and an appropriate amount of time (weeks) should be provided for the attainment of the objectives.

❓ARE YOU ABLE TO DO THE FOLLOWING:

- define cardiorespiratory fitness and state why it should be measured?

Tests of Cardiorespiratory Fitness

The best single measure of cardiorespiratory fitness is VO_2max, but performing this measurement requires expensive equipment (a treadmill or bicycle ergometer and direct gas analysis equipment) and trained personnel. Because of these requirements, VO_2max tests are rarely performed in physical education classes and in fitness centers only by certified individuals. Exercise physiology classes provide more detailed instructions about laboratory methods used to determine VO_2max. Cardiorespiratory fitness tests that require inexpensive equipment and that can be administered to large groups are presented here. However, validity, reliability, and objectivity coefficients are not available for all the tests presented.

We know that oxygen consumption has a direct linear relationship to heart rate; so, cardiorespiratory fitness can be estimated by measurement of the heart rate during and after testing. Though electronic measurement of the heart rate is preferred for accuracy, it is not practical or feasible in the testing of groups. In group testing, the heart rate is usually measured by counting the pulse rate at the radial artery in the wrist or at the carotid artery in the neck (lightly place the first two fingers at these sites). Because counting errors affect the validity of the test, it is essential that those individuals who are responsible for counting the pulse rate practice the procedure several times before the test is administered. Running tests (the timing of running a specified distance or the distance an individual can run in a stated time) are also highly correlated with maximum oxygen consumption. Scoring accuracy is greater with running tests, since it is necessary only to count the number of laps around a particular course or to record the time for running a specified distance.

Regardless of the type of cardiorespiratory test administered, many variables can influence cardiorespiratory functions. It has been found that exercise, age, gender, environmental temperature, humidity, altitude, digestion, loss of sleep, changes in body position, emotional and nervous conditions, body fat level, running efficiency, and motivation can influence cardiorespiratory fitness testing. It is not possible to control all of these variables, but you should be aware of them and recognize their influence on the tests. Also, all performers should be medically approved to take a cardiorespiratory fitness test, and you should recognize that good judgment may mean the postponement of cardiorespiratory fitness testing when the influence of any of these variables could jeopardize the health of the test performer.

12-Minute and 9-Minute Run
(AAHPERD 1980a)

Test Objective. To measure cardiorespiratory fitness.

Age Level. Junior high through adult for 12-minute run and ages five to college-age for 9-minute run.

Equipment. A stopwatch, whistle, and any flat, measured area. Sharp turns usually slow the runner, so it is best if the running course does not have them. If sharp turns are unavoidable, however, do not compare the running times for the curvy course with running times for a course that has no sharp turns. Different norms should be prepared for the course with sharp turns.

Validity. A validity coefficient of .90 has been reported when maximum oxygen consumption was used as the criterion.

Reliability. When the test-retest method was used, a coefficient of .94 was reported.

Norms. Tables 10.1 and 10.2 report norms for both runs. Cooper (1982) provides norms for ages thirteen through sixty and up for the 12-minute run.

Administration and Directions. All test performers should practice distance running and understand the advantage of maintaining a constant pace before attempting the test. The runners should be motivated to give their best effort, or the validity of the test will be affected. The running course should be marked so that the test administrator can determine with ease and promptness the exact distance in yards covered by the runner. Placing markers every 10 to 25 yards facilitates the scoring process. In addition, assigning a spotter to each runner makes the scoring process more efficient. After the test performers have warmed up, they gather behind a line, and on

the starting signal they run (walking is permitted) as many laps as possible around the course. The spotters count the number of laps for the runner, and when the signal (whistle) to stop is given, they run to the spot of the runner. The runners should be instructed to keep moving until they have cooled down.

Scoring. Both runs are scored to the nearest 10 yards. The importance of accurate counting of laps should be emphasized to the spotters.

1-Mile and 1.5-Mile Runs
(AAHPERD 1976a, 1980a)

Test Objective. To measure cardiorespiratory fitness.

Age Level. Five through adult for 1-mile run and thirteen through adult for 1.5-mile run.

Equipment. Stopwatch and a flat, measured area.

Validity and Reliability. Both runs are valid tests because they are related to maximum oxygen consumption. As do other similar tests, these runs have acceptable reliability when administered to properly prepared performers.

Norms. Table 10.3 reports norms for the 1-mile run, and table 10.1 reports norms for the 1.5-mile run. Cooper (1982) also provides norms for ages thirteen through sixty and up for the 1.5-mile run.

Administration and Directions. Again, all performers should practice distance running and understand the advantage of maintaining a constant pace before attempting the test. Assigning a partner, or spotter, to each runner aids in the recording of the scores. After the runners have warmed up, they gather behind a starting line, and on the signal to start, they run (walking is permitted) the distance as fast as possible. The partner of each runner is at the finish line and records the test time of the runner. The test administrator calls out the times as the runners cross the finish line.

TABLE 10.1 Norms for 12-Minute Run (Yards) and 1.5-Mile Run (Minutes and Seconds) for Ages Thirteen Through Eighteen

Percentile	Males		Females	
	12-Minute Run (Yards)	1.5-Mile Run (Time)	12-Minute Run (Yards)	1.5-Mile Run (Time)
95	3297	8:37	2448	12:17
75	2879	10:19	2100	15:03
50	2592	11:29	1861	16:57
25	2305	12:39	1622	18:50
5	1888	14:20	1274	21:36

Adapted from AAHPERD, *AAHPERD youth fitness test manual,* Reston, Va.: American Alliance for Health, Physical Education, Recreation and Dance, 1976.

TABLE 10.2 Norms in Yards for 9-Minute Run for Ages Five Through College-Age

Percentile	Age													
	5	6	7	8	9	10	11	12	13	14	15	16	17+	College
Males														
95	1760	1750	2020	2200	2175	2250	2250	2400	2402	2473	2544	2615	2615	2640
75	1320	1469	1683	1810	1835	1910	1925	1975	2096	2167	2238	2309	2380	2349
50	1170	1280	1440	1595	1660	1690	1725	1760	1885	1956	2027	2098	2169	2200
25	990	1090	1243	1380	1440	1487	1540	1500	1674	1745	1816	1887	1958	1945
5	600	816	990	1053	1104	1110	1170	1000	1368	1439	1510	1581	1652	1652
Females														
95	1540	1700	1900	1860	2050	2067	2000	2175	2085	2123	2161	2199	2237	2230
75	1300	1440	1540	1540	1650	1650	1723	1760	1785	1823	1861	1899	1937	1870
50	1140	1208	1344	1358	1425	1460	1480	1590	1577	1615	1653	1691	1729	1755
25	950	1017	1150	1225	1243	1250	1345	1356	1369	1407	1445	1483	1521	1460
5	700	750	860	970	960	940	904	1000	1069	1107	1145	1183	1221	1101

Adapted from *AAHPERD health related physical fitness test manual*, Reston, Va.: American Alliance for Health, Physical Education, Recreation and Dance, 1980; and R. R. Pate, *Norms for college students: Health related physical fitness test*, Reston, Va.: AAHPERD, 1985.

TABLE 10.3 Norms in Minutes and Seconds for 1-Mile Run for Ages Five Through College-Age

Percentile	Age													
	5	6	7	8	9	10	11	12	13	14	15	16	17+	College
Males														
95	9:02	9:06	8:06	7:58	7:17	6:56	6:50	6:27	6:11	5:51	6:01	5:48	6:01	5:30
75	11:32	10:55	9:37	9:14	8:36	8:10	8:00	7:24	6:52	6:36	6:35	6:28	6:36	6:12
50	13:46	12:29	11:25	11:00	9:56	9:19	9:06	8:20	7:27	7:10	7:14	7:11	7:25	6:49
25	16:05	15:10	14:02	13:29	12:00	11:05	11:31	10:00	8:35	8:02	8:04	8:07	8:26	7:32
5	18:25	17:38	17:17	16:19	15:44	14:28	15:25	13:41	10:23	10:32	10:37	10:40	10:56	9:47
Females														
95	9:45	9:18	8:48	8:45	8:24	7:59	7:46	7:26	7:10	7:18	7:39	7:07	7:26	7:02
75	13:09	11:24	10:55	10:35	9:58	9:30	9:12	8:36	8:18	8:13	8:42	9:00	9:03	8:15
50	15:08	13:48	12:30	12:00	11:12	11:06	10:27	9:47	9:27	9:35	10:05	10:45	9:47	9:22
25	17:59	15:27	14:30	14:16	13:18	12:54	12:10	11:35	10:56	11:43	12:21	13:00	11:28	10:41
5	19:00	18:50	17:44	16:58	16:42	17:00	16:56	14:46	14:55	16:59	16:22	15:30	15:24	12:43

Adapted from *AAHPERD health related physical fitness test manual*, Reston, Va.: American Alliance for Health, Physical Education, Recreation and Dance, 1980; and R. R. Pate, *Norms for college students: Health related physical fitness test*, Reston, Va.: AAHPERD, 1985.

Cardiorespiratory Fitness   **119**

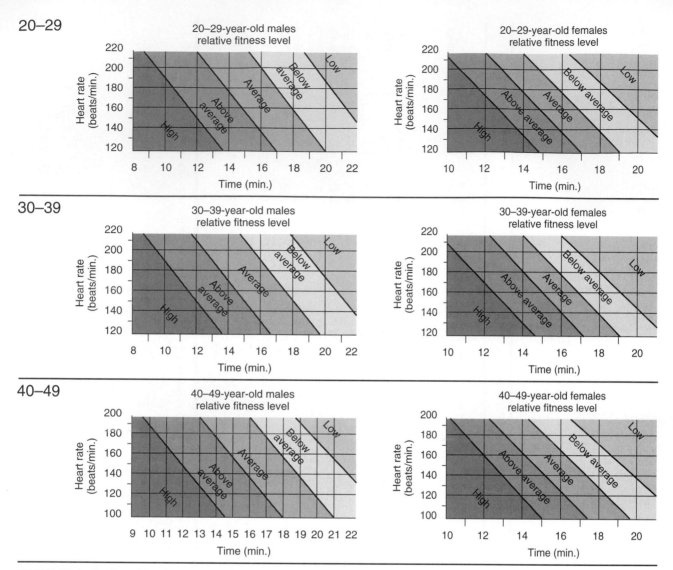

FIGURE 10.1 1-mile walking fitness chart.

All charts and tables taken from the *One Mile Walk Test* by Dr. James Rippe and colleagues. Reprinted with authors' permission.

Scoring. The score is the time in minutes and seconds to complete the run.

▦ 1-Mile Walking Test
(Kline et al. 1987; Rippe 1991)

Test Objective. To measure cardiorespiratory fitness through walking.

Age Level. Twenty through sixty-plus.

Validity. Coefficients of .79 for ages 20–29 and .92 for ages 30–69 have been reported.

Reliability. A coefficient of .98 was found for ages 30–69 years.

Equipment. Flat, measured surface and a stopwatch.

Norms. Fitness level charts for gender and age groups are provided in figure 10.1. The charts are based on weights of 170 pounds for men and 125 pounds for women. If the test taker weighs substantially less, his or her relative

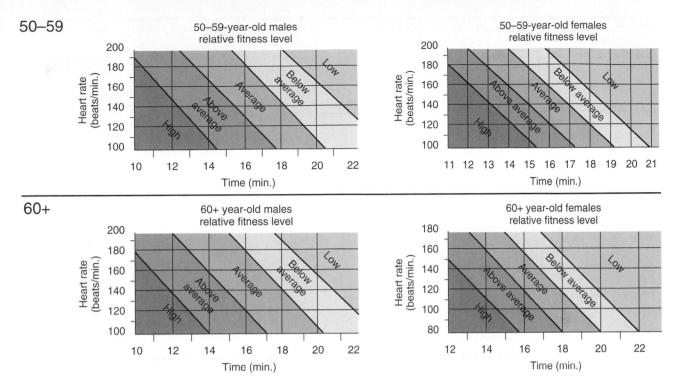

FIGURE 10.1 1-mile walking fitness chart (continued).

cardiorespiratory fitness level will be slightly underestimated. If the test taker weighs substantially more, his or her cardiorespiratory fitness will be slightly overestimated.

Administration and Directions. All test performers should practice counting their pulse at the radial or carotid artery before taking the test. After stretching for 5–10 minutes, the participants gather behind the starting line. On the signal to start, they walk 1 mile as fast as possible. Immediately at the end of the 1-mile walk, the test performers count their pulse for 15 seconds.

Scoring. The heart rate is multiplied by four, recorded, and located on the appropriate fitness test chart in figure 10.1. The point where the 1-mile time (horizontal axis) and the recorded heart rate (vertical axis) cross is the fitness score.

■ 3-Mile Walking Test (No Running)
(Cooper 1982)

Test Objective. To measure cardiorespiratory fitness through walking.

Age Level. Thirteen through sixty-plus.

Validity. Accepted because of linear relationship between workload, heart rate, and VO₂max.

Reliability. Not reported.

Equipment. Flat, measured surface and stopwatch.

Norms. Cooper (1982) provides fitness standards for male and female age groups, age thirteen through sixty-plus. Table 10.4 reports the "good" classification standards for the 3-mile walking test. Lower times place the test performers in the excellent classification and higher times place them in the fair to very poor classifications.

Administration and Directions. All test performers should practice walking for speed and endurance before attempting the test. After warming up, the test performers gather behind the starting line. On the signal to start, they attempt to cover 3 miles in the fastest time possible, without running. A partner for each walker is at the finish line to record the finishing time as the test administrator calls it out.

Scoring. The time in minutes and seconds to walk the 3 miles is the score.

■ 12-Minute Swimming Test
(Cooper 1982)

Test Objective. To measure cardiorespiratory fitness through swimming.

Age Level. Thirteen through sixty-plus.

TABLE 10.4 Standards for Classification of Good Fitness for 3-Mile Walk, 12-Minute Swimming, and 12-Minute Cycling Tests for Ages Thirteen Through Sixty+

Test	Age					
	13–19	20–29	30–39	40–49	50–59	60+
	Males					
3-mile walking (minutes: seconds)	33:00 to 37:30	34:00 to 38:30	35:00 to 40:00	36:30 to 42:00	39:00 to 45:00	41:00 to 48:00
12-minute swimming (yards)	700 to 799	600 to 699	550 to 649	500 to 599	450 to 549	400 to 499
12-minute cycling (miles)	4.75 to 5.74	4.50 to 5.49	4.25 to 5.24	4.00 to 4.99	3.50 to 4.49	3.00 to 3.99
	Females					
3-mile walking (minutes: seconds)	35:00 to 39:30	36:00 to 40:30	37:30 to 42:00	39:00 to 44:00	42:00 to 47:00	45:00 to 51:00
12-minute swimming (yards)	600 to 699	500 to 599	450 to 549	400 to 499	350 to 449	300 to 399
12-minute cycling (miles)	3.75 to 4.74	3.50 to 4.49	3.25 to 4.24	3.00 to 3.99	2.50 to 3.49	2.00 to 2.99

Adapted from K. H. Cooper, *The aerobics program for total well-being*, New York: M. Evans & Company, 1982.
Note: Lower times or greater distances place the individual in the excellent fitness category, and higher times or lesser distances place the individual in the fair to very poor fitness categories.

Equipment. Swimming pool, stopwatch, and whistle.
Validity. Accepted because of linear relationship between workload, heart rate, and VO₂max.
Reliability. Not reported.
Norms. Cooper (1982) provides fitness standards for male and female age groups, age thirteen through sixty-plus. Table 10.4 reports the "good" classification standards. Greater distances place the test performers in the excellent classification, and lesser distances place them in the fair to very poor classification.
Administration and Directions. All test performers should practice swimming for distance and pacing before attempting the test. The swimming course performers gather at one end of the pool. Each performer is instructed to swim in an individual lane. On the signal to start, they push off from the side and swim as far as possible in 12 minutes, using any stroke and resting when necessary. A test partner counts the laps and observes where the swimmer is when the signal to stop is given. The swimmer continues to swim to cool down.
Scoring. The distance in yards swum is the score.

■ 12-Minute Cycling Test
(Cooper 1982)

Test Objective. To measure cardiorespiratory fitness through cycling.
Age Level. Thirteen through sixty-plus.
Equipment. A bicycle with no more than three gears and a flat, measured distance.
Validity. Accepted because of linear relationship between workload, heart rate, and VO₂max.
Reliability. Not reported.
Norms. Cooper (1982) provides fitness standards for male and female age groups, age 13 through 60-plus. Table 10.4 reports the "good" classification standards. Greater distances place the test performers in the excellent classification, and lesser distances place them in the fair to very poor classifications.
Administration and Directions. All test performers should practice cycling for distance and pacing before attempting the test. The cycling course should be on a hard, flat surface in an

area where traffic is not a problem. Every quarter-mile should be marked. On the day of the test the wind should be less than 10 mph. After warming up, the test performers gather at the starting line, and on the signal to start they attempt to cycle as far as possible in 12 minutes. A test partner spots the position of the cyclist when the signal to stop is given. All cyclists should continue to move until they have cooled down.

Scoring. The score is the distance in miles cycled.

■ Queens College Step Test
(Katch and McArdle 1977; McArdle et al. 1972)

Test Objective. To measure cardiorespiratory fitness with a submaximal step test.

Age Level. College.

Equipment. Gymnasium bleachers and a metronome. To facilitate testing, record the instructions and commands (cadence) on tape. It is helpful to the test performers if the cadence is maintained through the commands "up, up, down, down," rather than through the metronome. Recording the instructions and commands standardizes the administration of the test and permits you to circulate among the performers during the test.

Validity. When VO_2max was used as the criterion, correlation coefficients of $-.75$ and $-.72$ were found for college-age women and men, respectively.

TABLE 10.5 Norms for the Queens College Step Test for College Students

Percentile	Males		Females	
	Heart Rate	VO_2	Heart Rate	VO_2
95	124	59.3	140	40.0
75	144	50.9	158	36.6
50	156	45.8	166	35.1
25	168	40.8	176	33.3
5	184	34.1	196	29.6

Equations for predicting VO_2max

Males: VO_2max (ml/kg/min) = 111.33 − .42 (pulse rate; beats/min)

Females: VO_2max (ml/kg/min) = 65.81 − 0.1847 (pulse rate; beats/min)

Adapted from F. I. Katch and W. D. McArdle, *Nutrition, weight control, and exercise,* Boston: Houghton Mifflin, 1977.

Reliability. Coefficients of .92 and .89 were found for college-age women and men, respectively.

Norms. Table 10.5 reports norms.

Administration and Directions. Before administration of the test, provide all participants ample time to practice measuring the pulse rate by palpating the carotid artery for 15-second intervals. Test performers should have a partner to count the pulse rate. Since the test cadence is different for males and females, pair a male with a female, then you can test the males as a group and the females as a group. Demonstrate the test and allow the test performers a brief practice period (15 to 20 seconds) to learn the cadence. After the practice period, permit the participants to rest. To perform the test, all participants step up and down on the bleacher for 3 minutes. The cadence for males is 24 steps/minute (metronome set at 96 beats/minute), and the cadence for females is 22 steps/minute (metronome set at 88 beats/minute). At the end of 3 minutes, the test performers remain standing while the partners count their pulse rate for 15 seconds, beginning 5 seconds after the completion of the test. (Pulse count should be completed 20 seconds after test performer has completed test.)

Scoring. Multiply the 15-second pulse rate by four to obtain the performer's score in beats per minute. Katch and McArdle (1977) also developed regression equations to predict VO_2max from heart rate (beats per minute). They are included in table 10.5.

■ Harvard Step Test
(Brouha 1943)

Note: This is a strenuous test and should not be used on older individuals.

Test Objective. To estimate the capacity of the body to adjust to and recover from hard muscular work.

Age Level. College males.

Equipment. A bench or platform 20 inches high, a stopwatch, and a metronome. Recording the commands "up, up, down, down" helps the performers maintain the cadence and permits you to circulate among them.

Validity. Studies on Harvard undergraduates showed that athletes scored higher than nonathletes, and the scores of the athletes increased with more training and decreased after they stopped training.

Norms. Classification standards are given in the discussion of scoring.

Administration and Directions. Permit the test performers to practice counting their pulse at the radial or carotid artery. Pair up the test performers. Test performers step up and down on a bench 30 times/minute for 5 minutes, unless they must stop earlier because of fatigue. The body should be erect each time the performer steps onto the bench and the lead foot may be changed during the test. As soon as performers stop the test, they sit down and remain sitting throughout the pulse count. There are two forms of the test. In the long form, the pulse is counted for 30 seconds on three occasions: 1 minute after exercise (1 to 1½ minutes), 2 minutes after exercise (2 to 2½ minutes), and 3 minutes after exercise (3 to 3½ minutes). In the short form, the pulse is counted for only 30 seconds, 1 minute after exercise (1 to 1½ minutes).

Scoring. In the long form, a physical efficiency index (PEI) is computed with the formula

$$PEI = \frac{\text{duration of exercise in seconds} \times 100}{2 \times \text{sum of pulse counts in recovery}}$$

The PEI standards for the long form are as follows:

below 55 — poor
55 to 64 — low average
65 to 79 — high average
80 to 89 — good
above 89 — excellent

For individuals who do not complete the 5-minute test, the following scoring standards may be used:

less than 2 minutes	25
from 2 to 3 minutes	38
from 3 to 3½ minutes	48
from 3½ to 4 minutes	52
from 4 to 4½ minutes	55
from 4½ to 5 minutes	59

In the short form, the scoring formula is

$$PEI = \frac{\text{duration of exercise in seconds} \times 100}{5.5 \times \text{pulse count for 1 to } 1\frac{1}{2} \text{ minutes after exercise}}$$

The PEI standards for the short form are as follows:

below 50 — poor
50 to 80 — average
above 80 — good

Modifications of the Harvard Step Test have been made so that it may be used on both sexes in elementary grades through college.

■ Harvard Step Test for Junior and Senior High Males
(Gallagher and Brouha 1943)

Males twelve through eighteen years of age with a body surface area (based on height and weight) less than 1.85 square meters use an 18-inch bench, whereas males of the same age with a surface area of 1.85 square meters or more use a 20-inch bench. A nomogram for estimating body surface is provided in the reference. Both groups perform 30 steps/minute for 4 minutes. The sequence of pulse counts and the formula for scoring are the same as those used for college males. The classification standards for this test are as follows:

50 or less — very poor
51 to 60 — poor
61 to 70 — fair
71 to 80 — good
81 to 90 — excellent
92 or more — superior

■ Harvard Step Test for Junior High, Senior High, and College Females
(Skubic and Hodgkins 1963)

For this test the bench is 18 inches high, the sequence is 24 steps/minute, the duration of exercise is 3 minutes, and only one 30-second pulse count is taken 1 minute after exercise (1 to 1½ minutes). The cardiovascular efficiency score (CES) is determined through the formula

$$CES = \frac{\text{no. of seconds completed} \times 100}{\text{recovery pulse} \times 5.6}$$

Norms for the three female groups are reported in table 10.6.

■ Harvard Step Test for Elementary School Males and Females
(Brouha and Ball 1952)

For this test the bench is 14 inches high and the cadence is 30 steps/minute. The duration of the exercise is adjusted by ages: 3 minutes for ages eight through twelve and 2 minutes for age seven. The pulse count, scoring formula, and classification standards are the same as those used for the original Harvard Step Test.

■ YMCA 3-Minute Step Test
(Golding, Myers, and Sinning 1989)

Test Objective. To measure cardiorespiratory fitness with a submaximal step test.

Age Level. Eighteen through 65-plus.

Equipment. A bench 12 inches high, a stopwatch, and a metronome.

Validity. Accepted because of linear relationships between workload, heart rate, and VO_2max.

TABLE 10.6 Norms for Cardiovascular Efficiency Test (Step Test) for Junior High, Senior High, and College Females

Rating	Junior High*		Senior High*		College**	
	Cardiovascular Efficiency Score	30-Second Recovery Rate	Cardiovascular Efficiency Score	30-Second Recovery Rate	Cardiovascular Efficiency Score	30-Second Recovery Rate
Excellent	72–100	44 or less	71–100	45 or less	71–100	45 or less
Very good	62–71	45–52	60–70	46–54	60–70	46–54
Good	51–61	53–63	49–59	55–66	49–59	55–66
Fair	41–50	64–79	40–48	67–80	39–48	67–83
Poor	31–40	80–92	31–39	81–96	28–38	84–116
Very poor	0–30	93 & above	0–30	97 & above	0–27	117–120

*Source: V. Skubic and J. Hodgkins, Cardiovascular efficiency test scores for junior and senior high school girls in the United States, *Research Quarterly* 35:184–192, 1964.
**Source: J. Hodgkins and V. Skubic, Cardiovascular efficiency test scores for college women in the United States, *Research Quarterly* 34:454–461, 1963.

Reliability. Not reported.

Norms. Table 10.7 reports norms.

Administration and Directions. All test performers should have a partner to count the carotid pulse (allow time to practice counting a partner's carotid pulse). On the signal to begin, the test performer steps up with one foot, then the other; steps down with the first foot, then the other foot. The knees must straighten with the step on the bench. The complete step represents 4 counts (up, up, down, down). The step is done at a cadence of 96 counts/minute or 24 complete step executions/minute (one 4-count step every 2.5 seconds). At the conclusion of 3 minutes, the test performer quickly sits down, and the partner counts the pulse for 1 minute.

Scoring. The score is the total 1-minute posttest pulse count.

Development of Cardiorespiratory Fitness

Most individuals can initiate an exercise program of low to moderate intensity without medical clearance. Some individuals, however, should consult a physician before they begin an exercise program. The Physical Activity Readiness Questionnaire (PAR-Q) in figure 10.2 is designed to determine whether individuals should check with a physician before they become more physically active.

Cardiorespiratory fitness is developed through aerobic activities, such as running, walking, swimming, cross-country skiing, or bicycling for a relatively long distance or jumping rope for an extended period at an appropriate intensity. Individuals should select an aerobic activity or activities they enjoy and to which they can make a commitment to continue. Running is the most convenient aerobic activity for development and maintenance of cardiorespiratory fitness, though some people find it tedious. In addition, individuals with joint problems (in the back, knees, and ankles) and foot disorders are unable to run for an extended period. Though some sports activities and forms of training require intense effort for short periods of time, they are inappropriate for development of cardiorespiratory fitness because they are not aerobic. These activities can, however, provide other exercise benefits and are highly recommended for those benefits.

An exercise program designed to develop cardiorespiratory fitness should be performed a minimum of 3 or 4 (nonconsecutive) days a week. Many individuals exercise more than 4 days a week but prefer to modify the intensity or the duration on alternate days. They exercise with greater intensity or for a longer period every other day. The exercise sessions for the other days consist of light, rhythmic movement. The avoidance of two consecutive days of intense or long exercise sessions prevents chronic fatigue for most individuals.

Determining the intensity at which one should exercise is critical; however, if training effects are to occur, the principle of overload must be observed. Overload is a gradual increase in the intensity of the physical activity. For the cardiovascular and respiratory systems (or any other physiological components of fitness) to improve,

TABLE 10.7 Norms for YMCA 3-Minute Step Test for Ages Eighteen Through Sixty-Five+

Rating	Age					
	18–25	26–35	36–45	46–55	56–65	65+
	Males					
Excellent	70–78	73–79	72–81	78–84	72–82	72–86
Good	82–88	83–88	86–94	89–96	89–97	89–95
Above average	91–97	91–97	98–102	99–103	98–101	97–102
Average	101–104	101–106	105–111	109–115	105–111	104–113
Below average	107–114	109–116	113–118	118–121	113–118	114–119
Poor	118–126	119–126	120–128	124–130	122–128	122–128
Very poor	131–164	130–164	132–168	135–158	131–150	133–152
	Females					
Excellent	72–83	72–86	74–87	76–93	74–92	73–86
Good	88–97	91–97	93–101	96–102	97–103	93–100
Above average	100–106	103–110	104–109	106–113	106–111	104–114
Average	110–116	112–118	111–117	117–120	113–117	117–121
Below average	118–124	121–127	120–127	121–126	119–127	123–127
Poor	128–137	129–135	130–138	127–133	129–136	129–134
Very poor	142–155	141–154	143–152	138–152	142–151	135–151

Source: L. A. Golding, C. R. Myers, and W. E. Sinning, eds., *The Y's way to physical fitness,* 3d ed., Champaign, Ill.: Human Kinetics, 1989. Reprinted with permission of the YMCA of the USA, 101 N. Wacker Drive, Chicago, IL 60606.

they must work harder than they are used to working. Stress must be imposed upon them so that over a period of time they will be able to accommodate the additional stress. Sedentary persons who initiate an exercise program should begin at a relatively low intensity and gradually increase the level of exertion. With great expectations of physical development, many individuals undertake a program, but mistakenly begin their activity at an intensity that is too high for them. Their efforts result in soreness and discomfort, which hinder continuation of the program. Also, upon recovery from the soreness, these individuals have no desire to resume the exercise program.

Monitoring the heart rate is the easiest method of determining the intensity of exercise. Unless advised differently by a qualified physician, most individuals should exercise at 60% to 75% of their maximum heart rate range. This range may be found by completing the following steps:

1. Estimate the maximum heart rate (220 minus age).
2. Subtract the resting heart rate from the value found in step 1.
3. Multiply the value found in step 2 by .60.
4. Add the value found in step 3 to the resting heart rate (this value is the minimum target heart rate).
5. Multiply the value found in step 2 by .75 and add to the resting heart rate (this value is the maximum target heart rate).

Sedentary individuals should begin an exercise program at 50% to 60% of their maximum heart rate range and increase the percentage as cardiorespiratory fitness improves.

The exercise period should include 5 to 10 minutes of flexibility exercises and a minimum of 20 minutes of aerobic activity. As the level of fitness improves, the duration of the exercise period can be increased.

Physical Activity Readiness
Questionnaire - PAR-Q
(revised 1994)

PAR - Q & YOU

(A Questionnaire for People Aged 15 to 69)

Regular physical acitivity is fun and healthy, and increasingly more people are starting to become more active every day. Being more active is very safe for most people. However, some people should check with their doctor before they start becoming much more physically active.

If you are planning to become much more physically active than you are now, start by answering the seven questions in the box below. If you are between the ages of 15 and 69, the PAR-Q will tell you if you should check with your doctor before you start. If you are over 69 years of age, and you are not used to being very active, check with your doctor.

Common sense is your best guide when you answere these questions. Please read the questions carefully and answer each one honestly: check YES or NO.

YES	NO		
☐	☐	1.	Has your doctor ever said that you have a heart condition <u>and</u> that you should only do physical activity recommended by a doctor?
☐	☐	2.	Do you feel pain in your chest when you do physical activity?
☐	☐	3.	In the past month, have you had chest pain when you were not doing physical activity?
☐	☐	4.	Do you lose your balance because of dizziness or do you ever lose consciousness?
☐	☐	5.	Do you have a bone or joint problem that could be made worse by a change in your physical activity?
☐	☐	6.	Is your doctor currently prescribing drugs (for example, water pills) for your blood pressure or heart condition?
☐	☐	7.	Do you know of <u>any other reason</u> why you should not do physical activity?

If you answered

YES to one or more questions

Talk with your doctor by phone or in person BEFORE you start becoming much more physically active or BEFORE you have a fitness appraisal. Tell your doctor about the PAR-Q and which questions you answered YES.

- You may be able to do any activity you want—as long as you start slowly and build up gradually. Or, you may need to restrict your activities to those which are safe for you. Talk with your doctor about the kinds of activities you wish to participate in and follow his/her advice.
- Find out which community programs are safe and helpful for you.

NO to all questions

If you answered NO honestly to <u>all</u> PAR-Q questions, you can be reasonably sure that you can:
- start becoming much more phyically active — begin slowly and build up gradually. This is the safest and easiest way to go.
- take part in a fitness appraisal — this is an excellent way to determine your basic fitness so that you can plan the best way for you to live actively.

DELAY BECOMING MUCH MORE ACTIVE:
- if you are not feeling well because of a temporary illness such as a cold or a fever — wait until you feel better; or
- if you are or may be pregnant — talk to your doctor before you start becoming more active.

Please note: If your health changes so that you then answer YES to any of the above questions, tell your fitness or health professional. Ask whether you should change your phyical activity plan.

<u>Informed Use of the PAR-Q:</u> The Canadian Society for Exercise Physiology, Health Canada, and their agents assume no liability for persons who undertake physical activity, and if in doubt after completing this questionnaire, consult your doctor prior to phyical activity.

You are encouraged to copy the PAR-Q but only if you use the entire form

NOTE: If the PAR-Q is being given to a person before he or she participates in a physical activity program or a fitness appraisal this section may be used for legal or administrative purposes.

I have read, understood and completed this questionnaire. Any questions I had were answered to my full satisfaction.

NAME _____

SIGNATURE _____   DATE _____

SIGNATURE OF PARENT _____   WITNESS _____
or GUARDIAN (for participants under the age of majority)

© Canadian Society for Exercise Physiology
　Société canadienne de physiologie de l'exercice

Supported by: Health   Santé
Canada   Canada

1. Review additional step tests found in other textbooks. Note the groups for whom the tests are intended and the validity and reliability coefficients.

2. Administer one step test and one running test described in this chapter to several of your classmates. Ask them to provide constructive criticism of your test administration.

3. If possible, observe the administration of cardiorespiratory fitness tests at the health and fitness clubs in your community. Observe how the instructions are given, how the results are interpreted to the group, and what safety precautions are followed.

11 Flexibility

Upon completion of this chapter, you should be able to

1. Define and measure flexibility;

2. State why flexibility should be measured; and

3. Prescribe activities to improve flexibility.

Flexibility is the ability to move the body joints through a maximum range of motion without undue strain. It is not a general factor, but it is specific to given joints and to particular sports or physical activities. An individual with good flexibility in the shoulders may not have good flexibility in the lower back or posterior upper legs. Flexibility depends more on the soft tissues (ligaments, tendons, and muscles) of a joint than on the bony structure of the joint itself. However, the bony structures of certain joints do place limitations on flexibility, as illustrated by extension of the elbow or knee and hyperextension and abduction of the spinal column.

Flexibility also is related to body size, gender, age, and physical activity. Any increase in body fat usually decreases flexibility. In general, females are more flexible than males. Anatomical distinctions or differences in regular physical activity may account for these flexibility differences. During the early school years flexibility increases, but a leveling off or decrease begins in early adolescence. The dramatic loss of flexibility during the aging process is probably due to failure to maintain an active program of movement.

In general, active individuals are more flexible than inactive individuals. The soft tissues and joints tend to shrink, losing extensibility when the muscles are maintained in a shortened position. Habitual postures and chronic heavy work through restricted ranges of motion also can lead to adaptive shortening of muscles. Physical activity with wide ranges of movement helps prevent this loss of extensibility. In general, then, flexibility is more related to habitual movement patterns for each individual and for each joint than to age or to gender.

Why Measure Flexibility?

Flexibility is an important component of health-related fitness, and the lack of it can create functional problems or disorders for many individuals. Medical records indicate that low back pain is one of the most prevalent health complaints in the United States, and many low back disorders are caused by poor muscle tone, poor flexibility of the lower back, and inadequate abdominal muscle tone. In addition, anyone with a stiff spinal column is at a disadvantage in many physical activities and also fails to get full value from the shock-absorbing arrangement of the spine when walking, running, or jumping. Lack of flexibility in the back can be responsible for bad posture, compression of peripheral nerves, painful menstruation, and other ailments. Furthermore, short muscles limit work efficiency. They become sore when they perform physical exertion, and without a good range of movement, the individual is more likely to incur torn ligaments and muscles during physical activities.

Because individuals with good flexibility have greater ease of movement, less stiffness of muscles, enhancement of skill, and less chance of injury during movement, the measurement of flexibility should be included in all physical education and wellness programs. Individuals with poor flexibility should be identified, and the appropriate exercises and activities prescribed for them. Flexibility tests are usually administered to identify individuals with too little range of joint movement, but they also can be administered to determine if individuals have too much flexibility in certain joints. Too much range of movement can result in joint instability and can increase the possibility of injury.

Though flexibility is usually measured for diagnostic purposes, many physical educators believe it is acceptable to grade flexibility performance. However, since the degree of flexibility most desirable for health purposes has not been determined, the grading of flexibility is questionable. If flexibility performance is graded, the standards should be reasonable, and the students should be informed of the standards at the beginning of the unit.

⸮ARE YOU ABLE TO DO THE FOLLOWING:

- define flexibility and state why it should be measured?

Tests of Flexibility

For clinical assessment of flexibility, devices such as the Leighton Flexometer, the electrogoniometer, and the goniometer are used. There also are many valid, practical tests that may be used in physical education and wellness programs and that may be administered to both sexes. Such tests will be covered in this chapter. None of the tests that will be described pose risk of injury to the performer.

There are two types of flexibility tests. **Relative flexibility tests** are designed to be relative to the length or width of a specific body part. In these tests, the movement and the length, or width, of an influencing body part are measured. **Absolute flexibility tests** are designed to measure only the movement in relation to an absolute performance goal. Both types of test are presented.

Because the test performers will be stretching to their maximum, they should warm up before taking the flexibility tests. Also, warm-up exercises improve flexibility performance, thus improving the reliability of the scores. The warm-up should include slow, sustained static stretching of all joints to be tested.

■ Sit and Reach Test
(AAHPERD 1980)

Note: Other similar tests for measurement of lower back and posterior thigh flexibility may be used. The V-sit reach test included in the President's Challenge, the sit and reach test included in the AAU Physical Fitness Test, and the back saver sit-and-reach included in the FITNESSGRAM are appropriate tests. These tests are described in chapter 15.

Test Objective. To measure the flexibility of the lower back and posterior thighs.

Age Level. Five through adulthood.

Equipment. Figure 11.1 includes the specifications of the box used for this test. It is crucial that the 9-inch mark be exactly in line with the vertical panel against which the test performer's feet will be placed. This flexibility test and box are included in many fitness tests. Some tests, however, report the score in centimeters. If centimeters are used, the 23-centimeter line should be exactly in line with the vertical panel against which the test performer's feet will be placed. If the AAHPERD norms are used, the specially constructed box, or benches that are only 12 inches high, should be used when administering this test. If local norms are established, benches turned on their sides, or the bottom row of bleachers that are a few inches higher than 12 inches, may be used. Yardsticks may be taped to the benches or bleachers so that several students can be measured at the same time.

Validity. Logical validity has been claimed. The AAHPERD sit-and-reach test has been validated against several other tests, and coefficients ranging between 0.80 and 0.90 have been found.

Reliability. .70 or higher.

Objectivity. Not reported.

Norms. Table 11.1 includes norms for ages five through college-age. The AAHPERD test manuals provide percentile norms.

Administration and Directions. The test apparatus should be prevented from slipping (may be placed against a wall), and

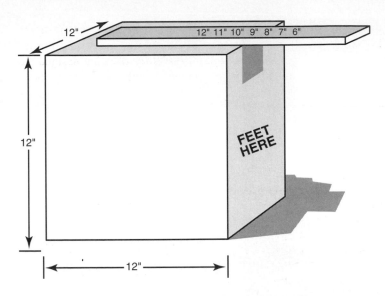

FIGURE 11.1 Sit and reach box.

TABLE 11.1 Norms in Inches for Sit-and-Reach Test for Ages Five Through College

Percentile	Age													
	5	6	7	8	9	10	11	12	13	14	15	16	17+	College
	Males													
95	12.50	13.50	13.00	13.50	13.50	13.00	13.50	13.75	14.25	15.50	16.25	16.50	17.75	17.75
75	11.50	11.50	11.00	11.50	11.50	11.00	11.50	11.50	12.00	13.00	13.50	14.25	15.75	15.50
50	10.00	10.25	10.00	10.00	10.00	10.00	10.00	10.25	10.25	11.00	12.00	12.00	13.50	13.50
25	8.75	8.75	8.75	8.75	8.75	8.00	8.25	8.25	8.00	9.00	9.50	10.00	11.00	11.50
5	6.75	6.25	6.25	6.25	4.75	4.75	5.25	4.75	4.75	6.00	5.25	4.50	6.00	7.50
	Femal es													
95	13.50	13.50	13.50	14.25	13.75	13.75	14.50	15.75	17.00	17.50	18.25	18.25	17.50	18.50
75	12.00	12.00	12.25	12.25	12.25	12.25	12.50	13.50	14.25	15.00	16.25	15.50	15.75	16.25
50	10.75	10.75	10.75	11.00	11.00	11.00	11.50	12.00	12.25	13.00	14.25	13.50	13.75	14.50
25	9.00	9.00	9.50	9.00	9.00	9.50	9.50	10.00	9.50	11.00	12.25	12.00	12.25	12.50
5	7.00	7.00	6.25	6.75	6.75	6.25	6.25	6.00	6.75	7.00	7.50	5.50	8.75	9.50

Adapted from *AAHPERD, Health related physical fitness test manual,* Reston, Va.: AAHPERD, 1980; and R. R. Pate, *Norms for college students: Health related physical fitness test,* Reston, Va.: American Alliance for Health, Physical Education, Recreation and Dance, 1985.

the test performer should not be wearing shoes. The performer (1) sits at the test apparatus with the knees fully extended and the feet shoulder-width apart, flat against the end of the board; (2) with the palms down and hands placed on top of each other, extends the arms forward; and (3) reaches directly forward four times and holds the position of the maximum reach on the fourth trial for one second (see figure 11.2). The test administrator may place a hand on the knees of the performer to discourage knee flexion, but the knees should not be hyperextended.

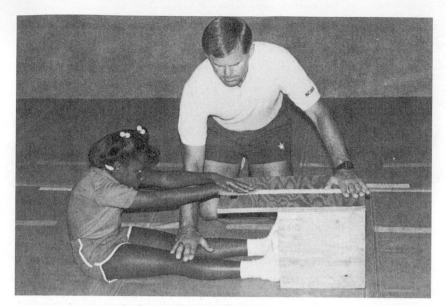

FIGURE 11.2 Sit and reach test.

Scoring. The score is the most distant point reached on the fourth trial, measured to the nearest ¼ inch or the nearest centimeter. The test administrator should be in a position to note the most distant line touched by the fingertips of both hands. If the hands reach unevenly, the position is not held for 1 second, or the knees bend, the test should be readministered. You should be aware that it is normal for many boys and girls not to reach the 9-inch level during the preadolescent and adolescent growth spurt (ages ten through fourteen). It is not unusual for the legs to become proportionately longer in relation to the trunk during this period. Flexibility exercises should be prescribed for individuals who score below P_{50}, as any score below this percentile represents poor flexibility in the posterior thigh, lower back, or posterior hip. Individuals who score below P_{25} have a critical lack of flexibility.

■ Sit and Reach Wall Test
(Robbins, Powers, and Burgess 1991)

The sit-and-reach wall test may be used to provide a quick estimate of lower back and posterior thigh flexibility. It only requires a wall and can be performed quickly by a large number of people.

Test Objective. To measure the flexibility of the lower back and posterior thighs.

Age Level. Junior high through college-age.

Equipment. A wall.

Validity. Logical validity.

Reliability and Objectivity. Not reported.

Norms. Table 11.2 includes norms for high school through college.

Administration and Directions. Individuals should be permitted to warm up before stretching. With shoes removed, the performer (1) sits facing a wall, with the knees straight and feet flat against the wall; (2) reaches as far as possible to touch fingertips, knuckles, or palms to the wall; and (3) holds position for 3 seconds.

Scoring. See table 11.2.

■ Trunk and Neck Extension
(Johnson and Nelson 1986)

Test Objective. To measure the ability to extend the trunk (relative flexibility).

TABLE 11.2 Norms for Sit and Reach Wall Test for High School and College Students

Performance Level	Score
Excellent	Palms touch wall
Good	Knuckles touch wall
Average	Fingertips touch wall
Poor	Cannot touch wall

Age Level. Six through college-age.

Equipment. Mat, and yardstick, or tape measure.

Validity. Face validity.

Reliability. .90 through test-retest.

Objectivity. .99.

Norms. Table 11.3 reports norms for college students.

Administration and Directions. The test performer should sit in a hard chair, and the test administrator should measure to the nearest ¼ inch the distance from the tip of the performer's nose to the seat of the chair in which the performer is sitting. (The chin must be level when the distance is measured.) The test performer then assumes a prone position on a mat, placing both hands on the lower back. With a partner holding the hips against the mat, the performer raises the trunk in a slow and controlled manner as high as possible from the mat. The distance from the tip of the nose to the mat is measured (see figure 11.3). If any back discomfort occurs, the test should be stopped immediately.

Scoring. The best of three lifts is subtracted from the trunk-and-neck length measurement. The closer the trunk lift is to the trunk-and-neck length, the better the score.

■ Trunk Extension
(Miller and Allen 1990)

The trunk extension test is very similar to the trunk-and-neck extension previously described. The difference is that this test measures absolute flexibility and does not require measurement of any body parts.

Age Level. Six through college-age.

Equipment. Mat, and yardstick, or tape measure.

Validity. Face validity.

Reliability and Objectivity. Not reported.

Norms. Table 11.3 reports norms for college students.

Administration and Directions. The test performer lies prone on a mat with a partner holding the hips against the mat.

TABLE 11.3 Norms in Inches for Trunk-and-Neck Extension and Trunk Extension Tests for College Students

Performance Level	Trunk and Neck Extension	Trunk Extension
Males		
Above average	6 to 0	19 and above
Average	8 to 6¼	16 to 18
Below average	8¼ and above	15 and less
Females		
Above average	5¾ to 0	21 and above
Average	7¾ to 6	18 to 20
Below average	8 and above	17 and less

Adapted from B. L. Johnson and J. K. Nelson, *Practical measurements for evaluation in physical education,* 4th ed., Edina, Minn.: Burgess Publishing, 1986; and D. K. Miller and T. E. Allen, *Fitness: A lifetime commitment,* 4th ed., New York: Macmillan Publishing, 1990.

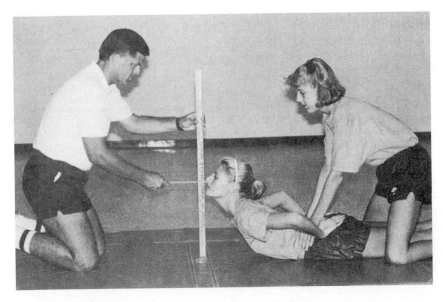

FIGURE 11.3 Trunk-and-neck extension test.

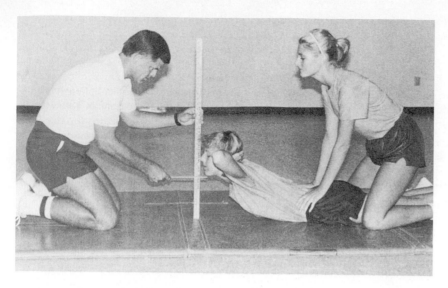

FIGURE 11.4 Trunk extension test.

The fingers are interlocked behind the neck, and the chest and head are raised in a slow and controlled manner off the mat as far as possible. The distance in inches is measured from the mat to the chin (see figure 11.4). If any back discomfort occurs, the test should be stopped immediately.

Scoring. The best of three lifts is the score.

■ Shoulder-and-Wrist Elevation
(Johnson and Nelson 1986)

Test Objective. To measure shoulder and wrist flexibility (relative flexibility).

Age Level. Six through college-age.

Equipment. Mat and two yardsticks, or one yardstick and a tape measure.

Validity. Face validity.

Reliability. .93 through test-retest.

Objectivity. .99.

Norms. Norms for college students are reported in table 11.4.

Administration and Directions. The arm length of the test performer should be measured from the acromion process (shoulder tip) to the middle fingertip, as the arms hang down. The test performer then assumes a prone position with the arms extended directly in front of the shoulders and holds a yardstick, with the hands about shoulder-width apart. The yardstick is raised upward as far as possible while keeping the chin on the floor. Because it is difficult to elevate the shoulders without extending the wrists, the movement of the two joints are combined for the test score. When the highest

TABLE 11.4 Norms in Inches for Shoulder-and-Wrist Elevation and Shoulder Lift for College Students

Performance Level	Shoulder-and-Wrist Elevation	Shoulder Lift
	Males	
Above average	8¼ to 0	22 and above
Average	11½ to 8½	17 to 21
Below average	11¾ and above	16 and less
	Females	
Above average	7½ to 0	23 and above
Average	10¾ to 7¾	19 to 22
Below average	11 and above	18 and less

Adapted from B. L. Johnson and J. K. Nelson, *Practical measurements for evaluation in physical education,* 4th ed., Edina, Minn.: Burgess Publishing, 1986; and D. K. Miller and T. E. Allen, *Fitness: A lifetime commitment,* 4th ed., New York: Macmillan Publishing, 1990.

point is reached, the distance is measured to the nearest ¼ inch. Though some individuals are extremely flexible and can move the yardstick beyond the highest vertical point, the measurement is still taken at the highest vertical point.

Scoring. The score is the best of three trials subtracted from the arm length. The closer the lift is to the arm measurement, the better the score.

Shoulder Lift
(Miller and Allen 1990)

The shoulder lift test is very similar to the shoulder-and-wrist elevation test, but it measures shoulder flexibility only. It measures absolute flexibility rather than relative flexibility.

Age Level. Six through college-age.

Equipment. Mat and two yardsticks, or one yardstick and a tape measure.

Validity. Face validity.

Reliability and Objectivity. Not reported.

Norms. Table 11.4 reports norms for college students.

Administration and Directions. The test performer lies prone on the mat with the chin to the mat and the arms extended forward directly in front of the shoulders. A yardstick is held with the hands about shoulder-width apart. The wrists and elbows are kept straight as the yardstick is raised upward as far as possible, with the chin touching the mat. The distance in inches is measured from the bottom of the yardstick to the mat (see figure 11.5).

Scoring. The score is the best of three trials.

Figures 11.6 through 11.13 (Jenson and Hirst 1980; Robbins, Powers, and Burgess 1991) illustrate observation measures of flexibility. No score is recorded, but the measures may be used to identify individuals with inadequate flexibility.

Exercises to Develop Flexibility

As previously stated, individuals with poor flexibility are susceptible to musculoskeletal problems as well as other ailments. Once these individuals have been identified, the appropriate flexibility exercises should be prescribed for them.

Three stretching techniques can be used to improve flexibility: static stretching, ballistic stretching, and proprioceptive neuromuscular facilitation (PNF). **Static stretching** involves slowly moving to a position to stretch the designated muscles and holding the position for a specified length of time. The recommended length of time for holding the stretch varies from 10 to 30 seconds, and the stretch for each muscle is repeated two or three times in each stretching session.

Ballistic stretching makes use of repetitive bouncing motions. Though ballistic stretching can improve flexibility, it is not often recommended as a stretching technique. If the force produced by the effort to stretch is greater than the extensibility the muscle tissues can tolerate, the muscle may be injured. In addition, the use of a fast, forceful, bobbing type of stretching induces the stretch reflex (the reflex contraction of a muscle in response to being suddenly stretched beyond its normal length). The purpose of this reflex action is to prevent injury caused by overstretching. The amount and rate of the stretch reflex contraction vary directly in proportion to the amount and rate of the movement causing the stretch. The faster and more forceful the stretch, the faster and more forceful the reflex contraction of the stretched muscle. As the individual is attempting to stretch the muscle through a bouncing action, the stretch reflex responds to

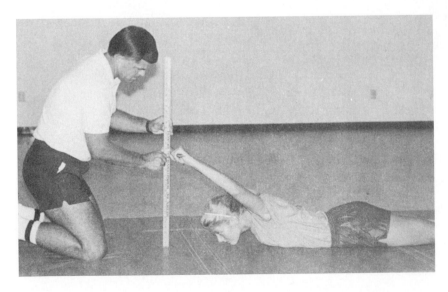

FIGURE 11.5 Shoulder lift test.

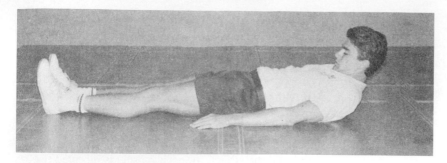

FIGURE 11.6 Normal flexibility for the neck allows the chin to move closer to the upper chest.

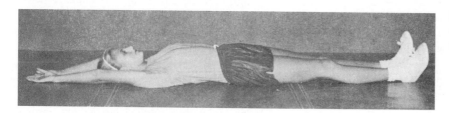

FIGURE 11.7 Normal flexibility of chest muscles allows arms to be flexed to 180° of shoulders.

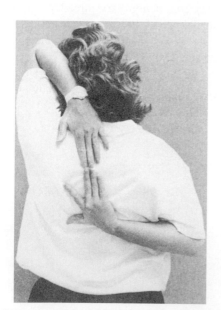

FIGURE 11.8 Normal flexibility of shoulder girdle allows fingertips to touch.

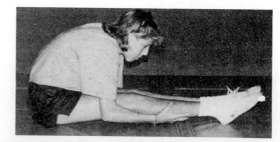

FIGURE 11.9 Normal flexibility in the hips and lower back allows for flexion to about 135°.

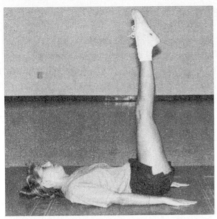

FIGURE 11.10 Normal flexibility of the hamstring muscles allows straight-leg lifting to 90° from supine position.

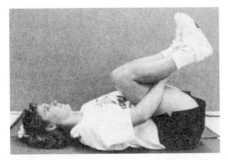

FIGURE 11.11 Normal flexibility of lower back allows thighs to touch chest.

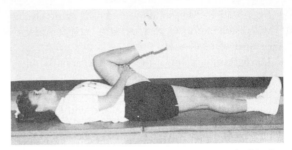

FIGURE 11.12 Normal flexibility of iliopsoas muscle (hip flexor) allows thigh to touch chest. Extended leg should remain on floor and straight.

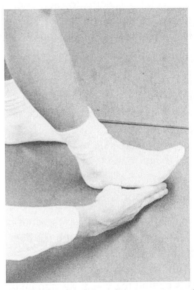

FIGURE 11.13 Normal flexibility of the gastrocnemius muscle (calf) allows the ball of the foot to clear the floor by a height equal to the width of two fingers.

prevent the muscle from being stretched. This combination may result in muscle injury.

There are a number of **PNF** techniques used for stretching, but all involve a combination of alternating contraction and relaxation of both agonist and antagonist muscles. The disadvantage of the PNF techniques is that they require the assistance of a partner.

Both static stretching and PNF techniques will improve flexibility, but there is lack of agreement regarding which technique is superior. It is difficult to compare flexibility studies, because different designs for training programs, length of stretch time, and number of PNF repetitions influence the results of the studies. Since it is accepted that static stretching improves flexibility and no partner is required to perform the exercises, only descrip-

tions of static stretching exercises will be provided in this text. The exercises are designed to improve flexibility throughout the body, but the most important areas to consider are neck and shoulder flexion, back extension, trunk and hip flexion (including lower back and posterior upper-leg muscles), and posterior lower-leg extension (ankle flexion). Unless stated otherwise, the following guidelines should be observed for best results when performing the exercises:

- Spend 20 to 30 seconds in a gentle, static stretch with each exercise, and perform each exercise two or three times.
- Increase the extent of the stretch gradually and progressively, with full extension, flexion, or both being placed on the joint.
- Breathe slowly, rhythmically, and with control.
- Stretch beyond the normal length of the muscle, but only to the point that a slight stretch pain is felt.
- Practice regularly; perform the exercises several times each day.

Flexibility is highly specific to each joint and activity; therefore, flexibility exercises should be performed for each joint in which increased flexibility is desired.

Neck

1. Place the hands behind the head and gradually press down; hold. The posterior neck muscles should feel stretched.
2. Bend the neck from side to side and then from front to back. Do not rotate the head.

Shoulder and Upper Chest

1. Stand in a doorway and grasp the door jamb above the head. Lean forward through the doorway until the stretch is felt.
2. Stand with the feet shoulder-width apart and lock the hands behind the waist. Straighten the arms, raise, and hold. Bending forward at the waist is a good variation.
3. Extend the arms overhead and interlace the fingers with the palms facing upward. Push upward and slightly backward.
4. Interlace the fingers in front of the chin with the palms turned out. Extend the arms forward.
5. Bring the right hand over the right shoulder to the upper back and reach down as far as possible. Bring the left hand under the left shoulder to the upper back. Grab the fingers and hold. If you are unable to grasp the fingers together, hold a towel between them. Gradually move the left hand up the towel. Reverse the hand positions and repeat.

Upper Back

1. Lie on the back with the knees bent and the feet flat on the floor. Interlace the fingers behind the head and gently pull forward until you feel a comfortable stretch. This stretch also may be performed while in the standing position.

Lower Back

1. Lie on the back with the knees bent and the feet flat on the floor. Place the hands under the knees and pull both thighs to the chest with your hands while simultaneously raising the head.
2. Sit on the floor with the legs crossed and the arms at the sides. Tuck the chin and curl forward. Slide the hands forward on the floor, allowing the back to be rounded.

Trunk

1. Stand with the feet shoulder-width apart and the toes pointed straight ahead. Extend both arms overhead; grasp the left hand with the right hand and bend slowly to the right. Pull the left arm over the head and down toward the ground with the right hand. Bend to the left, reversing the hand positions.
2. Stand and hold a towel overhead with the hands about 12 inches apart, the elbows straight, and the feet 18 to 24 inches apart. Bend to one side as far as possible, keeping the elbows straight. Repeat on the other side.
3. Sit on the floor with the right leg extended; cross the left foot over the right knee and place the foot flat on the floor. Place the left hand on the floor behind the hips and use the right hand to slowly twist the spine to the left. Look over the left shoulder. Repeat to the other side.

Posterior Hip, Upper Leg, and Lower Back

1. Sit on the floor with the legs straight and the feet together. Bend forward at the waist (do not dip the head or round the back) and slide the hands down the lateral sides of the legs. Try to place the chest on the thighs and grasp the outer borders of the

feet. Keep the toes pointed back to stretch the posterior lower-leg muscles.

2. Sit on the floor. Extend one leg and place the sole of the other foot against the knee of the extended leg. Lean forward at the waist and attempt to pull the toes of the extended leg back to exert a stretch in the calf and hamstrings. Repeat with the other leg.

3. Lie flat on the back. Raise one leg straight up with the knee extended and ankle flexed at 90°. Grasp the leg around the calf and pull toward the head. Repeat with the opposite leg.

Anterior Hip and Thigh

1. In a standing position, draw one knee (hands under knee) up to the chest and pull it tightly to the chest with the hands. Repeat with the other knee.

2. Support yourself by leaning against a wall with the right hand; stand on the right leg and bend the left knee. Grasp the ankle behind you with the left hand and gently pull backward; keep the knee pointed down. Repeat with the other leg.

3. Squat with the bent knee of one leg forward and the other leg extended behind you. Push forward until the knee of the front leg is directly over the ankle. The knee of the backward extended leg should be resting on the floor. Without changing the position of the legs and feet, lower the front of your hips downward to create an easy stretch. Reverse the position of the legs and repeat.

Groin Area

1. Sit on the floor. Put the soles of the feet together and grasp the toes. Gently pull yourself forward, bending at the hips.

2. Sit on the floor with the back pressed against a wall or anything that will give support. With the back straight and the soles of the feet together, gently push down on the inside of the thighs with the hands.

Posterior Lower Leg

1. Face a wall, standing approximately 3 to 4 feet away. Lean forward and place the palms against the

wall, with the arms straight and at shoulder height. Keep the feet flat and the body in a straight line. Allow the elbows to bend while leaning forward more. Do not allow the heels to rise off the floor.

2. Assume the same position as described in the previous exercise. Perform the same routine but also bend at the knees. Do not allow the heels to rise off the floor. You should feel the stretch in the area closer to the Achilles tendon.

Foot and Ankle

1. Sit on the floor with the left leg extended. Bend the right leg and provide support under the lower calf with the right hand. Grasp the right foot with the left hand and gently rotate the foot clockwise and counterclockwise through a complete range of motion. Repeat with the other foot.

2. Stand with the feet apart. Reach back with one foot and touch the floor with the upper side of the toes. Press down until a stretch is felt. Repeat with the other foot.

 REVIEW PROBLEMS

1. Review additional flexibility tests found in other textbooks. Note the groups for whom the tests are intended and the validity, reliability, and objectivity coefficients.

2. Administer one of the tests described in this chapter to several of your classmates. Ask them to provide constructive criticism of your test administration.

3. A physical education teacher administered the sit and reach test to twenty 15-year-old students. After the students followed a 10-week flexibility program for the lower back and posterior thighs, the teacher again administered the test. Determine if the students significantly improved their flexibility scores.

Student	Pretest Score	Posttest Score
A	17.50	18.25
B	16.75	17.50
C	17.00	17.75
D	15.50	16.25
E	15.00	15.75

Student	Pretest Score	Posttest Score	Student	Pretest Score	Posttest Score
F	18.50	18.50	N	15.75	16.50
G	18.00	18.50	O	15.50	16.25
H	14.25	16.25	P	16.25	16.25
I	17.00	17.25	Q	15.75	16.00
J	16.50	17.25	R	15.25	15.25
K	15.75	15.75	S	16.00	16.50
L	17.50	18.00	T	17.00	17.75
M	16.75	17.75			

12 Muscular Strength, Endurance, and Power

Upon completion of this chapter, you should be able to

1. Define muscular strength, dynamic strength, static strength, dynamic and static muscular endurance, and power;

2. State why muscular strength, endurance, and power should be measured;

3. Measure muscular strength, endurance, and power; and

4. Prescribe activities to improve muscular strength, endurance, and power.

Muscular strength is the ability of a muscle or muscle group to exert maximum force. **Dynamic strength** is force exerted by a muscle group as a body part moves. Dynamic strength also may be referred to as isotonic strengh. **Static strength** is the force exerted against an immovable object; that is, movement does not take place. This type of strength is also referred to as isometric strength. Both types of strengths are best measured by tests that require one maximum effort.

Muscular endurance is the ability of a muscle or muscle group to resist fatigue and to make repeated contractions against a defined submaximal resistance (**dynamic endurance**). It also may be the ability to maintain a certain degree of force over time (**static endurance**). Muscular strength and endurance are closely related, though weight-training methods for them are typically different. In general, strength is best developed through a high-resistance, low-repetition program, whereas endurance is improved through a low-resistance, high-repetition program. Strength and endurance can be improved through either program, however. Also, it is necessary to have some strength to develop endurance.

For example, to develop abdominal muscular endurance through sit-ups, you must have the strength to perform at least one sit-up. The inability to perform one sit-up is due to lack of strength, not to lack of endurance.

Muscular power is the ability to generate maximum force in the fastest possible time. It also may be defined as the ability to release maximum muscular force in an explosive manner. Power is equal to the product of force times velocity. Force is generated by muscle strength (strength is a component of power), and velocity is the speed at which the force is used. Although power is not considered an essential component of physical fitness or good health, it is often the characteristic of a good athlete. Power usually is measured by some type of jump, throw, or charge (the vertical jump, shot put, or a charge at a blocking sled).

Why Measure Muscular Strength, Endurance, and Power?

There are several reasons for measuring muscular strength and endurance. Strength is essential for high-level performance in many sports, and, though not to the same degree, it also is essential for good health. Strong muscles help protect the joints, making them less susceptible to sprains, strains, and other injuries. Strength is necessary for good posture. Such postural problems as sagging abdominal muscles, round shoulders, and low-back pain may be prevented if adequate strength is maintained. In addition, strength will enable you to perform routine tasks more efficiently and to experience more satisfaction from leisure sport participation.

The need for muscular endurance is demonstrated in many of our daily activities. Have you ever experienced occasions when it was necessary to "keep going," though your arms, legs, or entire body felt too tired to do so? Perhaps your arms felt this way when carrying the groceries from the car into the house. You had the strength to pick up the groceries, but they felt heavier and heavier the farther you carried them. This phenomenon can occur when a person is pushing a stalled car, carrying a heavy suitcase, or performing any task that involves sustained muscular contraction. Even if you do not lift and carry heavy loads, you probably lift light loads repeatedly or lift and move your body throughout the day. To avoid end-of-day fatigue, you need muscular endurance. Also, possessing adequate muscular endurance enables you to maintain good posture, thereby decreasing the likelihood that you will experience backaches and muscular injury while performing routine tasks.

As previously stated, muscular power is often a characteristic of a good athlete, but it is rarely necessary to have power when performing daily tasks. Because it is not considered to be an essential component of health and physical fitness, it is not usually emphasized in physical education and wellness programs. Occasionally, leisure sports participants feel that increasing their power will improve their sport performance.

? ARE YOU ABLE TO DO THE FOLLOWING:

- define muscular strength, dynamic and static muscular strength, dynamic and static muscular endurance, and power?
- state why muscular strength, muscular endurance, and muscular power should be measured?

Tests of Muscular Strength and Endurance

Though not required, dynamometers, cable tensiometers, electromechanical instruments, weight-training machines, and free weights may be used to test muscular strength and endurance. This equipment is expensive and is typically used in research studies when accuracy of measurement is essential. Two types of dynamometers are used to measure static strength, one for handgrip and one for back and leg strength. Cable tensiometers may be used to measure static strength of many different muscle groups. Electromechanical instruments measure static and dynamic strength, endurance, and power. Through measurement of the intensity and frequency (in terms of electrical activity) of muscle contractions, these instruments are capable of determining the maximum contraction of a muscle group at a constant speed throughout the entire range of the movement. Many public schools and fitness centers have weight-training machines and free weights, but few have dynamometers, cable tensiometers, and electromechanical instruments.

Tests with Weight-Training Equipment

If weight-training equipment is available, the measurement of dynamic muscular strength and endurance is a simple procedure. It is important, however, that handgrip, knee flexion, foot placement, and all other considerations that may influence test performance be standardized and enforced. In addition, since motivational factors can influence the test results, the test administration must be standardized for motivational considerations. Test participants should warm up, but avoid overworking, and safety precautions should be observed, especially if free weights are used.

Dynamic strength is measured with one repetition maximum (1-RM). Because a direct relationship exists between body weight and weight lifted (heavier individuals generally can lift more), the maximum weight that can be lifted should be interpreted in relation to the individual's weight. The 1-RM is determined through trial and error. A weight the individual can lift comfortably is first selected. After performing the lift, the test participant is permitted to rest for 2 to 3 minutes. The weight is increased by 5 to 15 pounds, and another lift is attempted.

With allowance for rest after each lift, this procedure is followed until the participant is unable to perform a successful lift. Although 1-RMs may be administered to measure most muscle groups, the body's major muscle groups may be tested with the bench press, standing press, arm curls, and leg press. Table 12.1 reports the optimal strength values for these lifts for the various body weights.

Muscular endurance tests may be relative or absolute. In a relative endurance test, the performer works with a weight that is proportionate to the maximum strength of a particular muscle group or to body weight. In an absolute endurance test, all performers work with the same amount of weight (the weight has no relationship to maximum strength or body weight of the test performer). In a

test for muscular endurance, the weight should be lifted and returned without jerky movements. A 3-second cadence may be used for each lift to encourage continuous, smooth movement. The score is the number of repetitions completed, and the test is completed when a lift can no longer be properly executed or performed with the cadence. Pollock, Wilmore, and Fox (1978) suggest that a fixed percentage of 70% of the maximum strength be used to test muscle endurance. This percentage would be the same for all muscle groups tested. No norms have been developed for this procedure, but on the basis of limited test data, the individual seeking health fitness should be able to perform 12 to 15 repetitions, and the competitive athlete should be able to perform 20 to 25 repetitions of each of the lifts tested.

Tests Requiring Limited Equipment

The following tests for muscular strength, endurance, and power are simple and practical, and they require little equipment for administration. However, reliability and objectivity coefficients are not reported for all the tests, and many of them are not appropriate for both sexes. If a test is designed primarily for one sex, that sex is indicated. Rest should be permitted when two or more test trials are administered.

■ Sit-Ups Test (Strength)
(Johnson and Nelson 1986)

Test Objective. To measure strength of abdominal and trunk flexion muscles.
Age Level. Twelve through college-age.
Equipment. A mat, weight bar, dumbbell bar, weight plates, and a 12-inch ruler.
Validity. Face validity.
Reliability. .91.
Objectivity. .98.
Norms. Johnson and Nelson (1986) provide norms (weight lifted divided by body weight) for college students.
Administration and Directions. The sit-up is performed with a weight plate, a dumbbell, or a barbell behind the neck. If a dumbbell or barbell is used, the attached weight plates must not have a greater circumference than standard 5-pound plates. The test performer (1) selects the amount of weight that is to be held during the sit-up; (2) assumes a supine position on a mat so the selected weight is behind the neck, flexes the knees, and places the feet flat on the mat; (3) with a

TABLE 12.1 Optimal Strength Values in Pounds for Various Body Weights (Based on 1-RM Test on Universal Gym Apparatus)

Body Weight	Bench Press	Standing Press	Arm Curl	Leg Press
Males				
80	80	53	40	160
100	100	67	50	200
120	120	80	60	240
140	140	93	70	280
160	160	107	80	320
180	180	120	90	360
200	200	133	100	400
220	220	147	110	440
240	240	160	120	480
Females				
80	56	37	28	112
100	70	47	35	140
120	84	56	42	168
140	98	65	49	196
160	112	75	56	224
180	126	84	63	252
200	140	93	70	280

Adapted from M. L. Pollock, J. H. Wilmore, and S. M. Fox, *Health and fitness through physical activity,* New York: John Wiley & Sons, 1978.

test partner holding a ruler under the knees, slides the feet toward the buttocks until the ruler can be held in place by the flexion of the lower legs; (4) slowly slides the feet forward until the ruler falls—at that point the test administrator marks the heel line and the buttocks line, indicating the distance that should remain between the heels and the buttocks during the test; and (5) as the partner holds the performer's feet firmly to floor, attempts to sit up while holding the weight behind the neck (see figure 12.1). The test administrator should be prepared to remove the weight at the completion of the sit-up.

Scoring. Two sit-ups are permitted, and the greatest amount of weight lifted is recorded. The test score may be (1) the amount of weight lifted or (2) the amount of weight lifted divided by body weight.

■ Sit-Ups Test (Endurance)
(AAHPERD 1980a; Pollock, Wilmore, and Fox 1978)

Test Objective. To measure abdominal strength and endurance.
Age Level. Five through adulthood.
Equipment. Mats and a stopwatch.
Validity. Logical validity.
Reliability. .68 to .94 for modified sit-ups test.
Norms. Tables 12.2 and 12.3 include norms.
Administration and Directions. Two types of sit-ups tests may be administered, but both are performed for 60 seconds. With the modified sit-ups test, the test performer assumes a supine position on the mat with the knees flexed, feet flat on the mat, and the heels between 12 and 18 inches from the buttocks. The arms are crossed on the chest with the hands on opposite shoulders. A test partner holds the feet of the test

performer to keep them in contact with the mat. On the signal, "Go," the test performer (1) curls to a sitting position and touches the thighs with the elbows while maintaining arm contact with the chest and keeping the chin tucked on the chest (see figure 12.2); (2) curls back to the floor until the midback contacts the mat; and (3) continues to perform as many sit-ups as possible in 60 seconds. The test administrator should use the signal, "Ready, Go," to begin the test, and the word, "Stop," to conclude the test at the end of 60 seconds. Pausing between sit-ups is permitted. Table 12.2 includes norms for this sit-ups test for ages five through college-age.

A second type of sit-ups test is administered in a similar procedure, except the hands are interlocked behind the performer's neck, the elbows are touched to the knees, and the performer must return to the full lying position before starting the next sit-up (see figure 12.3). The performer should be cautioned not to use the arms to thrust the body into a sitting position. Table 12.3 includes norms for ages twenty through sixty-nine for this sit-ups test.

Scoring. The score for both tests is the number of sit-ups correctly performed during the 60 seconds. Incorrect performance for the modified sit-ups test includes failure to curl up, failure to keep the arms against the chest, failure to touch the thighs with the elbows, and failure to touch the midback to the mat. The distance between the heels and the buttocks should be monitored continuously. Incorrect performance for the second type of sit-ups test includes failure to keep the hands interlocked behind the neck, failure to touch the knees with the elbows, and failure to return to the full lying position. If partners are permitted to count the number of sit-ups, the test administrator should observe to be sure the partners are counting only sit-ups that are performed correctly.

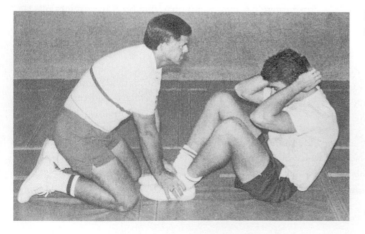

FIGURE 12.1 Sit-ups test for strength.

TABLE 12.2 Norms for Modified Sit-Ups Test for Ages Five Through College-Age

Percentile							Age							
	5	6	7	8	9	10	11	12	13	14	15	16	17+	College
							Males							
95	30	36	42	48	47	50	51	56	58	59	59	61	62	60
75	23	26	33	37	38	40	42	46	48	49	49	51	52	50
50	18	20	26	30	32	34	37	39	41	42	44	45	46	44
25	11	15	19	25	25	27	30	31	35	36	38	38	38	38
5	2	6	10	15	15	15	17	19	25	27	28	28	25	30
							Females							
95	28	35	40	44	44	47	50	52	51	51	56	54	54	53
75	24	28	31	35	35	39	40	41	41	42	43	42	44	42
50	19	22	25	29	29	32	34	36	35	35	37	33	37	35
25	12	14	20	22	23	25	28	30	29	30	30	29	31	30
5	2	6	10	12	14	15	19	19	18	20	20	20	19	21

Adapted from *AAHPERD health related physical fitness test manual,* Reston, Va.: American Alliance for Health, Physical Education, Recreation and Dance, 1980; and R. R. Pate, *Norms for college students: Health related physical fitness test,* Reston, Va.: AAHPERD, 1985.

TABLE 12.3 Norms for Sit-Ups Test with Hands Behind Neck (Muscular Endurance) for Ages Twenty Through Sixty-Nine

Performance Level	Age				
	20–29	30–39	40–49	50–59	60–69
	Males				
Above average	43 and above	35 and above	30 and above	25 and above	20 and above
Average	37 to 42	29 to 34	24 to 29	19 to 24	14 to 19
Below average	36 and below	28 and below	23 and below	18 and below	13 and below
	Females				
Above average	39 and above	31 and above	26 and above	21 and above	16 and above
Average	33 to 38	25 to 30	19 to 25	15 to 20	10 to 15
Below average	32 and below	24 and below	18 and below	14 and below	9 and below

Adapted from M. L. Pollock, J. H. Wilmore, and S. M. Fox, *Health and fitness through physical activity,* New York: John Wiley & Sons, 1978.

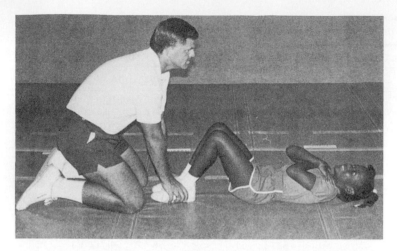

FIGURE 12.2 Modified sit-ups test.

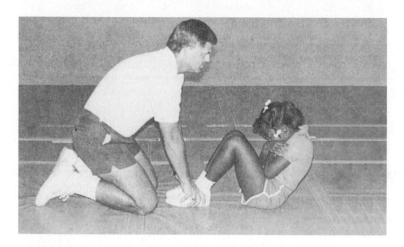

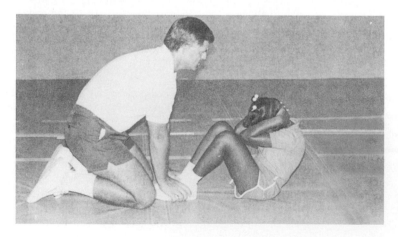

FIGURE 12.3 Sit-ups test (hands behind neck).

TABLE 12.4 Norms for Abdominal Curls for Ages Eighteen Through Thirty

	Males	Females
Excellent	96 and above	89 and above
Good	82–95	76–88
Average	68–81	63–75
Poor	54–67	49–62
Very poor	53 and below	48 and below

Source: G. Robbins, D. Powers, and S. Burgess, *A wellness way of life*, 2d ed., Dubuque, Iowa: Brown & Benchmark Publishers, 1994.

■ Abdominal Curls
(Robbins, Powers, and Burgess 1991)

Test Objective. To measure abdominal strength and endurance.
Age Level. Five through adulthood.
Equipment. Mats, tape, and stopwatch.
Validity. Logical validity.
Reliability. Not reported.
Norms. Table 12.4 includes norms for ages eighteen through thirty.
Administration and Directions. A strip of tape 3 inches wide is placed on the mat. The test performer assumes a supine position on the mat, with the fingertips at the edge of the strip. The knees are flexed, the feet are placed flat on the floor, and the heels are as close to the hips as possible. The test performer curls forward until the fingertips move forward 3 inches and curls backward until the shoulder blades touch the mat. The shoulder blades should lift from the mat with each curl, but the lower back should stay on the mat. The feet should not lift off the mat, and the feet *should not* be held down by a partner.
Scoring. The test score is the number of curls that can be performed in 1 minute.

■ Pull-Ups Test for Strength
(Johnson and Nelson 1986)

Test Objective. To measure arm and shoulder girdle strength.
Age Level. Twelve through college-age.
Equipment. A horizontal bar; 2½-, 5-, 10- and 25-pound weight plates; a rope or strap to secure the weights to the waist of the test performer; and a chair.
Validity. Face validity.
Reliability. .99.

Objectivity. .99.
Norms. Johnson and Nelson provide norms for college males.
Administration and Directions. The horizontal bar is raised to a height so that the test performer's feet will be off the floor. The test performer (1) secures the desired amount of weight to the waist and steps on the chair (test administrator should assist when the performer steps to and from the chair); (2) grasps the bar with the overhand grip (palms forward) and assumes a straight-arm hang (chair is removed); and (3) pulls upward until the chin is above the bar (chair is replaced under the feet). The performer may step down and readjust the weights before repeating the test.
Scoring. Two pull-ups are permitted, and the greatest amount of weight lifted is recorded. The test score is the amount of weight lifted divided by body weight. The test performer who cannot lift more than his or her own body weight receives a score of zero. No swinging action to move upward is permitted.

■ Pull-Ups Test for Endurance
(AAHPERD 1976a)

Test Objective. To measure arm and shoulder girdle strength and endurance.
Age Level. Nine through college-age.
Equipment. Metal or wooden bar approximately 1½ inches in diameter (inclined ladder may be used).
Validity. Face validity.
Reliability. .87.
Norms. Table 12.5 includes male norms for ages nine through seventeen-plus.
Administration and Directions. The test performer hangs from the bar using the overhand grip (palms forward) with the legs and arms fully extended. The feet should not touch the floor. The performer pulls upward until the chin is over the bar and then lowers the body to a full hang position. The pull-up is repeated as many times as possible.
Scoring. Only one trial is administered, unless it is obvious the performer can do better with a second attempt. The score is the number of completed pull-ups. The knees must not be flexed, and kicking, swinging, and snap-up motions are not permitted. The test administrator may prevent these actions by holding an extended arm across the front of the performer's thighs.

A test using the reverse grip (palms facing the body) is also administered to measure arm and shoulder girdle strength and endurance. This is an acceptable grip, but because the test performers will be able to complete more repetitions with this grip, the AAHPERD norms should not be used for scoring.

Percentile	Age							
	9–10	11	12	13	14	15	16	17+
95	9	8	9	10	12	15	14	15
75	3	4	4	5	7	9	10	10
50	1	2	2	3	4	6	7	7
25	0	0	0	1	2	3	4	4
15	0	0	0	0	1	1	3	2

Adapted from AAHPERD, *AAHPERD youth fitness test manual,* Reston, Va.: American Alliance for Health, Physical Education, Recreation and Dance, 1976.

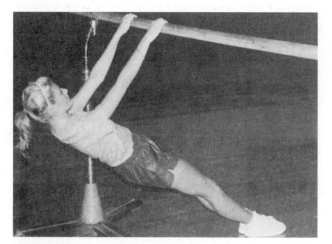
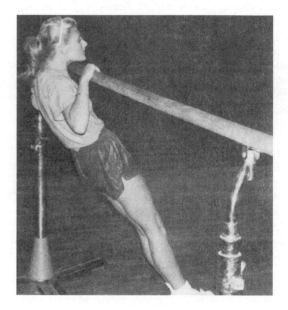

FIGURE 12.4 Modified pull-ups for females.

■ Modified Pull-Ups for Endurance

Note: Though designed for females, this test may be administered to males who are unable to perform the pull-ups previously described.

Test Objective. To measure arm and shoulder girdle endurance.

Age Level. Ten through college-age.

Equipment. Horizontal bar.

Validity. Face validity.

Norms. None.

Administration and Directions. The bar is adjusted to he height of the base of the performer's sternum when the performer is standing erect. The performer (1) grasps the bar with an overhand grip (palms forward) and slides the feet under the bar until the arms are straight and the angle between the arms and trunk is 90°; (2) keeps the body rigid and straight and brings the chin over the bar; and (3) completes as many pull-ups as possible (see figure 12.4).

Scoring. Only one trial is permitted, and the score is the number of correct pull-ups completed.

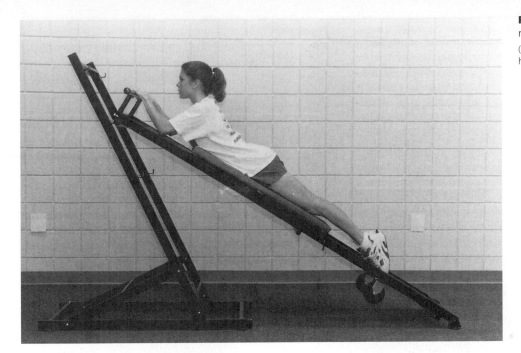

■ Baumgartner Modified Pull-Ups Test

(Baumgartner and Jackson 1982; Baumgartner et al. 1984)

Test Objective. To measure arm and shoulder girdle strength, endurance, or both.

Age Level. Elementary school through college.

Equipment. The necessary equipment is sold commercially, or it may be constructed locally with inexpensive parts. The equipment consists of an inclined board with a rail system for a scooter board to slide on (see figure 12.5).

Validity. Face validity and construct validity, since males performed significantly better than females.

Reliability. Reliability coefficients of .89 to .98 have been reported.

Norms. Table 12.6 reports norms for ages six through college-age.

Administration and Directions. The test performer lies prone on the scooter board and grasps the bar with an overhand grip, hands shoulder-width apart. The arms should be fully extended. The test is then performed like the regular pull-ups test, pulling the chin over the bar and returning to a straight-arm hanging position. The performer should pull evenly with both arms and not drag the toes.

Scoring. The score is the completed number of repetitions.

■ Modified Pull-Ups Test

(Pate et al. 1987)

Test Objective. To measure upper body muscular strength and endurance.

Age Level. Five through eighteen.

Equipment. Modified pull-up stand or a low pull-up bar that allows for adjustment of height and elastic bands.

Administration and Directions. The test performer lies on the back with the shoulders between the uprights and reaches straight up as high as possible (head and shoulders remain flat on floor). The tester sets the bar approximately 2 inches above the performer's outstretched hands and places the elastic band 7 to 8 inches below the bar. The performer raises the body high enough to grasp the bar with the palms forward (see figure 12.6a). In the starting position, the heels are on the floor, the buttocks are off the floor, and the arms and legs are straight. The pull-up is completed when the chin is hooked over the elastic band (see figure 12.6b). The performer returns to the full extension of the arms and repeats as many times as possible. The body is to remain straight throughout the test.

Scoring. The score is the completed number of repetitions. No norms have been reported.

TABLE 12.6 Norms for Baumgartner's Modified Pull-Ups Test

Performance Level	Age									
	6	7	8	9–11	**	14	15	16	17–18	College
	Males									
Above average	18 and above	23 and above	26 and above	32 and above		30 and above	31 and above	35 and above	33 and above	34 and above
Average (40% to 60%)	13 to 17	18 to 22	19 to 25	25 to 31		25 to 29	27 to 30	30 to 34	29 to 32	28 to 33
Below average	12 and below	17 and below	18 and below	24 and below		24 and below	26 and below	29 and below	28 and below	27 and below

Performance Level	Age						
	6	7	8	9–11	**	14–15	**	College
	Females						
Above average	18 and above	21 and above	19 and above	24 and above		14 and above		13 and above
Average (40% to 60%)	13 to 17	15 to 20	14 to 18	18 to 23		10 to 13		10 to 12
Below average	12 and below	14 and below	13 and below	17 and below		9 and below		9 and below

Adapted from A. Jackson et al., Baumgartner's modified pull-up test for male and female elementary school aged children, *Research Quarterly for Exercise and Sport* 53:163–164, 1982; and T. A. Baumgartner et al., Equipment improvements and additional norms for the modified pull-ups test, *Research Quarterly for Exercise and Sport* 55:64–68, 1984.
**Norms not reported for males ages twelve through thirteen, or for females ages twelve through thirteen and sixteen through eighteen.

■ Flexed-Arm Hang
(AAHPERD 1976a)

Test Objective. To measure arm and shoulder girdle endurance.
Age Level. Nine through college-age.
Equipment. A horizontal bar 1½ inches in diameter and a stopwatch.
Validity. Face validity.
Reliability. .90.
Objectivity. .99.
Norms. Table 12.7 includes female norms for ages nine through seventeen-plus.
Administration and Directions. The bar should be at a height that does not allow the test performer to touch the floor from the flexed-arm position. With the assistance of two spotters and using an overhand grip, the performer raises the body off the floor so that the chin is above the bar and the elbows are flexed. This position is held for as long as possible.

Scoring. The score is the number of seconds the proper position is maintained. The test administrator should begin the time as soon as the performer is in the flexed-arm position and should stop the time when the chin touches the bar, tilts backward, or drops below the bar. Though developed for females, this test may be used for males who are unable to perform the pull-ups test.

■ Dip Test for Strength
(Johnson and Nelson 1986)

Test Objective. To measure arm and shoulder girdle strength.
Age Level. Twelve through college-age.
Equipment. Parallel bars, weight plates, straps, and a chair.
Validity. Face validity.
Reliability. .98.
Objectivity. .99.
Norms. Johnson and Nelson (1986) provide norms for college males.

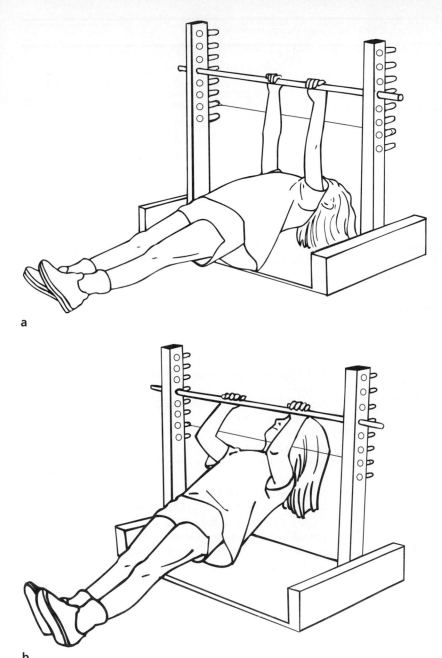

a

b

FIGURE 12.6 Modified pull-ups.

Muscular Strength, Endurance, and Power   **151**

TABLE 12.7   Norms in Seconds for Flexed-Arm Hang for Females Ages Nine Through Seventeen+

Percentile	Age							
	9–10	11	12	13	14	15	16	17+
95	42	39	33	34	35	36	31	34
75	18	20	18	16	21	18	15	17
50	9	10	9	8	9	9	7	8
25	3	3	3	3	3	4	3	3
15	1	2	1	1	2	2	1	2

Adapted from AAHPERD, *AAHPERD youth fitness test manual,* Reston, Va.: American Alliance for Health, Physical Education, Recreation and Dance, 1976.

Administration and Directions. The bars should be at a height that allows the test performer to be freely above the floor while in the lowered bent-arm support position. After securing the desired amount of weight to the waist, the test performer (1) steps on the chair and takes a secure grip on the bars (he or she should be assisted when stepping to and from the chair); (2) assumes a straight-arm support position (the chair is removed); (3) lowers himself or herself until the elbows form a right angle; and (4) pushes to a straight-arm support position (chair is replaced). The performer may step down and readjust the weights before attempting the exercise again.

Scoring. Two dips are permitted. The greatest amount of weight lifted is recorded. The test score is the amount of weight lifted divided by body weight. The test performer is not permitted to swing or kick in returning to the straight-arm support position.

■ **Dips Test for Endurance**
(*Johnson and Nelson 1986*)

Test Objective. To measure arm and shoulder girdle endurance.
Age Level. Ten through college-age.
Equipment. Parallel bars.
Validity. Face validity.
Reliability. .90.
Objectivity. Not reported.
Norms. None reported.
Administration and Directions. The bars should be at a height that allows the test performer to be freely above the floor while in the lowered bent-arm support position. The performer (1) jumps to a straight-arm support position between the bars; (2) lowers the body until the angle at the

elbows is a right angle or less; and (3) completes the exercise as many times as possible.
Scoring. The score is the number of correct dips completed. Resting between dips and kicking or swinging are not permitted.

■ **Push-Ups**
(*Johnson and Nelson 1986*)

Test Objective. To measure arm and shoulder girdle endurance.
Age Level. Ten through adulthood.
Equipment. None required; mats may be used.
Validity. Face validity.
Objectivity. .99.
Norms. Table 12.8 reports norms for males and females (modified push-ups) ages twenty through sixty-nine.
Administration and Directions. The test performer (1) lies face down on the floor with the body straight, arms bent, and hands flat on the floor beneath the shoulders; (2) pushes upward to a straight-arm position; (3) lowers the body until the chest touches the floor; and (4) repeats the exercise as many times as possible, without rest. The body must stay rigid (not sag or pike upward) throughout the test. A sponge that is 2 inches high may be placed on the floor for the performer to touch with the chest.
Scoring. The score is the number of correct push-ups completed.

■ **Modified Push-Ups**

Test Objective. To measure arm and shoulder girdle endurance.
Age Level. Ten through adulthood.
Equipment. None required; mats may be used.
Validity. Face validity.

Performance Level	Age				
	20–29	30–39	40–49	50–59	60–69
	Males				
Above average	45 and above	35 and above	30 and above	25 and above	20 and above
Average	35 to 44	25 to 34	20 to 29	15 to 24	10 to 19
Below average	34 and below	24 and below	19 and below	14 and below	9 and below
	Females (Modified Push-Ups)				
Above average	34 and above	25 and above	20 and above	15 and above	5 and above
Average	17 to 33	12 to 24	8 to 19	6 to 14	3 to 4
Below average	16 and below	11 and below	7 and below	5 and below	2 and below

Adapted from M. L. Pollock, J. H. Wilmore, and S. M. Fox, *Health and fitness through physical activity,* New York: John Wiley & Sons, 1978.

Reliability. .93 (Johnson and Nelson 1986).

Objectivity. Not reported.

Norms. Table 12.8 provides norms for females ages twenty through sixty-nine.

Administration and Directions. The test performer (1) lies face down on the floor with the body trunk straight, knees bent at right angles, arms bent, and hands flat on the floor beneath the shoulders; (2) pushes upward to a straight-arm position (see figure 12.7); (3) lowers the body until the chest touches the floor; and (4) repeats the exercise as many times as possible without rest. The body trunk must remain straight throughout the test. Modified push-ups also may be performed with a bench. The push-up is performed in the same manner as regular push-ups (weight supported on hands and toes) except the hands are placed on a bench that is approximately 15 inches high and 15 inches long.

Scoring. The score is the number of correct push-ups completed.

Muscular Power

Two types of muscular power may be measured: athletic power and work power. The distance the body or an object can be propelled through space indicates athletic power (vertical jump and medicine ball put). If work power is to be measured, extraneous movements are controlled or eliminated, so that maximum effort must be put forth by the muscle groups being tested. For example, if the vertical jump is used to measure work power, the test performer is not permitted to swing the arms. Because power is rarely measured to determine the health or physical fitness status of an individual, only two athletic power tests will be presented.

■ Vertical Jump
(Sargent 1921)

Test Objective. To measure explosive leg power.

Age Level. Nine through adulthood.

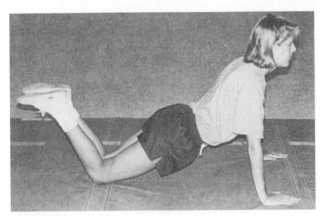

FIGURE 12.7 Modified push-ups.

Muscular Strength, Endurance, and Power   **153**

Percentile	Age							
	10	11	12	13	14	15	16	17+
				Males				
95	15.5	16.5	17.5	19.0	20.5	21.5	22.5	24.0
75	12.5	13.5	14.5	16.0	17.5	18.5	19.5	21.0
50	11.0	12.0	13.0	14.5	16.0	17.0	18.0	19.5
25	9.0	10.0	11.0	12.5	14.0	15.0	16.0	17.5
5	6.0	7.0	7.0	8.5	10.0	11.0	12.0	13.5
				Females				
95	14.0	14.5	15.0	15.5	16.0	17.0	17.0	17.0
75	11.5	12.0	12.5	13.0	13.5	14.5	14.5	14.5
50	10.0	10.5	11.0	11.5	12.0	13.0	13.0	13.0
25	8.5	9.0	9.5	10.0	10.5	11.5	11.5	11.5
5	6.0	6.5	7.0	7.5	8.0	9.0	9.0	9.0

Adapted from *Physical fitness—motor ability test,* Austin, Tex.: Texas Governor's Commission on Physical Fitness, 1973.

Equipment. A yardstick or measuring tape, chalk, and a wall of sufficient height.

Validity. .78 using a criterion test of four power events in track and field.

Reliability. .93.

Objectivity. Coefficients >.90 have been reported.

Norms. Table 12.9 reports norms for ages ten through seventeen-plus.

Administration and Directions. A yardstick or tape measure is taped to the wall to measure the distance between two chalk marks. The test performer (1) stands with the dominant side toward the wall and feet flat on the floor; (2) holding a piece of chalk (1 inch in length) in the dominant hand, reaches as high as possible and makes a mark on the wall; and (3) jumps as high as possible and makes another mark at the height of the jump. Three trials are administered. (Rather than using a piece of chalk to make the mark, chalk can be placed on the fingertips.) All test performers should practice the jump until it can be executed correctly before attempting the test.

Scoring. For each jump the score is the distance between the two chalk marks, measured to the nearest half inch. The greatest distance is the test score.

■ **Standing Broad Jump**
(AAHPERD 1976a)

Test Objective. To measure explosive leg power.

Age Level. Six through college-age.

Equipment. A yardstick, tape, and tape measure; mat is optional.

Validity. Face validity.

Reliability. Coefficients ranging from .83 to .99 have been reported.

Norms. Table 12.10 reports norms for ages nine through seventeen-plus.

Administration and Directions. A tape measure should be taped to the floor or mat close to and parallel with the area where the jump will be performed. The test performer (1) stands behind the restraining line with the feet parallel and several inches apart; (2) bends the knees and swings the arms forward; and (3) jumps forward as far as possible. The test administrator marks the landing point of the nearest heel to the restraining line with the yardstick (yardstick is placed perpendicular to tape measure). All test performers should be permitted to practice the jump until they can perform it correctly. Three trials are administered.

TABLE 12.10 Norms in Feet and Inches for Standing Broad Jump for Ages Nine Through Seventeen+

Percentile	Age							
	9–10	11	12	13	14	15	16	17+
	Males							
95	6' 0"	6' 2"	6' 6"	7' 1"	7' 6"	8' 0"	8' 2"	8' 5"
75	5' 4"	5' 7"	5' 9"	6' 3"	6' 8"	7' 2"	7' 6"	7' 9"
50	4' 11"	5' 2"	5' 5"	5' 9"	6' 2"	6' 8"	7' 0"	7' 2"
25	4' 6"	4' 8"	5' 0"	5' 2"	5' 6"	6' 1"	6' 6"	6' 6"
5	3' 10"	4' 0"	4' 2"	4' 4"	4' 8"	5' 2"	5' 5"	5' 3"
	Females							
95	5' 10"	6' 0"	6' 2"	6' 5"	6' 8"	6' 7"	6' 6"	6' 9"
75	5' 2"	5' 4"	5' 6"	5' 9"	5' 11"	5' 10"	5' 9"	6' 0"
50	4' 8"	4' 11"	5' 0"	5' 3"	5' 4"	5' 5"	5' 3"	5' 5"
25	4' 1"	4' 4"	4' 6"	4' 9"	4' 10"	4' 11"	4' 9"	4' 11"
5	3' 5"	3' 8"	3' 10"	4' 0"	4' 0"	4' 2"	4' 0"	4' 1"

Adapted from AAHPERD, *AAHPERD youth fitness test manual,* Reston, Va.: American Alliance for Health, Physical Education, Recreation and Dance, 1976.

Scoring. The score is the number of inches between the restraining line and the nearest heel on landing. If the test performer falls backward on landing, the measurement is made from the restraining line to the nearest part of the body touching the floor or mat.

Exercises to Develop Muscular Strength and Endurance

Muscular strength and endurance will improve within a few weeks if the correct exercises are done on a regular basis. Though weight-training programs typically involve the use of free weights, Universal Gym, or Nautilus equipment, muscular strength and endurance can be improved without the use of expensive equipment or a special room. Avoiding extreme soreness or injury when the following, and similar, exercises are performed requires that certain guidelines be observed:

1. Perform stretching and warm-up exercises before attempting muscular effort.

2. Since some exercises are more difficult than others, perform the ones that provide a mild overload and gradually progress to the more difficult ones.
3. Unless otherwise indicated, begin with ten repetitions and add two or three repetitions each week until the desired number is reached. If unable to perform ten repetitions, begin with a lower number.
4. Perform the exercises 3 to 5 days per week.

Posterior Upper Arms, Shoulders, Chest, and Upper Back

Chair Push-Up. (1) Place hands shoulder-width apart with fingertips forward on chair or bench, feet on the floor, and weight supported on the toes; (2) straighten arms with chin up and chest forward; (3) bend arms and lower chest within 1 to 2 inches of chair; and (4) push back to starting position.

Modified Push-Up. Perform in same manner as modified push-up (page 152).

Muscular Strength, Endurance, and Power **155**

Push Up. Perform in same manner as push-up (page 152).

Advanced Push-Up. Perform in same manner as regular push-up, but place feet on a bench or chair.

Anterior Upper Arms, Shoulders, Chest, and Upper Back

Modified Pull-Up. Perform in same manner as modified pull-up (page 148).

Pull-Up. Perform in same manner as pull-up (page 147).

Pull-Up with Weight. (1) Fill two plastic milk or bleach bottles with equal amounts of water or sand, and tie a bottle to each end of a rope that is 24 to 36 inches long; (2) hang the bottles around the shoulders so that they are in front of the body (may place padding between the rope and neck); and (3) perform the pull-ups.

Arm Curls. (1) Fill two plastic milk or bleach bottles with equal amounts of water or sand, and tie a bottle to each end of a bar or heavy stick that is approximately 36 to 40 inches long; (2) stand erect with arms fully extended downward and grasp bar with palms up and shoulder-width apart; (3) raise bar to chest by bending arms (elbows should remain at sides and back should remain straight); and (4) perform two or three sets of six to ten repetitions.

Abdomen

To perform these exercises, lie on the back with the knees bent and feet flat on the floor.

Trunk Curl. (1) Clasp hands on top of head (placing the hands behind head may cause the head to jerk forward, straining the neck muscles); (2) roll head and shoulders forward and upward enough to feel tension; and (3) return to starting position.

Reverse Sit-Up. (1) Place arms at sides and lift knees to chest, raising hips off the floor, and (2) return to starting position.

Assisted Flexed Knee Sit-Up. Perform sit-up with hands under thighs to help pull the upper body up to position where no resistance is encountered.

Flexed Knee Sit-Up. Perform sit-up with arms at sides, arms folded across chest, or hands clasped on top of head.

Sit-Up with Feet Elevated. Begin in same position as previous sit-ups but place feet on seat of chair, bed, or bench; knees remain bent, and arms may be placed in any position.

Lateral Trunk

Side Bender. (1) Stand with feet shoulder-width apart and hands clasped behind head, and (2) alternate bending to right and left while maintaining straight back and legs. Perform the same number of repetitions for each side. Exercise may be made more difficult by extending arms overhead or extending at sides, holding a weight in each hand.

Lower Back and Buttocks

Back Tightener. (1) Lie facedown with hands behind lower back, and (2) raise head and chest slightly off floor, tensing lower back and buttocks muscles. Do not overextend.

Leg Raise. (1) With body supported on hands and knees, extend and raise one leg behind the body. (2) Perform the same number of repetitions with each leg. Wearing heavy shoes or adding weight to ankles will increase resistance.

Back Leg Raise. (1) Lie facedown, hands clasped behind head, and (2) lift straight legs a few inches off floor. Hold head and chest down.

Back Extension. (1) Lie on a bench facedown and extend body from waist up over the edge of bench (will be necessary to strap feet down or have someone hold them). (2) With hands clasped behind head, lift head and trunk. Do not overextend.

Lateral Hips and Thighs

Side Leg Raise. (1) Using the arms to maintain balance, lie on right side with legs straight; (2) lift left leg straight up from side as high as possible; (3) return to starting position; and (4) perform the same number of repetitions with each leg. Wearing heavy shoes or adding weight to ankles will increase resistance.

Leg Raise. (1) Lie on back with arms at sides and lift legs until they are perpendicular to floor; (2) open legs to a wide V-shape; and (3) close the V and return to starting position. May use heavy shoes or weights for added resistance.

Upper Legs

Two-Leg Squat. (1) Stand with feet 12 inches apart, with arms extended in front and parallel to floor; (2) squat until knees are bent at a 90° angle (do not go beyond this point; place a chair behind the legs to prevent squatting past 90°); and (3) return to standing position.

Single Leg Knee Dip (with Assistance). (1) Stand facing a partner and hold right hands as if shaking hands (if necessary may use table or chair); (2) keeping left leg extended in front, squat down on right foot until knee is at a 90° angle (partner remains standing); (3) grab partner's hand with both hands to return to standing position; and (4) perform the same number of dips with each leg, though attempt no more than five to seven dips when first performing this exercise. Using partner's hand only for balance throughout exercise will increase difficulty.

Lower Legs

Heel Raises. (1) Stand on a board, book, or something similar, with heels resting off the edge; (2) using arms for balance, rise up onto toes; and (3) return to starting position. Hanging weights around shoulders will increase resistance.

Jumps in Place. (1) With feet parallel, 12 inches apart, jump in place. (2) Maintain a steady pace. Do not attempt to jump too high, and try to perform on a soft surface (mats, or wood floor with carpet).

▶ REVIEW PROBLEMS ◀

1. Review additional muscular strength, endurance, and power tests found in other textbooks. Note the groups for whom the tests are intended and the validity, reliability, and objectivity coefficients.
2. Administer one of the muscular strength and one of the endurance tests described in this chapter to several of your classmates. Ask them to provide constructive criticism of your test administration.
3. Interview individuals responsible for weight-training programs at fitness or wellness centers. Inquire about tests that are used to measure muscular strength and endurance, interpretation of tests results, and programs prescribed for development of muscular strength and endurance.
4. A physical education teacher administered the modified sit-ups test to students in the second grade. The scores listed below are for the fifty girls in the second grade. Determine the mode, median, mean, and standard deviation for the scores. Refer to table 12.2, and compare the group with national norms.

15	34	20	31	22
29	16	39	27	31
23	33	24	30	32
21	35	15	38	20
37	18	21	33	22
29	37	40	22	6
19	18	24	30	22
20	29	18	28	14
36	22	18	29	28
25	18	38	17	31

13

Anthropometry and Body Composition

Upon completion of this chapter, you should be able to

1. Define the terms *anthropometry, somatotype, body composition, overfat, obese,* and *lean body weight;*

2. State why body structure and composition should be measured;

3. Describe the major characteristics of Sheldon's classification of body types;

4. Correctly interpret height-weight tables;

5. Classify body frames;

6. State the problems associated with the use of height-weight tables to determine desirable weight;

7. Describe eight acceptable sites for skinfold measurements;

8. Perform skinfold measurements, estimate percent body fat, and advise individuals of optimal percent fat ranges;

9. Calculate an individual's desirable body weight on the basis of an acceptable percent body fat; and

10. Determine body mass index (BMI) and waist-to-hip ratio and advise individuals of BMI values and waist-to-hip ratios associated with the lowest risk of health problems.

Anthropometry, the measurement of the structure and proportions of the body, is one of the earliest forms of measurement in physical education. It may include measurement of height and weight; measurement of circumferences, diameters, and lengths of body segments; and **somatotyping** (body typing).

Body composition refers to the component parts of the body. Though there are many component parts, for measurement purposes body composition is interpreted as referring to body fat weight and lean body weight. Because **lean body weight** is found by subtracting the weight of body fat from the total body weight, it is often interpreted as fat-free weight. Technically, however, it in-

cludes a small amount of essential lipid that is associated with a variety of tissues in the body, such as the nerve sheaths, the brain, and the cell membranes. Depending on body size, about 1.5% to 3% of the weight of the lean body is essential lipids, and 40% to 50% is composed of muscle weight or mass. Organs and tissues, such as skin and bones, make up the remaining portion.

Why Measure Body Structure and Composition?

Research involving somatotyping requires accurate body type classification, but understanding the concept of somatotyping and being able to roughly determine body types can be of value to coaches, physical education teachers, and fitness instructors. The values found in most weight tables are grouped into height and body type categories. Estimation of desirable weight through a height-weight table is not ideal, because no estimation of percent body fat can be made. If this method is used, however, individuals should realistically determine their body type. In addition, body type classification may be useful when planning obtainable fitness goals. For example, individuals with a thick abdomen, wide hips, heavy buttocks, and short, heavy legs (endomorphic body type characteristics) usually do not perform as well on running tests as individuals with a slender abdomen and hips and lean or muscular legs. This does not mean that certain individuals are to avoid running for health benefits, but it does mean that their running goals should be realistic in terms of their body type.

Height and weight measurements may be recorded for diagnostic purposes. Great differences exist in the physiological maturity of boys and girls, and not all individuals of the same age are expected to have identical heights and weights. The recording of these variables during the growing and developing years may serve to prevent the occurrence of long-term health problems. Young people who significantly deviate from either height or weight range, or both, for their ages probably should be observed to determine that no health problems exist. (This determination should be done in a way that is not embarrassing to the individuals.) Height and weight measurements also may be used for homogeneous grouping of youth for sports participation. Classification indexes based on height, weight, and age were developed in the 1930s for this purpose, but currently, they are not extensively used.

The measurement of body composition is of importance to all physical educators. It has been estimated that more than 80 million Americans are **overfat** in that their percentage of body fat exceeds a desirable level. Possibly, over 40 million adults are **obese,** which means their body fat content exceeds 25% (men) or 30% (women) of the total body weight. This excess fat is not limited to the older population. The percentage of overweight children and adolescents has doubled in the last 30 years, and over 20% of teenagers are overfat. Indeed, overfatness is a national problem.

In an effort to combat overfatness, millions of Americans undertake weight-loss diets. They fail, however, to understand the difference between the loss of body fat and lean body weight, and the role of exercise in weight management. In addition, they mistakenly use weight as indicated on scales to determine the success or lack of success of their diet. Physical educators need to assume a leadership role in counseling individuals who are attempting to lose weight. We should be prepared to measure body composition and to advise individuals how to correctly lose body fat.

Furthermore, some people attempt to lose weight, though their percent body fat is acceptable. For example, some athletes, especially amateur wrestlers and gymnasts, have unrealistic images of what their weight should be, and they do not realize the implications of changes in their body composition. Many distance runners also attempt to get their weight too low, with the belief that their running times will improve. This problem is not limited to athletes, however. Other individuals create health problems for themselves because they have an incorrect perception of a slender body. Many of these people have emotional problems and need professional counseling to overcome those problems, but possibly some would discontinue efforts to lose weight if they understood the relationship of body fat and good health.

⍰ARE YOU ABLE TO DO THE FOLLOWING:

- define anthropometry, somatotype, body composition, overfat, obese, and lean body weight?
- state why body structure and composition should be measured?

Body Type Classification (Somatotyping)

There are several methods of body type classification, but the classification described by Sheldon, Stevens, and Tucker (1970) is the best known. Sheldon's morphological classification includes the ectomorph, the mesomorph, and the endomorph. An **ectomorph** is a slender person with a light frame—the arms and legs are slender and long, the neck appears long, and muscle tissue has little definition. A **mesomorph** is an athletic-looking individual—the shoulders are broad, the hips are narrow, and muscle tissue is predominant. An **endomorph** is a thick individual—the arms and legs are short compared with the torso, the chest and waist are about the same size, and the neck is thick.

Three numbers are used to designate the components of each of the three types, with 7 as the highest and 1 as the lowest rating for each. The first number refers to endomorphic, the second to mesomorphic, and the third to ectomorphic characteristics. The rating 7–1–1 designates a pure endomorph; 1–7–1, a pure mesomorph; and 1–1–7, a pure ectomorph. Such extreme ratings are rare, however; usually, at least two components of each type are present in an individual. A 2–5–4 designation indicates a less than average number of endomorphic characteristics, a more than average number of mesomorphic characteristics, and an average number of ectomorphic characteristics. Simplified modifications of Sheldon's classification have been developed, but unless you are involved in research, rarely will it be necessary for you to use a numbering system to designate body types.

By knowing the major characteristics of each body type, one can estimate the two dominant body types of each individual and put the estimate to practical use. For example, a relationship exists between somatotype and certain sports. A football lineman with a low center of gravity and wide hips and shoulders has an advantage in blocking. Football linemen, therefore, usually rate high on the mesomorph and endomorph scales and low on the ectomorph scale. On the other hand, individuals who play center on college or professional basketball teams, as well as long distance runners, rate high on the ectomorph scale. When advising individuals about the relationship of physical activity and body types, you should emphasize that training may result in improved performance, but it will not result in a change of body type.

Height-Weight Tables

Since 1959 many individuals have used the Metropolitan Life Insurance Company height-weight tables to determine their desirable weight. In 1983, the company released revised tables that were said to represent the weights associated with the lowest death rates among approximately 4,200,000 people observed for 22 years (see table 13.1).

However, when the new tables were released, the American Heart Association (AHA) encouraged Americans to continue to use the 1959 recommendations (see table 13.2). The AHA took this position because the new tables list average weight range increases of 13 pounds for short men and 10 pounds for short women, little increases for medium-height men and women, and insignificant increases for tall men and women. The AHA noted that merely looking at death rates obscured health risks associated with the increased weights. The AHA also stated that few health problems are improved by gaining weight, pointing out that the incidence of heart disease, high blood pressure, and diabetes increases in relation to weight gained. Also, the new acceptable weights most likely are skewed upward by the fact that cigarette smokers, who tend to be thinner than nonsmokers and who die at significantly younger ages, were not taken into account in calculating the new tables. Another controversy occurred in 1990 when the U.S. Departments of Agriculture and Health and Human Services released their booklet *Nutrition and Your Health: Dietary Guidelines for Americans.* The nutritional guidelines provided in this booklet were endorsed by nutritionists and the medical community, but the suggested weights for Americans were not accepted by all. Many medical personnel believed that the booklet's weight chart permitted too much weight gain during the aging process. The arguments against the chart were the same as those opposing the 1983 charts of the Metropolitan Life Insurance Company.

The major problem associated with the use of height-weight tables is that they reveal nothing about body composition. Two individuals may be the same height and weight but have entirely different body composition. One individual may be overfat; the other individual may be very muscular. With this limitation, however, the tables have value as a screening device. If individuals are more than 10% below the midpoint of the weight range for their height and weight, they may be underweight. If individuals are more than 10% above the midpoint of the weight range, they may be overfat. For such individuals, an appropriate method for determination of body composition should be performed before any decision is made about their fatness or leanness.

A major drawback to all height-weight tables is that some individuals do not correctly determine their frame size when selecting an appropriate weight range. Many small- or medium-framed overfat individuals consider themselves large-framed and do not realistically examine

TABLE 13.1 1983 Metropolitan Height and Weight Tables for Men and Women of Ages Twenty-Five Through Fifty-Nine

Height (with Shoes on; 1-in. Heels)	Small Frame (lb)	Medium Frame (lb)	Large Frame (lb)
Men (Indoor Clothing Weighing 5 lb)			
5 ft 2 in.	128–134	131–141	138–150
5 ft 3 in.	130–136	133–143	140–153
5 ft 4 in.	132–138	135–145	142–156
5 ft 5 in.	134–140	137–148	144–160
5 ft 6 in.	136–142	139–151	146–164
5 ft 7 in.	138–145	142–154	149–168
5 ft 8 in.	140–148	145–157	152–172
5 ft 9 in.	142–151	148–160	155–176
5 ft 10 in.	144–154	151–163	158–180
5 ft 11 in.	146–157	154–166	161–184
6 ft 0 in.	149–160	157–170	164–188
6 ft 1 in.	152–164	160–174	168–192
6 ft 2 in.	155–168	164–178	172–197
6 ft 3 in.	158–172	167–182	176–202
6 ft 4 in.	162–176	171–187	181–207
Women (Indoor Clothing Weighing 3 lb)			
4 ft 10 in.	102–111	109–121	118–131
4 ft 11 in.	103–113	111–123	120–134
5 ft 0 in.	104–115	113–126	122–137
5 ft 1 in.	106–118	115–129	125–140
5 ft 2 in.	108–121	118–132	128–143
5 ft 3 in.	111–124	121–135	131–147
5 ft 4 in.	114–127	124–138	134–151
5 ft 5 in.	117–130	127–141	137–155
5 ft 6 in.	120–133	130–144	140–159
5 ft 7 in.	123–136	133–147	143–163
5 ft 8 in.	126–139	136–150	146–167
5 ft 9 in.	129–142	139–153	149–170
5 ft 10 in.	132–145	142–156	152–173
5 ft 11 in.	135–148	145–159	155–176
6 ft 0 in.	138–151	148–162	158–179

Source of basic data: Society of Actuaries and Association of Life Insurance Medical Directors of America, *1979 build study,* New York: Metropolitan Life Insurance Company, 1980.

TABLE 13.2 1959 Metropolitan Life Insurance Company Table of Desirable Weights (in Pounds) for Men and Women of Ages Twenty-Five and Over (Indoor Clothing)

Height (with Shoes on; 1-in Heels)	Small Frame (lb)	Medium Frame (lb)	Large Frame (lb)
Men			
5 ft 2 in.	112–120	118–129	126–141
5 ft 3 in.	115–123	121–133	129–144
5 ft 4 in.	118–126	124–136	132–148
5 ft 5 in.	121–129	127–139	135–152
5 ft 6 in.	124–133	130–143	138–156
5 ft 7 in.	128–137	134–147	142–161
5 ft 8 in.	132–141	138–152	147–166
5 ft 9 in.	136–145	142–156	151–170
5 ft 10 in.	140–150	146–160	155–174
5 ft 11 in.	144–154	150–165	159–179
6 ft 0 in.	148–158	154–170	164–184
6 ft 1 in.	152–162	158–175	168–189
6 ft 2 in.	156–167	162–180	173–194
6 ft 3 in.	160–171	167–185	178–199
6 ft 4 in.	164–175	172–190	182–204
Women			
4 ft 10 in.	92–98	96–107	104–119
4 ft 11 in.	94–101	98–110	106–122
5 ft 0 in.	96–104	101–113	109–125
5 ft 1 in.	99–107	104–116	112–128
5 ft 2 in.	102–110	107–119	115–131
5 ft 3 in.	105–113	110–122	118–134
5 ft 4 in.	108–116	113–126	121–138
5 ft 5 in.	111–119	116–130	125–142
5 ft 6 in.	114–123	120–135	129–146
5 ft 7 in.	118–127	124–139	133–150
5 ft 8 in.	122–131	128–143	137–154
5 ft 9 in.	126–135	132–147	141–158
5 ft 10 in.	130–140	136–151	145–163
5 ft 11 in.	134–144	140–155	149–168
6 ft 0 in.	138–148	144–149	153–173

Source of basic data: Society of Actuaries, *Build and blood pressure study,* New York: Metropolitan Life Insurance Company, 1959.
Note: For those between 18 and 25, subtract 1 pound for each year under 25.

TABLE 13.3 Standards for Estimating Medium Frame Using Elbow Breadth and Height

	Males			Females	
Height (inches)*	Elbow Breadth** (inches)		Height (inches)*	Elbow Breadth** (inches)	
61 to 62	2½ to 2⅞		57 to 58	2¼ to 2½	
63 to 66	2⅝ to 2⅞		59 to 62	2¼ to 2½	
67 to 70	2¾ to 3		63 to 66	2⅜ to 2⅝	
71 to 74	2¾ to 3⅛		67 to 70	2⅜ to 2⅝	
75 and above	2⅞ to 3¼		71 and above	2½ to 2¾	

Source of basic data: Society of Actuaries and Association of Life Insurance Medical Directors of America, *1979 build study,* New York: Metropolitan Life Insurance Company, 1980.
*Height without shoes.
**Measurements lower than those listed indicate a small frame, and higher measurements indicate a large frame.

their weight problem. On the other hand, some medium- or large-framed individuals with an acceptable percent body fat view themselves as small-framed and mistakenly attempt to lose weight. Determination of body frame is best performed by trained personnel, but the following practical methods may be used.

Elbow Breadth

Extend the right arm and bend the forearm upward at a 90° angle. Keep the fingers straight and turn the palm away from the body. Place the thumb and index finger of the left hand on the two prominent bones on either side of the right elbow, and measure the space between the thumb and index finger of the left hand with a ruler or tape measure. Record the measurement and compare with the standards in table 13.3.

TABLE 13.4 Standards for Estimating Body Frame Size from Ankle Girth (Inches)

Sex	Small	Medium	Large
Male	Less than 8	8 to 9.25	More than 9.25
Female	Less than 7.5	7.5 to 8.75	More than 8.75

Source: P. B. Johnson et al., *Sport, exercise and you,* New York: Holt, Rinehart & Winston, 1975.

Ankle Girth

Pulling the tape as snug as possible, measure the girth of the right ankle at the smallest point, just above the bony prominences. Record the measurement and compare with the standards in table 13.4.

? ARE YOU ABLE TO DO THE FOLLOWING:

- describe the major characteristics of Sheldon's classification of body types?
- correctly interpret height-weight tables and classify body frames?
- state the problems associated with the use of height-weight tables to determine desirable weight?

Body Composition

Several methods are available for measurement of body composition. Most methods are expensive and are limited to research or medical purposes. A method that is popular in health promotion environments is bioelectrical impedance analysis (BIA). BIA is based on the difference between the resistance of lean tissue to an electrical current and the resistance of fat tissue. With this method, electrodes are attached to the body, and a tiny electrical current is sent through the body. The amount of water in the body affects the flow of the current. Lean-body mass is approximately 70% water, whereas fat tissue is less than 10% water. The less the recorded resistance, the greater is the water content and hence the greater the lean tissue.

Underwater weighing, as demonstrated in figure 13.1, is one of the most valid methods for measurement of body composition. The objective of underwater weighing, also called hydrostatic weighing, is to determine body volume, which is then used to calculate body density. This method is based on the Archimedes principle for measuring the density of a body. According to the Archimedes principle, when a body (person) is submerged under water, the weight a body loses underwater equals the weight of the water it displaces.

That is:

weight of the water displaced = weight of body in air—weight of body under water

The weight of the water displaced divided by the density of the water equals the volume of the water, and the volume of the water equals the volume of the body submerged. For individuals, this volume is referred to as body volume. The density of the water, determined with the appropriate formula, is a function of its temperature. Before determining body density, residual lung volume (the amount of air remaining in the lungs after maximal exhalation) also must be measured. With body volume, water density, and residual lung volume determined, the appropriate mathematical equation is then used to calculate body density. After body density is calculated another equation is used to estimate the percentage of body fat. Lean tissue (bone and muscle) has a greater density than fat tissue. Thus, the higher the body density of an individual, the lower the percentage of body fat for that individual.

Obviously, the estimation of body fat through underwater weighing is costly and requires more time and trained personnel than other methods. For these reasons, it is rarely used to test large groups.

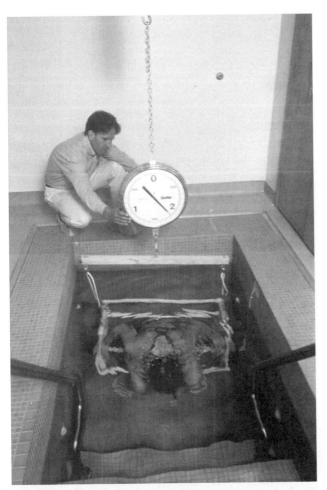

FIGURE 13.1 Underwater weighing technique.

Photograph provided by Richard G. Israel, Human Performance/Clinical Research Lab, Department of Health and Exercise, Colorado State University.

Skinfold Tests

The measurement of body composition may also be done through the measurement of subcutaneous body fat with skinfold calipers. The use of a skinfold caliper involves pinching a fold away from the underlying muscle and applying the caliper to the fold. All measurements are taken on the right side of the body, and they should not be taken immediately after exercise because the shift of body fluid to the skin will increase the skinfold size. The directions for skinfold testing are as follows:

1. Grasp the skinfold firmly between the thumb and index finger about ½ inch from the site at which the caliper is to be applied. Since the thickness of the fold reflects the percentage of body fat, it should be great enough to include two thicknesses of skin with intervening fat, but it should not include muscle or fascia. The test administrator may ask the

Anthropometry and Body Composition **165**

subject to tense the underlying muscles to determine if muscle tissue is included in the fold.

2. While continuing to hold the fold, apply the caliper to the fold above or below the finger and slowly release the caliper grip so that full tension is exerted on the fold. The measurement is read to the nearest 0.5 millimeter about 1 to 2 seconds after the grip is released.

3. Take a minimum of two measurements at each site, and if they vary by more than 1 millimeter, take a third measurement. Specific test instructions sometimes differ in this step. For example, one test may use the median score of three measurements, while another test may require that two consecutive measurements agree within 0.5 millimeters. It is best to follow the instructions of the test being administered. Complete a measurement at one site before going to another site, but if consecutive measurements become smaller and smaller at the same site, complete the measurements at the other sites. Later, return to the trouble site. Consecutive measurements are sometimes smaller because of the compression of fat.

Skinfold measurements may be taken in several places, eight of which are described here. To ensure accuracy and consistency, you can mark the sites with a grease pencil. Figures 13.2 through 13.9 present the measurement sites.

1. Chest: a diagonal fold half of the distance between the anterior axillary line and nipple.
2. Axilla: a vertical fold on the midaxillary line at the level of the xiphoid process of the sternum.
3. Triceps: a vertical fold over the triceps muscle, halfway between the acromion and olecranon processes (arm should be extended and relaxed).
4. Subscapula: a diagonal fold parallel to the axillary border at the inferior angle of the scapula.
5. Abdominal: a vertical fold approximately ½ to 1 inch to the right of the navel.
6. Suprailium: a slightly diagonal fold on the crest of the ilium at the midaxillary line.
7. Thigh: a vertical fold on the anterior right thigh midway between the hip and knee joints (weight should be on left foot).
8. Calf: a vertical fold on the inside of the calf; right foot is placed flat on bench with knee flexed to 90°;

vertical fold of skin is grasped just above the largest part of calf girth and fold of skin is measured at the largest part of girth.

Skinfold measurements rarely are performed outside the laboratory setting for two reasons: the expense of the skinfold calipers and the lack of confidence in the reliability of the measurements. A study by Lohman and Pollock (1981) concluded that the less expensive calipers may be suitable for a mass testing setting, if the test administrator is well trained. Differences between the scores of experienced and inexperienced testers occurred less often when an expensive metal caliper was used. However, Lohman and Pollack also found that when inexperienced testers were trained, similar scores were obtained when using a plastic caliper with a spring and a caliper with a uniform tension independent of skinfold thickness. The major requirement for a skinfold caliper is that it exert a constant force of 10 g/mm^2 at the skinfold site, regardless of the skinfold thickness. Inexpensive calipers are capable of exerting this force if the springs in them are not weakened.

Skinfold measurements can be reliable if testers are willing to practice performing the measurements. Consistency of measurement is obtained only through practice. Testers who are willing to measure many individuals can develop the skill to perform skinfold measurements with accuracy and consistency. As a physical educator, you should seek to develop this skill.

Estimating Percent Body Fat

Many regression equations with functions to predict hydrostatically measured body density from skinfold measurements have been published. These equations are termed **population-specific** or **generalized.** Population-specific equations were developed from homogeneous samples, meaning their application is limited to a similar sample (age and gender, for instance). Generalized equations that can be used with samples varying in age and body fatness have been developed to eliminate that problem. The generalized equations were based on large heterogeneous samples. Regression models that account for age and the nonlinear relationship between skinfold fat and body density were then developed. The generalized approach makes it possible to use one equation rather than several, without a loss in prediction accuracy.

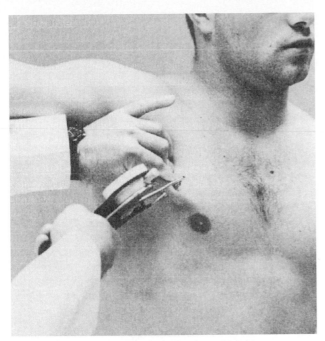

FIGURE 13.2 Caliper placement for chest skinfold measurement.

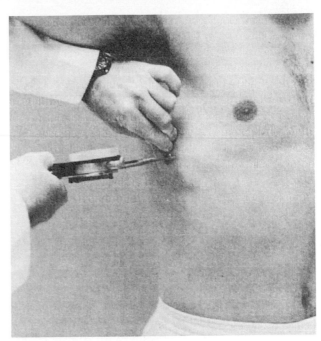

FIGURE 13.3 Caliper placement for axilla skinfold measurement.

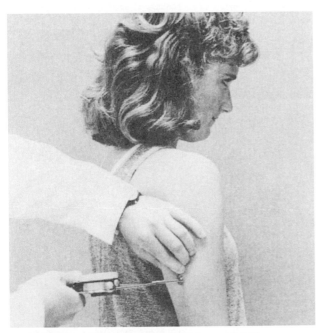

FIGURE 13.4 Caliper placement for triceps skinfold measurement.

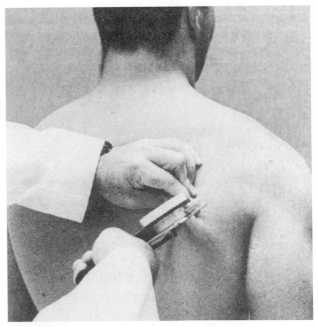

FIGURE 13.5 Caliper placement for subscapular skinfold measurement.

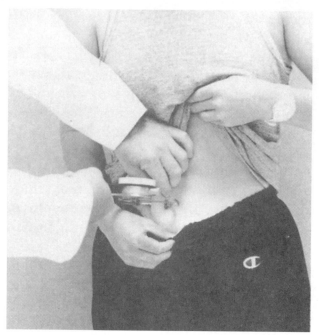

FIGURE 13.6 Caliper placement for abdominal skinfold measurement.

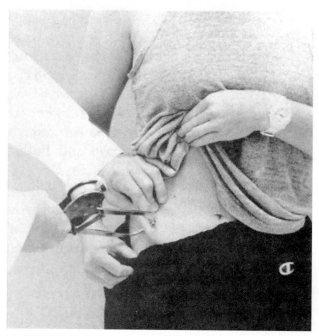

FIGURE 13.7 Caliper placement for suprailium skinfold measurement.

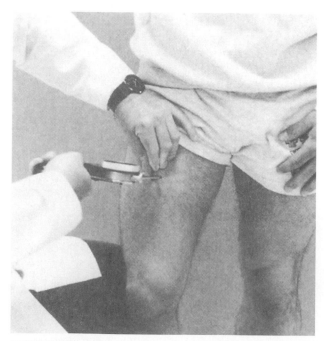

FIGURE 13.8 Caliper placement for thigh skinfold measurement.

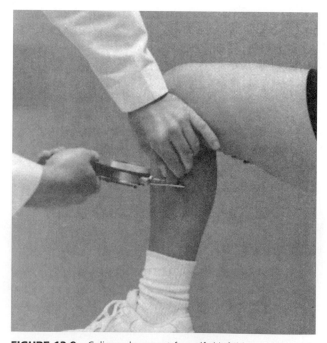

FIGURE 13.9 Caliper placement for calf skinfold measurement.

Computer and microcomputer programs are available, or may be developed, to determine body density and percent body fat after the skinfold measurements have been completed. However, computer-generated tables that provide percent body fat estimates have been developed, eliminating the need for calculations by the test administrator. Values published by Jackson and Pollock (1985) are presented in tables 13.5 through 13.8. Jackson and Pollock found that two different sums of three skinfolds for males and females were highly correlated with the sum of seven of the skinfolds previously described. For males, chest, abdomen, and thigh skinfolds were used, and for females, triceps, suprailium, and thigh skinfolds were used. The researchers also found that the sums of triceps, chest, and subscapular skinfolds for males and triceps, abdomen, and suprailium for females were similarly accurate. The test administrator has the option of using either combination, but the latter skinfolds may be more practical.

✇ARE YOU ABLE TO DO THE FOLLOWING:

- list and describe eight sites for skinfold measurements?
- perform skinfold measurements, estimate percent body fat, and advise individuals of optimal percent fat ranges?

Optimal Percent Body Fat and Desirable Body Weight

Health-related physical fitness tests, which include a body composition component, are included in chapter 15. Health standards for percent fat or sum of skinfold measurements for children and youth are provided with the tests; some tests include standards for adults. Though skinfolds are related to body fatness in children, the absolute amount of body fat cannot be accurately determined. The relation of skinfold fat to body fatness differs by sex and also changes as children mature. Therefore, a given skinfold thickness does not correspond to the same body fat content for 7-year-olds as it does for 17-year-olds.

What is a desirable percent fat for children and adults? As stated previously, being overfat, and certainly being obese, increases your risk of health problems. On the other hand, the loss of too much body fat may affect your health. Different optimal limits of percent body fat have been reported, but it is difficult to compare standards because studies do not always group age ranges in the same way. The FITNESSGRAM (Cooper Institute for Aerobics Research 1999), described in chapter 15, reports the optimal range of body fatness for males and females, ages 5 to 25, as 10% to 20% and 15% to 25%, respectively. For children above the age of 12 years, the FITNESSGRAM considers males with less than 8% and females with less than 13% fat to be very lean, and being this lean may not be best for health. The YMCA Physical Fitness Test (Golding, Myers, and Sinning 1989), also described in chapter 15, reports the "good" standard for percent fat for males, ages 26 to 35, as 13% to 15%. For females of the same age group the range is 19% to 21%. Ross and Jackson (1990) report that for the age group 30 to 39, the optimal range for percent fat is 12% to 22% for males and 16% to 26% for females. T. G. Lohman (1982) reports that a 10% to 22% fat content in men and a 20% to 32% fat content in women seems satisfactory. For the nonathlete, the percent body fat probably should be no lower than between 5% and 10% for males and between 15% and 18% for females.

In some sports, a low percent body fat is desirable. The average percent body fat for highly trained male endurance athletes (e.g., distance runners) is 4% to 10%. For highly trained female endurance athletes, it is 13% to 18%. The recommended minimal percent fat for male athletes is 3% to 7%, and for female athletes it is 10% to 18%.

Although they are not the same, the optimal percent fat ranges for the tests reported in chapter 15 are acceptable by health experts. Your selection of one of these tests to use in a professional setting need not be determined by the percent fat standards. If your professional responsibilities are in the school environment and you perform skinfold measurements, you should use an acceptable standardized physical fitness test and its health-related percent fat standards. If your professional responsibilities are elsewhere and you choose not to use an acceptable standardized physical fitness test, the upper limit of percent body fat probably should be no more than 15% to 18% for adult males and 22% to 26% for adult females. Once the percent body fat has been estimated, desirable

TABLE 13.5 Percent Fat Estimate for Men: Sum of Chest, Abdomen, and Thigh Skinfolds

Sum of Skinfolds (mm)	Age to Last Year*								
	Under 22	23–27	28–32	33–37	38–42	43–47	48–52	53–57	Over 57
8–10	1.3	1.8	2.3	2.9	3.4	3.9	4.5	5.0	5.5
11–13	2.2	2.8	3.3	3.9	4.4	4.9	5.5	6.0	6.5
14–16	3.2	3.8	4.3	4.8	5.4	5.9	6.4	7.0	7.5
17–19	4.2	4.7	5.3	5.8	6.3	6.9	7.4	8.0	8.5
20–22	5.1	5.7	6.2	6.8	7.3	7.9	8.4	8.9	9.5
23–25	6.1	6.6	7.2	7.7	8.3	8.8	9.4	9.9	10.5
26–28	7.0	7.6	8.1	8.7	9.2	9.8	10.3	10.9	11.4
29–31	8.0	8.5	9.1	9.6	10.2	10.7	11.3	11.8	12.4
32–34	8.9	9.4	10.0	10.5	11.1	11.6	12.2	12.8	13.3
35–37	9.8	10.4	10.9	11.5	12.0	12.6	13.1	13.7	14.3
38–40	10.7	11.3	11.8	12.4	12.9	13.5	14.1	14.6	15.2
41–43	11.6	12.2	12.7	13.3	13.8	14.4	15.0	15.5	16.1
44–46	12.5	13.1	13.6	14.2	14.7	15.3	15.9	16.4	17.0
47–49	13.4	13.9	14.5	15.1	15.6	16.2	16.8	17.3	17.9
50–52	14.3	14.8	15.4	15.9	16.5	17.1	17.6	18.2	18.8
53–55	15.1	15.7	16.2	16.8	17.4	17.9	18.5	19.1	19.7
56–58	16.0	16.5	17.1	17.7	18.2	18.8	19.4	20.0	20.5
59–61	16.9	17.4	17.9	18.5	19.1	19.7	20.2	20.8	21.4
62–64	17.6	18.2	18.8	19.4	19.9	20.5	21.1	21.7	22.2
65–67	18.5	19.0	19.6	20.2	20.8	21.3	21.9	22.5	23.1
68–70	19.3	19.9	20.4	21.0	21.6	22.2	22.7	23.3	23.9
71–73	20.1	20.7	21.2	21.8	22.4	23.0	23.6	24.1	24.7
74–76	20.9	21.5	22.0	22.6	23.2	23.8	24.4	25.0	25.5
77–79	21.7	22.2	22.8	23.4	24.0	24.6	25.2	25.8	26.3
80–82	22.4	23.0	23.6	24.2	24.8	25.4	25.9	26.5	27.1
83–85	23.2	23.8	24.4	25.0	25.5	26.1	26.7	27.3	27.9
86–88	24.0	24.5	25.1	25.7	26.3	26.9	27.5	28.1	28.7
89–91	24.7	25.3	25.9	26.5	27.1	27.6	28.2	28.8	29.4
92–94	25.4	26.0	26.6	27.2	27.8	28.4	29.0	29.6	30.2
95–97	26.1	26.7	27.3	27.9	28.5	29.1	29.7	30.3	30.9
98–100	26.9	27.4	28.0	28.6	29.2	29.8	30.4	31.0	31.6
101–103	27.5	28.1	28.7	29.3	29.9	30.5	31.1	31.7	32.3
104–106	28.2	28.8	29.4	30.0	30.6	31.2	31.8	32.4	33.0
107–109	28.9	29.5	30.1	30.7	31.3	31.9	32.5	33.1	33.7
110–112	29.6	30.2	30.8	31.4	32.0	32.6	33.2	33.8	34.4
113–115	30.2	30.8	31.4	32.0	32.6	33.2	33.8	34.5	35.1
116–118	30.9	31.5	32.1	32.7	33.3	33.9	34.5	35.1	35.7
119–121	31.5	32.1	32.7	33.3	33.9	34.5	35.1	35.7	36.4
122–124	32.1	32.7	33.3	33.9	34.5	35.1	35.8	36.4	37.0
125–127	32.7	33.3	33.9	34.5	35.1	35.8	36.4	37.0	37.6

Source: A. S. Jackson and M. L. Pollock, Practical assessment of body composition, *The Physician and Sportsmedicine* 13(5):76–90, 1985.
*Last calendar birthday.

TABLE 13.6 Percent Fat Estimate for Women: Sum of Triceps, Suprailium, and Thigh Skinfolds

Sum of Skinfolds (mm)	Age to Last Year*								
	Under 22	23–27	28–32	33–37	38–42	43–47	48–52	53–57	Over 57
23–25	9.7	9.9	10.2	10.4	10.7	10.9	11.2	11.4	11.7
26–28	11.0	11.2	11.5	11.7	12.0	12.3	12.5	12.7	13.0
29–31	12.3	12.5	12.8	13.0	13.3	13.5	13.8	14.0	14.3
32–34	13.6	13.8	14.0	14.3	14.5	14.8	15.0	15.3	15.5
35–37	14.8	15.0	15.3	15.5	15.8	16.0	16.3	16.5	16.8
38–40	16.0	16.3	16.5	16.7	17.0	17.2	17.5	17.7	18.0
41–43	17.2	17.4	17.7	17.9	18.2	18.4	18.7	18.9	19.2
44–46	18.3	18.6	18.8	19.1	19.3	19.6	19.8	20.1	20.3
47–49	19.5	19.7	20.0	20.2	20.5	20.7	21.0	21.2	21.5
50–52	20.6	20.8	21.1	21.3	21.6	21.8	22.1	22.3	22.6
53–55	21.7	21.9	22.1	22.4	22.6	22.9	23.1	23.4	23.6
56–58	22.7	23.0	23.2	23.4	23.7	23.9	24.2	24.4	24.7
59–61	23.7	24.0	24.2	24.5	24.7	25.0	25.2	25.5	25.7
62–64	24.7	25.0	25.2	25.5	25.7	26.0	26.7	26.4	26.7
65–67	25.7	25.9	26.2	26.4	26.7	26.9	27.2	27.4	27.7
68–70	26.6	26.9	27.1	27.4	27.6	27.9	28.1	28.4	28.6
71–73	27.5	27.8	28.0	28.3	28.5	28.8	29.0	29.3	29.5
74–76	28.4	28.7	28.9	29.2	29.4	29.7	29.9	30.2	30.4
77–79	29.3	29.5	29.8	30.0	30.3	30.5	30.8	31.0	31.3
80–82	30.1	30.4	30.6	30.9	31.1	31.4	31.6	31.9	32.1
83–85	30.9	31.2	31.4	31.7	31.9	32.2	32.4	32.7	32.9
86–88	31.7	32.0	32.2	32.5	32.7	32.9	33.2	33.4	33.7
89–91	32.5	32.7	33.0	33.2	33.5	33.7	33.9	34.2	34.4
92–94	33.2	33.4	33.7	33.9	34.2	34.4	34.7	34.9	35.2
95–97	33.9	34.1	34.4	34.6	34.9	35.1	35.4	35.6	35.9
98–100	34.6	34.8	35.1	35.3	35.5	35.8	36.0	36.3	36.5
101–103	35.3	35.4	35.7	35.9	36.2	36.4	36.7	36.9	37.2
104–106	35.8	36.1	36.3	36.6	36.8	37.1	37.3	37.5	37.8
107–109	36.4	36.7	36.9	37.1	37.4	37.6	37.9	38.1	38.4
110–112	37.0	37.2	37.5	37.7	38.0	38.2	38.5	38.7	38.9
113–115	37.5	37.8	38.0	38.2	38.5	38.7	39.0	39.2	39.5
116–118	38.0	38.3	38.5	38.8	39.0	39.3	39.5	39.7	40.0
119–121	38.5	38.7	39.0	39.2	39.5	39.7	40.0	40.2	40.5
122–124	39.0	39.2	39.4	39.7	39.9	40.2	40.4	40.7	40.9
125–127	39.4	39.6	39.9	40.1	40.4	40.6	40.9	41.1	41.4
128–130	39.8	40.0	40.3	40.5	40.8	41.0	41.3	41.5	41.8

Source: A. S. Jackson and M. L. Pollock, Practical assessment of body composition, *The Physician and Sportsmedicine* 13(5):76–90, 1985.
*Last calendar birthday.

TABLE 13.7 Percent Fat Estimate for Men: Sum of Triceps, Chest, and Subscapular Skinfolds

Sum of Skinfolds (mm)	Age to Last Year*								
	Under 22	23–27	28–32	33–37	38–42	43–47	48–52	53–57	Over 57
8–10	1.5	2.0	2.5	3.1	3.6	4.1	4.6	5.1	5.6
11–13	3.0	3.5	4.0	4.5	5.1	5.6	6.1	6.6	7.1
14–16	4.5	5.0	5.5	6.0	6.5	7.0	7.6	8.1	8.6
17–19	5.9	6.4	6.9	7.4	8.0	8.5	9.0	9.5	10.0
20–22	7.3	7.8	8.3	8.8	9.4	9.9	10.4	10.9	11.4
23–25	8.6	9.2	9.7	10.2	10.7	11.2	11.8	12.3	12.8
26–28	10.0	10.5	11.0	11.5	12.1	12.6	13.1	13.6	14.2
29–31	11.2	11.8	12.3	12.8	13.4	13.9	14.4	14.9	15.5
32–34	12.5	13.0	13.5	14.1	14.6	15.1	15.7	16.2	16.7
35–37	13.7	14.2	14.8	15.3	15.8	16.4	16.9	17.4	18.0
38–40	14.9	15.4	15.9	16.5	17.0	17.6	18.1	18.6	19.2
41–43	16.0	16.6	17.1	17.6	18.2	18.7	19.3	19.8	20.3
44–46	17.1	17.7	18.2	18.7	19.3	19.8	20.4	20.9	21.5
47–49	18.2	18.7	19.3	19.8	20.4	20.9	21.4	22.0	22.5
50–52	19.2	19.7	20.3	20.8	21.4	21.9	22.5	23.0	23.6
53–55	20.2	20.7	21.3	21.8	22.4	22.9	23.5	24.0	24.6
56–58	21.1	21.7	22.2	22.8	23.3	23.9	24.4	25.0	25.5
59–61	22.0	22.6	23.1	23.7	24.2	24.8	25.3	25.9	26.5
62–64	22.9	23.4	24.0	24.5	25.1	25.7	26.2	26.8	27.3
65–67	23.7	24.3	24.8	25.4	25.9	26.5	27.1	27.6	28.2
68–70	24.5	25.0	25.6	26.2	26.7	27.3	27.8	28.4	29.0
71–73	25.2	25.8	26.3	26.9	27.5	28.0	28.6	29.1	29.7
74–76	25.9	26.5	27.0	27.6	28.2	28.7	29.3	29.9	30.4
77–79	26.6	27.1	27.7	28.2	28.8	29.4	29.9	30.5	31.1
80–82	27.2	27.7	28.3	28.9	29.4	30.0	30.6	31.1	31.7
83–85	27.7	28.3	28.8	29.4	30.0	30.5	31.1	31.7	32.3
86–88	28.2	28.8	29.4	29.9	30.5	31.1	31.6	32.2	32.8
89–91	28.7	29.3	29.8	30.4	31.0	31.5	32.1	32.7	33.3
92–94	29.1	29.7	30.3	30.8	31.4	32.0	32.6	33.1	33.4
95–97	29.5	30.1	30.6	31.2	31.8	32.4	32.9	33.5	34.1
98–100	29.8	30.4	31.0	31.6	32.1	32.7	33.3	33.9	34.4
101–103	30.1	30.7	31.3	31.8	32.4	33.0	33.6	34.1	34.7
104–106	30.4	30.9	31.5	32.1	32.7	33.2	33.8	34.4	35.0
107–109	30.6	31.1	31.7	32.3	32.9	33.4	34.0	34.6	35.2
110–112	30.7	31.3	31.9	32.4	33.0	33.6	34.2	34.7	35.3
113–115	30.8	31.4	32.0	32.5	33.1	33.7	34.3	34.9	35.4
116–118	30.9	31.5	32.0	32.6	33.2	33.8	34.3	34.9	35.5

Source: A. S. Jackson and M. L. Pollock, Practical assessment of body composition, *The Physician and Sportsmedicine* 13(5):76–90, 1985.
*Last calendar birthday.

TABLE 13.8 Percent Fat Estimate for Women: Sum of Triceps, Abdomen, and Suprailium Skinfolds

Sum of Skinfolds (mm)	Age to Last Year*								
	Under 22	23–27	28–32	33–37	38–42	43–47	48–52	53–57	Over 57
8–12	8.8	9.0	9.2	9.4	9.5	9.7	9.9	10.1	10.3
13–17	10.8	10.9	11.1	11.3	11.5	11.7	11.8	12.0	12.2
18–22	12.6	12.8	13.0	13.2	13.4	13.5	13.7	13.9	14.1
23–27	14.5	14.6	14.8	15.0	15.2	15.4	15.6	15.7	15.9
28–32	16.2	16.4	16.6	16.8	17.0	17.1	17.3	17.5	17.7
33–37	17.9	18.1	18.3	18.5	18.7	18.9	19.0	19.2	19.4
38–42	19.6	19.8	20.0	20.2	20.3	20.5	20.7	20.9	21.1
43–47	21.2	21.4	21.6	21.8	21.9	22.1	22.3	22.5	22.7
48–52	22.8	22.9	23.1	23.3	23.5	23.7	23.8	24.0	24.2
53–57	24.2	24.4	24.6	24.8	25.0	25.2	25.3	25.5	25.7
58–62	25.7	25.9	26.0	26.2	26.4	26.6	26.8	27.0	27.1
63–67	27.1	27.2	27.4	27.6	27.8	28.0	28.2	28.3	28.5
68–72	28.4	28.6	28.7	28.9	29.1	29.3	29.5	29.7	29.8
73–77	29.6	29.8	30.0	30.2	30.4	30.6	30.7	30.9	31.1
78–82	30.9	31.0	31.2	31.4	31.6	31.8	31.9	32.1	32.3
83–87	32.0	32.2	32.4	32.6	32.7	32.9	33.1	33.3	33.5
88–92	33.1	33.3	33.5	33.7	33.8	34.0	34.2	34.4	34.6
93–97	34.1	34.3	34.5	34.7	34.9	35.1	35.2	35.4	35.6
98–102	35.1	35.3	35.5	35.7	35.9	36.0	36.2	36.4	36.6
103–107	36.1	36.2	36.4	36.6	36.8	37.0	37.2	37.3	37.5
108–112	36.9	37.1	37.3	37.5	37.7	37.9	38.0	38.2	38.4
113–117	37.8	37.9	38.1	38.3	39.2	39.4	39.6	39.8	39.2
118–122	38.5	38.7	38.9	39.1	39.4	39.6	39.8	40.0	40.0
123–127	39.2	39.4	39.6	39.8	40.0	40.1	40.3	40.5	40.7
128–132	39.9	40.1	40.2	40.4	40.6	40.8	41.0	41.2	41.3
133–137	40.5	40.7	40.8	41.0	41.2	41.4	41.6	41.7	41.9
138–142	41.0	41.2	41.4	41.6	41.7	41.9	42.1	42.3	42.5
143–147	41.5	41.7	41.9	42.0	42.2	42.4	42.6	42.8	43.0
148–152	41.9	42.1	42.3	42.8	42.6	42.8	43.0	43.2	43.4
153–157	42.3	42.5	42.6	42.8	43.0	43.2	43.4	43.6	43.7
158–162	42.6	42.8	43.0	43.1	43.3	43.5	43.7	43.9	44.1
163–167	42.9	43.0	43.2	43.4	43.6	43.8	44.0	44.1	44.3
168–172	43.1	43.2	43.4	43.6	43.8	44.0	44.2	44.3	44.5
173–177	43.2	43.4	43.6	43.8	43.9	44.1	44.3	44.5	44.7
178–182	43.3	43.5	43.7	43.8	44.0	44.2	44.4	44.6	44.8

Source: A. S. Jackson and M. L. Pollock, Practical assessment of body composition, *The Physician and Sportsmedicine* 13(5):76–90, 1985.
*Last calendar birthday.

weight can be determined. The desired weight is calculated from lean weight.

A sample calculation is provided.

Given: Body weight = 200 pounds; % fat = 24%.

Calculation of fat weight (FW)

$$FW = body\ weight \times (\%\ fat \div 100)$$

$$= 200 \times (24\% \div 100)$$

$$= 200 \times .24$$

$$FW = 48\ pounds$$

Calculation of lean body weight (LBW)

$$LBW = body\ weight - FW$$

$$= 200 - 48$$

$$LBW = 152\ pounds$$

Calculation of desirable body weight (DBW)

$$DBW = \frac{LBW}{1.00 - (desired\ \%\ fat \div 100)}$$

$$= \frac{152}{1.00 - (19\% \div 100)}$$

$$= \frac{152}{1.00 - .19}$$

$$= \frac{152}{.81}$$

$$DBW = 187.7\ pounds$$

Because measurement errors may occur, when you are estimating body density it is best to determine desirable body weight ranges. As stated previously, the upper limit of ideal weight for adult males probably should include no more than 15% to 18% fat, and for adult females, 22% to 26%. Values above these percentages indicate overfatness. Body fat content in excess of 25% and 30% indicates obesity for males and females, respectively.

Cooper Method for Determining Ideal Weight

When body fat cannot be estimated through skinfold measurements, the Cooper (1982) method may be used to calculate the ideal weight for men and women. Men multiply their height in inches by 4, and then subtract 128.

Women multiply their height in inches by 3.5, and then subtract 108. The resulting values will give men of average build a weight with roughly 15% to 19% body fat, and women of average build a weight with roughly 18% to 22% body fat. Large-boned individuals should add 10% to the calculated figure to determine their ideal weight, and small-boned individuals should subtract 10%.

Body Mass Index (BMI)

The **body mass index** (BMI) provides an indication of the relationship of weight to height. Because it does not provide an estimate of percent body fat, BMI is not a recommended procedure for determining body composition. The BMI has been found to be correlated with health risks, however, and can be used when body fat estimates are not available. The BMI is computed with the following equation:

$$BMI = \frac{weight\ in\ kilograms}{(height\ in\ meters)^2}$$

(1 kilogram = 2.2046 pounds; 1 meter = 39.37 inches)

In general, a BMI of 20 to 25 is associated with the lowest risk of health problems, and health risks increase as the BMI increases. BMI values above 27.3 for females and 27.8 for males are indicators of excessive weight and have been associated with increased risks for several health problems, including high blood pressure and diabetes. Individuals with a BMI greater than 30 are considered obese, and anyone with a BMI greater than 40 is considered morbidly obese and in need of medical attention.

Fat Distribution

Research shows that body shape, as well as body fat, is important to health. Excess body fat concentrated in the abdominal area may be a greater health risk than fat found around the thighs and hips. It appears that abdominal fat is more easily broken down than fat in other places. This broken-down fat goes straight to the liver, which may lead to dangerous elevations in blood fat and insulin levels.

A favorable **waist-to-hip ratio** may decrease the risk of diseases associated with excess weight. To determine the waist-to-hip ratio, perform the following steps:

1. Measure around the waist where it is the smallest; stand relaxed and do not pull in the stomach.
2. Measure the hips where they are the largest.
3. Divide the waist measurement by the hips measurement to obtain waist-to-hip ratio.

Ratios above .80 for females and .90 for males are linked to greater health risks.

?ARE YOU ABLE TO DO THE FOLLOWING:

- calculate an individual's desirable weight on the basis of an acceptable percent body fat?
- determine the body mass index (BMI) and waist-to-hip ratio and advise individuals of BMI values and waist-to-hip ratios associated with the lowest risk of health problems?

Weight-Loss Programs

The best approach to reduction of body fat is through a program involving exercise and a modest decrease in caloric intake. With only a modest decrease in caloric intake, a permanent change in eating behavior is more eas-ily made than with a great decrease in caloric intake. When exercise and diet changes are combined, 80% to 95% of the weight loss is through loss of fat tissue. If weight loss is accomplished strictly through dieting, 30% to 45% of the weight reduction is through loss of lean tissue. Unsound gimmicks or diets should be avoided, and weight reduction should be gradual, with a loss of no more than 1 to 2 pounds/week. For weight reduction purposes, exercise does not have to be intense. For example, walking a mile expends almost the same amount of calories as running a mile. If possible, percent body fat should be monitored during weight loss to be sure the body composition is not being altered in the wrong way.

▶ REVIEW PROBLEMS ◀

1. If skinfold calipers are available, perform skinfold measurements on several of your classmates. Use different types of calipers, if possible, on the same individuals and compare the results. Do you obtain similar measurements with different calipers?
2. Ask the directors of several local health or fitness clubs how they estimate percent body fat for their members.

14 Posture and Body Mechanics

Upon completion of this chapter, you should be able to

1. Define proper posture and body mechanics;

2. State why posture and body mechanics should be measured;

3. Measure for proper posture while an individual is sitting, standing, walking, running for speed, running for distance, lifting heavy objects, or walking with heavy objects; and

4. Prescribe activities and exercises for development of proper posture and movement mechanics.

Proper posture is the correct alignment of body parts and a balance of forces that, with minimal effort, will provide maximum support; the least amount of strain on the muscles, tendons, ligaments, and joints; and the greatest mechanical efficiency. Good posture depends on good body mechanics. **Body mechanics** is the application of physical laws to the human body. The bones of the body act as levers (simple machines), and the muscles supply the force to move them. Therefore, through the application of mechanical laws, efficient movement can be accomplished while avoiding strain or injury.

The postures that are maintained for various positions and movements are the result of conscious and unconscious practice, which usually lead to the formation of postural habits. As a person repeatedly assumes a given body alignment during work, play, and relaxation, postural habits are developed. When a person maintains a position for extended periods of time, a response is established in the neuromuscular system. This response be-

comes habitual; it is produced when the person is unconscious of posture. The habitual postural response occurs regardless of good or bad habit, and many individuals mistakenly feel comfortable in a position that actually places a strain on the joints.

Posture is influenced by general health, emotions, body build, gender, strength and endurance, visual and kinesthetic awareness, personal habits, and the demands of work. The following examples illustrate how these factors influence posture: Obese people often lean backward to shift the center of gravity backward over the feet (women in late pregnancy sometimes do the same thing); frail or tired individuals assume the "fatigue slouch," placing stress on the ligaments rather than the muscles; young, tall girls sometimes slouch to make themselves appear shorter (short men tend to stand in good posture to make themselves appear taller); and depressed and unhappy people usually slouch, whereas happy ones stand tall.

Why Measure Posture and Body Mechanics?

Poor posture can cause a number of health problems, including the following:

1. Dysmenorrhea can occur with a swayback posture, with greater severity among college women.
2. A low but significant relationship exists between posture and trunk strength imbalance.
3. Dysmenorrhea, constipation, and back pain are found with increased inclination of the pelvis.
4. Diseases and cardiac and pulmonary problems occur more often among elementary children with poor posture.
5. Protruding abdomen and lumbar lordosis may contribute to painful menstruation, susceptibility to back injury, and backache.
6. Rounded shoulders may impair respiratory capacity.
7. Hyperextended knees may lead to knee injury.
8. Unbalanced postural lines can cause tension in muscle groups, produce joint strain, and stretch ligaments.
9. A forward lean of the head can cause headache and neck and shoulder pain.
10. Improper foot alignment and footwear cause most of the foot problems that occur.
11. Habitual misalignment of body parts can lead to structural changes in the skeletal system and can restrict joint motion.

On the positive side, good posture contributes to a pleasing appearance and can make a favorable first impression. It gives the appearance of alertness and confidence and prevents the health problems associated with poor posture.

Children in the elementary grades should be measured for postural deviations. The earlier the postural problems are identified, the less complicated the correction. Most individuals with incorrect posture and movement mechanics have minimal structural deviations. Their postural problems are primarily due to faults in body alignment. To correct their faulty posture, individuals must know (1) the mechanics of good posture, (2) their postural faults, and (3) activities and exercises to perform in order to improve their posture and movement mechanics. Postural faults can be identified through the measurement and evaluation of posture. However, knowledge alone is not always enough for individuals to work to improve their postural faults. Many must be motivated to correct their faults. Unfortunately, posture evaluation sometimes identifies individuals with serious structural deviation. These individuals need to be treated by medical specialists.

Finally, evaluation of posture may encourage all tested individuals to be more posture-conscious, thereby possibly preventing future problems.

?ARE YOU ABLE TO DO THE FOLLOWING:

- define posture and body mechanics and state why they should be measured?

Measures of Posture

Numerous instruments and scales have been developed to measure posture. Though many of these instruments and scales have made positive contributions to posture evaluation, it is a mistake to expect all individuals to conform to the same postural standards. The variety of body types make it difficult to apply the same postural standards to everyone. Therefore, although certain body relationships are desirable and mechanical principles should be observed, there is probably no one best posture for all individuals. Use the standards provided here to diagnose possible postural problems, but do not insist that everyone conform to identical standards.

The only test with a numerical rating scale included in this group of tests is the New York State Posture Rating Test. Since the primary purpose of postural screening is to identify postural deviations, you should not be concerned with the obtaining of scores for comparison purposes.

■ New York State Posture Rating Test
(The University of the State of New York 1966)

Test Objective. To evaluate posture.
Age Level. Grades 4 through 12.
Equipment. Screen, rating chart, and plumb line.
Validity. Logical validity.
Reliability. .93 to .98 for boys and girls at different grade levels.

Norms. Norms are provided by grade and gender in the reference.

Administration and Directions. The posture rating chart in figure 14.1 is used to assess thirteen areas of the body. The rating chart shows three profiles for each area: the correct position, a slight deviation, and a pronounced deviation. The individual stands on a line that is 3 feet in front of a screen (parallel to the screen). A plumb line is suspended just in front of the line so that the individual is standing between the plumb line and the screen. Another line is drawn at a right angle to the first line and extended 10 feet farther back from the screen. The total distance from the screen to the end of the line is 13 feet. The test administrator stands at this point.

The student, while standing comfortably and naturally, is rated from two viewpoints. In one position, the student stands facing the screen with the plumb line bisecting the head and spine and passing down between the legs and feet. From this position, six areas of the body are rated.

The student then turns one quarter turn to the left (right side to the screen) so that the plumb line passes in a line through the ear, shoulder, hip, knee, and ankle. Seven areas of the body are rated from this position.

Scoring. Each of the thirteen areas is rated. For the correct position, 5 points are scored; for a slight deviation, 3 points are scored; and for a pronounced deviation, 1 point is scored. The total point value is the score, with a score of 65 being a perfect score.

Standing Posture Measurement

The subject backs up to a flat wall with the head, shoulders, hips, calves, and heels touching the wall. The test administrator attempts to place a hand in the space between the wall and the small of the subject's back. The space should accommodate the fingers but not the palm. If the space is greater than the thickness of the hand, the subject probably has lordosis, with shortened lumbar and hip flexor muscles.

Foot Alignment Measurement

An estimated 80% of the adult population experiences some type of foot problem. The two major causes of foot problems are improper foot alignment and footwear. Improper foot alignment may be due to toeing in, toeing out, flat feet, foot pronation, or congenital deformity. As with other postural deviations, it is important to initiate correction of improper foot alignment at an early age.

You can measure foot alignment by looking at the front of the body. A straight line should run from the knee cap, through the center of the ankle, and to the second toe. From the rear, a straight line should pass through the center of the Achilles tendon.

Descriptions of Proper Posture and Body Mechanics

The following descriptions of the proper techniques for standing, walking, running for speed, running for distance, sitting, lifting heavy objects, carrying heavy objects, and lying may be used to check posture and body mechanics. Remember, not everyone is expected to have identical posture, but if you discover postural deviations that may create health problems, you should attempt to correct them or advise the individual to seek medical help.

Standing

1. The head and chin are centered over the trunk and are held in a relaxed position at a right angle to the front of the neck.
2. The shoulders are free and easy and are not forward, back, or elevated.
3. The shoulder blades are drawn down and flat on the back.
4. The chest is held up, not too high or leaning, and is not sagging.
5. The trunk is within normal limits of curves, not too straight and flat or too round and hollow.
6. The abdomen is up and in and is not relaxed or protruding.
7. The hips are in line with the trunk and are not leading or thrust back.
8. The arms hang naturally and relaxed at the sides and are not held rigidly or too relaxed.
9. The knees are free and easy and are not bent or thrust back.
10. The feet are parallel and slightly apart.
11. The weight falls ahead of the outer anklebone and is distributed toward the outside of each foot.

From the front view, the weight should be evenly distributed about a vertical line through the midpoint of the body. From the side view, a vertical line should pass through the earlobe, through the middle of the shoulder, and through the middle of the hip, slightly behind the kneecap and

POSTURE RATING CHART

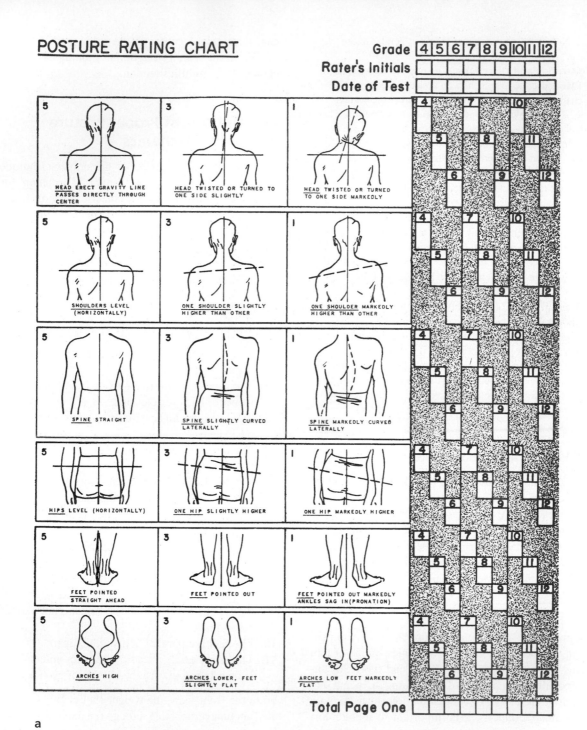

a

FIGURE 14.1 New York State Posture Rating Chart.

Courtesy of the University of the State of New York.

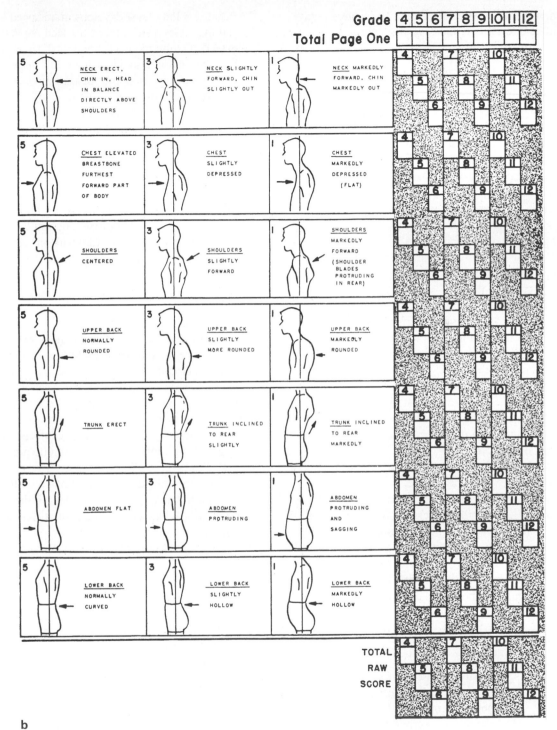

b

FIGURE 14.1 New York State Posture Rating Chart (continued).

slightly in front of the outer anklebone. The center of gravity should be directly over the base of support.

Walking

1. The upper body (head, chin, shoulders, and chest) is balanced on the trunk; it is not dragged forward by the pull of gravity.
2. The trunk is balanced in the pelvic basin. It does not come to an erect, rigid position between steps but remains slightly forward to keep it in line with the extended rear leg at the time of the push-off. The center of gravity remains within the base of support.
3. Motion originates in the hip joint, as the leading leg swings ahead of the body.
4. The leading leg is always parallel to or in advance of the trunk, so a new base of support is always ready to receive the body weight.
5. As a new base of support is established, the upper body remains in line with the axis of the rear leg.
6. The supporting and pushing leg applies its force directly through the center of gravity along the line of resistance of the trunk. This leg begins to push off before the front foot strikes the ground.
7. The heel strikes the ground first, directly in line with the direction of walk. The weight is transferred through the outer border of the foot to the ball of the foot.
8. The ankle joint is extended, as the final push, or thrust, is made with the big toe.
9. The weight shift of the alternate foot causes the pelvic girdle to oscillate back and forth. The arms and shoulders swing slightly to compensate for this oscillation and to keep the body weight evenly distributed.
10. The leg muscles supply most of the energy for locomotion so the body makes as few extraneous motions as possible.

Running for Speed

1. At slower speeds, runners are more erect, whereas at full speed, the typical sprinter leans forward at about 15° from the perpendicular. Forward lean comes naturally with most sprinters, and conscious attempts to increase lean are not usually necessary.

2. Because a long lever develops more speed at the end than does a short lever, the lead leg is fully extended at the moment of the push from the rear leg. This action also enables the full force of the push to be converted into forward movement.
3. Any vertical movement is great enough to counteract the downward pull of gravity, but because the forward speed of the runner is decreasing, it is not great enough to produce an unnecessary bounce. The higher the center of gravity rises, the longer the body is off the ground.
4. As the foot leaves the ground after a vigorous push, the knee is bent. The faster the leg moves, the more the knee is bent and the higher the foot is raised. By this action, the knee moves forward with greater angular velocity owing to the shorter radius of the arc through which the leg swings. The swing of the leg from the hip is in a straight forward and backward line.
5. The faster the runner moves, the higher the knee is raised in front. This movement delays the placing of the foot on the ground for its next thrust and permits the lead leg to reach full extension.
6. The runner lands on the ball of the foot. Landing on the heel of the foot causes the center of gravity to fall behind the contact foot, creating a retarding effect.
7. The faster the speed, the longer the stride. However, if the stride is too long, the foot contacts the ground ahead of the center of gravity, thereby producing a braking action.
8. The swing of the arms is coordinated with that of the legs to balance the rotary effect of the leg swing on the trunk. The elbows are bent at right angles with the arms close to the sides.
9. Shoulder motion is kept to a minimum, and the hands are relaxed.

Running for Distance

1. The head remains up, avoiding the tendency to watch the feet.
2. The back is straight but naturally comfortable. The shoulders are not thrown back, nor is the chest stuck out.
3. The buttocks are tucked in. In this position, a hypothetical line drawn through the shoulders and the hips is vertical, or nearly so.

4. The elbows are bent and held slightly away from the body. The arms are not placed out like wings, nor are they pressed to the chest. They are carried slightly above hip level.
5. The body is straight, as the legs move freely from the hips. The legs are lifted from the knees; the ankles are relaxed. The runner does not overstride; each foot falls just under the knee.
6. Using the heel-to-toe method for footstrike, the runner lands on the heel, then rocks forward to take off from the ball of the foot. This method is the least tiring over long distances and is the least wearing because the heel cushions the landing and the forward rocking distributes the pressure.
7. In the flat-foot method for footstrike, the foot falls under the knee in a quick, light action, with the entire foot landing on the ground at the same time. This type of landing provides a wide surface area to cushion the footstrike. The foot is not driven down but is allowed to pass beneath the body.

Sitting

1. The head, neck, and shoulders are in the same position as standing.
2. The backs of the buttocks touch the back of the chair.
3. The feet and knees are close together with one foot slightly in the lead, or the feet are together with both legs slanted to one side or crossed at the ankles. Regardless of feet and leg positions, the hips remain toward the back of the chair.
4. If the person is writing or reading while sitting at a table, the chair is brought well under the table, so that the edge of the table almost touches the front of the body. The body is all the way back in the chair and the trunk slants forward slightly from the hip joint to bring the eyes in line with the work. The head-neck-trunk line is kept as straight as possible for maximum support of the head.

Lifting Heavy Objects

1. The lifter should stand close to the object being lifted.
2. The knees are bent; the back remains straight.
3. The feet are spread at about shoulder width.

4. The hands grasp the object with the fingers widely spaced under the object to provide the upward force.
5. The lifting is performed by straightening the legs.

Lifting an Object from a Height

1. Heavy objects should not be lifted down from a height without assistance.
2. One leg is placed in front of the other in a stride position.
3. As the object is lifted down, the body weight shifts to the rear leg.

Carrying Heavy Objects

1. The center of gravity is always above the base of support.
2. The body alignment is altered as little as possible.
3. The object is carried as close to the body's center of gravity as possible and no higher than waist level.

Lying

1. If the person is lying on the back, a pillow is placed under the knees to help prevent exaggerated curvature of the lower back. The head is elevated slightly.
2. If the person is lying on the side, one or both knees are drawn up to relieve lower back strain.
3. If the person is lying on the stomach, a pillow is placed under the stomach and hips to help keep the back straight.

Exercises to Correct Postural Deviations

Only a few exercises for several postural deviations (from French and Jansma 1982) will be described. You should refer to a source that describes the deviations in greater detail and includes exercises for possible correction of the deviations. Textbooks dealing with physical education for special populations include this material, and physical therapists also can advise you about appropriate exercises to prescribe.

Lumbar Lordosis

Lumbar lordosis is an increase in the lumbar curve. The exaggerated curve places a strain on the abdomen, causing it to weaken and become more prominent. The lower back muscles and hip flexors are shortened; the hamstrings and gluteal muscles may be weakened; the knees are hyperextended; and the pelvis may be tilted forward and downward. Straight-leg sit-ups and leg raises should not be performed by the lordotic individual. However, these individuals can do the following:

1. Lie on the back with arms outstretched, press spine down until it is flat on the floor, tighten and hold stomach and seat muscles, and then relax.
2. Stand with feet apart, knees bent and hands on knees like a baseball player. Tighten seat and tuck in, drop head and round back, and relax. Repeat.
3. Stand erect against a wall with heels 4 inches from the wall, contract abdominal muscles, and push the lower back against the wall. Repeat.
4. Lie on the back with knees drawn to chest and arms wrapped under the knees to hold legs close to the body. Rock forward and backward trying to come to a sitting position.
5. Lie on the back with knees bent, feet flat on the floor, arms at the sides; lift arms 6 to 10 inches, and roll the head and neck forward, then the shoulders. Roll as far forward as possible without lifting the lower back off the floor, hold the position, and return to starting position. Repeat. As this exercise becomes easier, cross the arms with hands on the shoulders and roll up, touching the elbows to the knees. Do not anchor feet or place hands behind the head.

Kyphosis

Kyphosis involves an abnormal increase in the cervical curvature of the upper back. Round shoulders and forward head usually accompany this condition. The upper back extensors and the trapezius are weakened; the pectoral and intercostal muscles are shortened. Individuals with kyphosis should not perform push-ups. However, these individuals can do the following:

1. Lie on stomach with hands behind the neck, pinch the shoulder blades together, and lift head and chest slightly above the floor. Lower the head and chest to the floor and repeat.
2. Stand tall and slowly swing both arms forward and upward, reaching overhead to a full stretch. At the same time, rise high on the toes, turn the palms outward, and lower arms sideward and downward while forcefully pressing them back. Pull chin in, hold head high, and let heels drop to the floor. Avoid excessive arching of the back.
3. Lie on stomach with arms extended sideways. Lift arms while keeping the head, trunk, and legs in contact with the floor. Slowly lower arms to floor and repeat.

Winged Scapula

Winged scapula is the postural deviation of one or both shoulder blades farther than normal from the spinal column. This deviation may be caused by weakened rhomboids and trapezius or tightened pectorals. Individuals with this deviation can do the following:

1. Lie on back with knees bent and feet flat on the floor, holding a medicine ball in the hands. Raise the ball toward the ceiling, keeping feet together, body in correct alignment, and back flat as possible. Repeat.
2. Lie on back with knees bent, feet flat on the floor, arms out to side, and elbows bent. Pinch shoulder blades together while pressing arms, wrists, neck, and lower back to floor. Repeat.

Scoliosis

Scoliosis is an abnormal lateral curvature of the vertebral column. There may be a single curve, known as a C curve or a reverse C curve. This condition also may involve two or more curves in different directions. A double curve is usually shaped like an S. Persons afflicted with scoliosis can do the following:

1. Hang by both arms, or the arm of the lower shoulder, from a bar with an overhand grip.
2. Lie on back with legs extended and arms stretched overhead as far as possible.
3. Stand with the arm of the low shoulder raised directly overhead; slowly bend to the long side as far as possible for 6 seconds and return.
4. Facing a wall, stand erect, with feet approximately 18 inches apart. Reach up the wall with hand on the

concave side of the scoliotic curve and down the wall with the opposite hand. Repeat.

Knock-Knee

Knock-knee occurs when the knees are medially together (turned in), or even overlap. Usually, the medial ligaments of the knee are stretched; the external rotator muscles are weak; the tensor fasciae latae are tight; and the feet are flat and everted. Correction of knock-knee is possible if the condition is functional and is more effective if the condition is treated at a young age. Knock-kneed individuals can do the following:

1. Stand with knees relaxed and feet parallel; bend the knees and turn both outward. Repeat.
2. Stand with knees relaxed and feet parallel; turn the knees out and pull the thighs and calves inward. Repeat.

Bowlegs

When the knees are laterally separated (turned out) while the feet are together, the individual has bowlegs. Faulty posture due to outer rotation of the legs is usually the cause of bowlegs in children. Persons with bowlegs can do the following:

1. Sit on the floor with back against a wall and legs extended. Roll the legs inward, and turn the feet outward. Repeat.
2. Lie on back with a pillow between the ankles. Spread straightened legs, and rapidly bring them together against the pillow. Repeat.

Toeing In and Toeing Out

When the feet are pointed inward while an individual is standing or moving, the condition is toeing in. Toeing out occurs when the feet are pointed outward while the person is standing or moving. Usually, exercise is beneficial only in very mild, functional cases of these conditions. Individuals afflicted with toeing in or toeing out can do the following:

1. While sitting on the floor with the legs extended, slightly raise one leg (may use the hand to elevate the leg), fully extend the foot, and perform circles. Repeat with the foot flexed. Perform with other leg.

2. Sit in a chair with feet flat on the floor about 24 inches apart; rotate feet outward and inward without moving the heels.
3. Roller skate.

Flatfeet

Flatfeet is a congenital or acquired condition in which the longitudinal arch is lower than normal. Acquired flatfeet in children usually is caused by poor functional posture. Fallen arches occur in later life, as the muscle strength and elasticity decrease and the musculature is unable to support the bony arches. Having flatfeet is not necessarily a serious problem, as only a few people experience pain with fallen arches. In cases of flatfeet in which no structural damage has occurred, exercise may be of remedial value. Individuals can try to do the following:

1. Sit in a chair and attempt to pick up pencils or marbles with the toes and feet.
2. Sit in a chair with a tennis ball between the feet. Roll it back and forth with the soles of the feet.
3. Sit on the floor with legs extended forward. Flex the toes while extending the feet as far away from the body as possible. Repeat.

Foot Pronation

Foot pronation occurs when the body weight is carried over the inner border of the foot. This act weakens the foot because downward force is exerted over the longitudinal arch, where there is not supporting contact with the floor. Symptoms of pronation include lowering of the arch height, protrusion of the inner anklebones, and deviation of the heel cords from a vertical line when viewed from the rear. Individuals with pronation can do the following:

1. Sit barefoot with the soles of the feet on the floor. While holding the toes flat with the fingers, attempt to elevate the balls of the feet so the tendons stand out down the instep. The heels must remain on the floor, and the toes must not curl.
2. Sit in a chair and attempt to pick up pencils or marbles with the toes and feet.
3. Stand with the feet 4 inches apart and parallel. Curl the toes and shift the weight to the outside of the feet, hold 6 seconds, and relax. Repeat.

1. Ask several friends to stand side by side. Compare body type, limb length, weight, neck length, spinal curve, and posture. Are their postures different? If they are, what factors might contribute to the differences?
2. Observe the posture and body mechanics of students as they walk around the campus. Are there many individuals with poor posture and body mechanics?
3. Observe joggers for their posture and body mechanics. Are most mechanically sound in their jogging techniques?
4. Administer the New York State Posture Rating Test to one of your friends. Make note of any problems you experience in the test administration.

15 Physical Fitness

Upon completion of this chapter, you should be able to

1. Define and measure health-related physical fitness and skill-related physical fitness;

2. State why physical fitness should be measured;

3. List six guidelines for the administration and use of physical fitness tests;

4. Contrast norm-referenced and criterion-referenced fitness standards and state how both may be used appropriately in testing for physical fitness; and

5. Prescribe activities and exercises for the development of physical fitness.

The terms **fitness** and **physical fitness** are often used interchangeably. Though both terms involve quality of life, they do not mean the same thing. Fitness includes emotional, mental, spiritual, and social fitness, as well as physical fitness. Currently, a popular term for fitness is *wellness.* Everyone should be concerned with total fitness, but the responsibilities of physical educators are more related to physical fitness.

Different people and groups interpret physical fitness in different ways. It is sometimes defined as the capacity for sustained physical activity without excessive fatigue or as the capacity to perform everyday activities with reserve energy for emergency situations. By these definitions many persons incorrectly classify themselves as physically fit. It is especially incorrect to accept these definitions when the relations between inactivity and health are considered. Some individuals consider physical fitness synonymous with cardiorespiratory fitness, whereas other groups limit their perception of physical fitness to muscular strength and endurance.

When one is defining physical fitness, it may be best to describe two types of physical fitness: **health-related, and skill-related.** Both types require regular exercise, and both require proper nutrition and rest. However, health-related physical fitness includes cardiorespiratory fitness, muscular strength, muscular endurance, flexibility, and body composition (leanness/fatness). Health-related physical fitness means the organic systems of the body are healthy and function efficiently, so you are able to engage in vigorous tasks and leisure activities. It exerts a positive influence on several risk factors associated with cardiovascular diseases, and it is effective in reducing the risk of back pain, diabetes, osteoporosis, and obesity. In addition, it is an effective way to manage emotional stress. In other words, health-related fitness enables you to look better, feel better, and enjoy a healthy, happy, and full life.

Skill-related physical fitness may provide the same benefits as health-related physical fitness, but it also renders motor skills required in sports and specific types of jobs. For this reason, skill-related fitness is sometimes referred to as athletic-performance–related physical fitness, or motor fitness. In addition to the five components—cardiorespiratory fitness, muscular strength, muscular endurance, flexibility, and body composition—skill-related physical fitness includes agility, balance, coordination, power, reaction time, and speed.

Exercise programs for the maintenance and development of health-related physical fitness are usually different from programs for skill-related physical fitness, particularly if the purpose of the program is to prepare the individual for athletic competition. Too often exercise programs for athletes place little emphasis on health-related components. In fact, because they have not made a commitment to health-related fitness, many athletes fail to continue an exercise program after they cease to participate in sports.

Why Measure Physical Fitness?

The relationship of good health and cardiorespiratory fitness, muscular strength, muscular endurance, flexibility, and body composition has been described previously. The development of these components should be a primary objective in all school physical education programs as well as all fitness programs. As a physical educator, you should be prepared to measure them, interpret the test results, and prescribe the appropriate activities for the development of health-related physical fitness. In addition, test results can be used to teach the concepts of fitness, to motivate for self-improvement, and to help individuals plan fitness goals.

Though sports participation is not essential for a healthy lifestyle, many individuals enjoy taking part in sports, and the enjoyment is usually greater for individuals possessing skill-related physical fitness. The skills of agility, balance, coordination, power, reaction time, and speed are important components of sports performance. These motor skills also are related to the performance of many types of occupations and daily activities. Testing for skill-related physical fitness can serve to motivate high-ability individuals to perform at even higher levels. In addition, diagnostic testing will enable the physical educator to prescribe the appropriate activities for individuals who do not possess adequate skill-related fitness.

It is doubtful that performance on fitness tests should be used for grading purposes. A poor performance on a fitness test, resulting in an unwanted grade, may have a negative effect on an individual. Rather than being motivated to move toward an active lifestyle, the individual may become even more inactive. In the school environment, use fitness tests for the previously described reasons.

Guidelines for the Administration and Use of Fitness Tests

Fitness testing can be an important part of any school physical education or fitness programs. The following guidelines (from Corbin 1987; Franks, Morrow, and Plowman 1988), however, should be observed when fitness tests are administered:

1. Measure fitness components that the public and research experts agree are the most important. Focus on health and self-improvement rather than on comparison with others.
2. In the school environment, fitness tests should be a part of the total educational program. Attention should be given to the knowledge and understanding of fitness concepts, and students should be held accountable for class work. Written test items should measure the students' understanding of the concepts.
3. Fitness test results should be kept confidential; careful attention should be given to ensure that the test results do not embarrass a student or threaten his or her self-image.
4. Teach students how to take fitness tests; give ample time for practice of the test components.
5. Fitness awards should encourage lifetime activity rather than a one-time performance.
6. Take care to provide necessary, sufficient, and valid information regarding test results to parents and students.

Norm-Referenced Standards Versus Criterion-Referenced Standards

Although criterion-referenced standards and norm-referenced standards have been discussed previously, it is important to consider them again in the discussion of fitness testing. Both standards may be used appropriately.

The discussion in this section is based on Going and Williams (1989) and Cureton and Warren (1990).

Recall that comparison of an individual's performance with that of other individuals having common characteristics is called norm-referenced measurement. Norm-referenced tests are well suited for the measurement of skill-related physical fitness if the goal is to motivate individuals to achieve a high level of fitness. On the other hand, the use of norm-referenced fitness standards with physically inactive and low-fit individuals may be inadvisable. When norm-referenced fitness standards (percentiles) are used without consideration of the absolute score, improvements in student performance may not be noted and individuals may be discouraged rather than encouraged to seek improvement.

Criterion-referenced standards are used when individual differences are unimportant and performance is judged relative to some standard that reflects a satisfactory level of the attribute being measured. In contrast to norm-referenced testing, a score higher than another score at or above the standard is not necessarily better. Criterion-referenced standards for health-related physical fitness tests purportedly represent the minimum level of an attribute or function that is consistent with good health. The standards are used as goals for low-fit individuals, and, unless limited physically, most individuals are capable of attaining the standards. A criticism of such standards, however, is that because they represent desired minimum levels of fitness, they do not serve to motivate individuals to seek a higher level of fitness.

Both types of standards are included in the tests described in this chapter. The purpose of testing should determine the test and standards that you choose to use.

⁇ARE YOU ABLE TO DO THE FOLLOWING:

- define health-related and skill-related physical fitness and state why they should be measured?
- list six guidelines for the administration and use of fitness tests?
- contrast norm-referenced and criterion-referenced standards and state when each standard may be used appropriately?

Tests of Health-Related Physical Fitness

Establishing a single test battery that measures all components of health-related or skill-related physical fitness is difficult. Since there is no one item that measures total-body muscular strength, muscular endurance, or flexibility, a decision must be made as to which parts of the body are to be measured for these components. Some tests include items that measure arm and shoulder girdle strength and endurance. Strength and endurance of the abdominal region and low-back–posterior-thigh flexibility are often included in these tests because of their importance in prevention of low-back disorders. Rather than selecting a single test battery, however, you may choose to measure physical fitness through a combination of test items presented in previous chapters. This approach is acceptable if you use items intended for the group (age and gender) you are testing.

When reviewing the health-related and skill-related physical fitness tests described in this chapter, note that not all the sit-up tests are performed in the same manner. If you plan to use the norms of a particular test, it is important to administer all items in the manner described in the test. Also note that some criterion-referenced standards vary for the health-related physical fitness test items.

Discussions about the possibility of a national youth fitness test have been held among representatives of various groups. Health-related physical fitness tests are similar because most experts agree upon the components of health-related physical fitness and the various test items that can be used to measure the components. There is not agreement upon the health-related standards, however. In addition, some groups feel that a physical fitness test should include both health-related and skill-related physical fitness items. Developing a national test requires agreement about these concerns as well as awards, computer software, promotion, and title. In 1993, two highly respected national groups reached an agreement regarding these concerns. The American Alliance for Health, Physical Education, Recreation and Dance (AAHPERD) and the Cooper Institute for Aerobics Research (CIAR) merged their fitness programs and began to use the same fitness test items and educational materials. With this agreement, the AAHPERD provides the educational component of health fitness, and FITNESSGRAM of the CIAR assesses fitness.

(Cooper Institute for Aerobics Research 1999)

The FITNESSGRAM, developed by the Cooper Institute for Aerobics Research (CIAR), is a comprehensive health-related fitness activity assessment and computerized reporting system. FITNESSGRAM was endorsed in 1993 by the American Alliance for Health, Physical Education, Recreation and Dance (AAHPERD) as a replacement for the Physical Best fitness battery. This assessment and health promotion program is now promoted by the American Fitness Alliance, which consists of the CIAR, AAHPERD, and Human Kinetics Publishers.

The goals of FITNESSGRAM are to promote enjoyable regular physical activity and to provide comprehensive physical fitness and activity asssessments and reporting programs for children and adolescents. The criterion-referenced standards for the FITNESSGRAM test items represent a level of fitness that offers some degree of protection against health problems that result from sedentary living. Performance is classified in two general areas: "Needs Improvement" and "Healthy Fitness Zone (HFZ)." The HFZ includes lower-end and upper-end standards. The lower end (good) standards of the HFZ are provided in table 15.1. FITNESSGRAM does not advocate a recognition program that focuses primarily on fitness performance. The recognition is designed to reinforce the establishment of activity behaviors that will lead to fitness development. *You Stay Alive!*, the recommended recognition program, is a goal-setting system that can be used to acknowledge individual performance level based on personal goals. FITNESSGRAM also includes two opportunities to assess physical activity patterns. These assessments may be done through the FITNESSGRAM Physical Activity Questionnaire and the ACTIVITYGRAM Physical Activity Recall. With the ACTIVITYGRAM component of the software, the participant's activity habits are entered and prescriptive feedback about how active the participant should be is provided. The FITNESSGRAM manual includes test modifications for measurement of special populations. These modifications are described in chapter 17.

Information about FITNESSGRAM may be found at the Web site of the American Fitness Alliance: www.americanfitness.net. You also may write to the American Fitness Alliance, P. O. Box 5076, Champaign, IL 61825-5076, or you may call at 800-747-4457.

Age Level. Five through seventeen-plus.

Equipment. Stopwatch, flat running surface, pencils, score sheets, nonslippery surface at least 20 meters long, cassette player, measuring tape, marker cones, gym mats, cardboard measuring strips (30" × 3" and 30" × 4½"), yardstick, modified pull-up apparatus, sit and reach box, horizontal bar, scale that measures both height and weight, and skinfold caliper.

Test Components

1. Aerobic capacity: Three test options are provided.

   The PACER. The test objective is to run as long as possible back and forth across a 20-meter distance at a specified pace that gets faster each minute (initial pace is easy, but progresses to a harder pace). Two lines, 20 meters apart, are marked on the floor. On the start command, participants run across the area and touch the line by the time a beep sounds. At the sound of the beep, they run back to the starting line. Participants who get to a line before the beep must wait for the beep before running in the other direction. The participants continue in this manner until they can no longer reach a line before the beep sounds. The first time a participant does not reach the line by the beep, the participant reverses direction immediately. The participant is allowed to catch up with the pace, but the test is completed when the participant fails to reach the line by the beep for the second time. Set to music, this test can provide a valid, fun alternative to the distance run for measuring aerobic capacity. The PACER is recommended for all ages, but its use is strongly encouraged for grades K–3. Typically, in these grades the test will only last a few minutes. A lap is one 20-meter distance (from one end to the other). The recorded score is the total number of laps completed by the participant.

   1-mile run/1-mile run (alternative). Students are instructed to run 1 mile as fast as possible. Performance standards for students in grades K–3 have purposely not been established. These students are instructed to complete the distance at a comfortable pace. The run is scored in minutes and seconds.

   Walk test (alternative). This test is to be used with participants ages 13 years and older. The participants are instructed to walk 1 mile as quickly as possible while maintaining a constant walking pace the entire distance. At the conclusion of the 1-mile walk, the participants count their heart rate for 15 seconds. The walk time and the heart rate are entered into the FITNESSGRAM software, and an estimated VO_2 max is calculated.

2. Body composition: The sum of the triceps and medial-calf skinfold measurements for grades K–12. For college students, the formula to calculate percent body fat includes the abdominal skinfold measurement as well as the triceps and calf skinfold measurements. Each measurement should be taken three times, with the recorded score being the middle measurement value. Body mass index is calculated if skinfold measurements are not provided. The

TABLE 15.1 The FITNESSGRAM—Lower End (Good) Standards of the Healthy Fitness Zone

Test Item	5	6	7	8	9	10	11	12	13	14	15	16	17	17+
Males														
1-mile run (min:sec)*						11:30	11:00	10:30	10:00	9:30	9:00	8:30	8:30	8:30
PACER (laps)**						17	23	29	35	41	46	52	57	57
Percent fat	25	25	25	25	25	25	25	25	25	25	25	25	25	25
Body mass index	20	20	20	20	20	21	21	22	23	24.5	25	26.5	27	27.8
Curl-up	2	2	4	6	9	12	15	18	21	24	24	24	24	24
Trunk lift (in.)	6	6	6	6	6	9	9	9	9	9	9	9	9	9
Push-up	3	3	4	5	6	7	8	10	12	14	16	18	18	18
Modified pull-up	2	2	3	4	5	5	6	7	8	9	10	12	14	14
Pull-up	1	1	1	1	1	1	1	1	1	2	3	5	5	5
Flexed-arm hang (sec)	2	2	3	3	4	4	6	10	12	15	15	15	15	15
Back-saver sit and reach***	8	8	8	8	8	8	8	8	8	8	8	8	8	8
Shoulder stretch****														
Females														
1-mile run (min:sec)*						12:30	12:00	12:00	11:30	11:00	10:30	10:00	10:00	10:00
PACER (laps)**						7	9	13	15	18	23	28	34	34
Percent fat	32	32	32	32	32	32	32	32	32	32	32	32	32	32
Body mass index	21	21	22	22	23	23.5	24	24.5	24.5	25	25	25	26	27.3
Curl-up	2	2	4	6	9	12	15	18	18	18	18	18	18	18
Trunk lift (in.)	6	6	6	6	6	9	9	9	9	9	9	9	9	9
Push-up	3	3	4	5	6	7	7	7	7	7	7	7	7	7
Modified pull-up	2	2	3	4	4	4	4	4	4	4	4	4	4	4
Pull-up	1	1	1	1	1	1	1	1	1	1	1	1	1	1
Flexed-arm hang (sec)	2	2	3	3	4	4	6	7	8	8	8	8	8	8
Back-saver sit and reach***	9	9	9	9	9	10	10	10	10	10	12	12	12	12
Shoulder stretch****														

Source: Cooper Institute for Aerobics Research, *FITNESSGRAM Test Administration Manual*, Champaigr., Ill.: Human Kinetics, 1999.
*For ages 5–9 time standards not recommended. Completion of distance is recognized.
**For ages 5–9 lap count standards not recommended. Participation in run recognized.
***Test score Pass/Fail; must reach this distance to pass.
****Passing = Touching the fingers together behind the back.

index is determined with the following formula: Weight (kg)/Height^2(m).

3. Abdominal strength and endurance: The curl-up. Students perform in groups of three. One performs the curl-ups, another will place his or her hands under the head of the student doing the curl-ups and count, and the third will secure the measuring strip so that it does not move. The test performer lies in a supine position on a mat, knees bent at an angle of approximately 140°, feet flat on the floor, legs slightly apart, and arms straight and parallel to the trunk, with palms of hands resting on the mat. After the test performer assumes the correct position, the measuring strip (30" × 3" for grades K–4 and 30" × 4½" for grades 5–12) is placed under the knees on the mat so that the fingertips are just resting on the edge of the measuring strip. Keeping the feet in contact with the mat, the test performer curls up slowly until the fingertips reach the other side of the measuring strip, then curls back down until the head touches the partner's hands (on the mat). Movement should be slow and controlled to the specified cadence of about twenty curl-ups per minute (one curl every 3 seconds). The teacher should call a cadence or use a prerecorded cadence. The test is completed when the student can no longer continue or performs a maximum number of seventy-five curl-ups.

4. Trunk extensor strength and flexibility: Trunk lift. The student being tested lies on the mat in a prone position, with the toes in a pointed position and the hands placed under the thighs. The student lifts the upper body off the mat, in a very slow and controlled manner, to a maximum height of 12 inches. The position is held long enough to allow the tester to measure the distance of the student's chin from the floor. The score is recorded to the nearest inch, and distances above 12 inches are recorded as 12 inches.

5. Upper body strength and endurance: Several test items are available to measure this component. Both extensor and flexor muscles should be measured.

Push-up. The student performs as many push-ups as possible at a rate of twenty per minute (one push-up every 3 seconds),

Modified pull-up. The necessary equipment and test procedure are shown in figure 12.6 on page 151. The student attempts to perform as many modified pull-ups as possible.

Pull-up (palms facing away from the body). This test item should be administered only to students who are able to perform correct pull-ups. The student attempts to correctly complete as many pull-ups as possible.

Flexed-arm hang. The student attempts to hang the chin above the bar as long as possible.

6. Flexibility: Two items are used to measure different body areas.

Back-saver sit and reach. This item is similar to the traditional sit and reach except that it is performed on one side at a time. Measurement of only one side prevents possible hyperextension at the knees. The test is performed with the sit and reach box described on page 130. With the shoes removed, the student sits down at the test box. One leg is fully extended with the foot flat against the end of the box. The other knee is bent, with the sole of the foot flat on the floor and 2 to 3 inches to the side of the straight knee. The arms are extended forward over the measuring scale with the hands placed one on top of the other. With palms down, the student reaches directly forward with both hands along the scale four times and holds the position of the fourth reach for at least 1 second. After measuring one side, the student switches the position of the legs and reaches again. If necessary, the student may allow the bent knee to move to the side as the body moves by it. The recorded score is the last whole inch reached on each side to a maximum of 12 inches. The FITNESSGRAM will report this score as pass/fail depending on the distance reached as it compares with the appropriate standard.

Shoulder stretch. To test the right shoulder, the student reaches with the right hand over the right shoulder and down the back as if to pull up a zipper. At the same time, the left hand is placed behind the back and reaches up, trying to touch the fingers of the right hand. A partner observes if fingers touch. The left shoulder is measured by the movement of the arms reversing. The test is scored as pass/fail for each shoulder; the fingers must touch to pass.

■ AAHPERD Health-Related Physical Fitness Test for College Students
(AAHPERD 1980; Pate 1985)

The AAHPERD Health-Related Fitness Test was developed originally for use with students ages 6–17. Because the American Alliance for Health, Physical Education, Recreation and Dance (AAHPERD) is now a member of the American Fitness Alliance and promotes the FITNESSGRAM, the AAHPERD no longer promotes the Health-Related Fitness Test. In 1985, college-student norms were developed for this test. For this reason, it is a useful test for college physical education classes. Table 15.2 includes percentile norms for the test.

Age Level. College-age.

Equipment. Stopwatch, any flat measured area, skinfold caliper, sit and reach box.

Test Components

1. Cardiorespiratory functional capacity and endurance: 1-mile run or 9-minute run. The test performers are instructed to run 1 mile as fast as possible or to cover as much distance as possible in 9 minutes.
2. Body composition: The sum of the triceps and subscapular skinfold measurements.
3. Abdominal muscular strength and endurance: Modified sit-ups (arms crossed on chest). This test is described on page 144.
4. Flexibility (extensibility) of the low back and hamstrings: Sit and reach. The sit and reach box and test procedure are described on page 130.

■ South Carolina Physical Fitness Test
(Pate 1983)

The South Carolina test includes both criterion- and norm-referenced standards for students and criterion-referenced standards for adults. Table 15.3 includes the criterion-referenced standards.

Age Level. Nine through adult.

Equipment. Flat running surface, skinfold caliper, mat, yardstick, bench, and stopwatch.

Test Components

1. Cardiorespiratory function: 1-mile run or 9-minute run for distance. Test performers are instructed to run 1 mile as fast as possible or to cover as much distance as possible in 9 minutes.
2. Muscular strength and muscular endurance of the abdominal musculature: 1-minute bent-knee sit-ups. Sit-ups are performed with fingers interlaced behind the neck and partner holding feet. When the performer sits up, both elbows should touch the knees, and when the performer returns to the lying position after each sit-up, both elbows must touch the mat.
3. Low-back/hamstring muscle flexibility: Sit and reach. Test is administered with sit and reach box described on page 130.
4. Body composition: The sum of the triceps and abdominal skinfold measurements.

■ Fit Youth Today
(American Health and Fitness Foundation 1986)

Fit Youth Today (FYT) is a complete program of health-related fitness for school-age youth. The program, founded on the principle that there is an acceptable level of fitness that

TABLE 15.2 College-Age Norms for the AAHPERD Health-Related Physical Fitness Test

Percentile	1-mile run (min:sec)	9-Minute Run (yards)	Sum of SF	Percent Fat	Sit-ups	Sit and Reach
			Males			
95	5:30	2640	12	3.9	60	17.75
75	6:12	2349	16	6.6	50	15.50
50	6:49	2200	21	9.4	44	13.50
25	7:32	1945	26	13.1	38	11.50
5	9:47	1652	40	20.4	30	7.50
			Females			
95	7:02	2230	17	13.7	53	18.50
75	8:15	1870	24	19.0	42	16.25
50	9:22	1755	30	22.8	35	14.50
25	10:41	1460	37	27.1	30	12.50
5	12:43	1101	51	33.7	21	9.50

Source: Adapted from AAHPERD, *Norms for College Students—Health Related Physical Fitness Test,* Reston, VA: American Alliance for Health, Physical Education, Recreation and Dance, 1985.

TABLE 15.3   Criterion-Referenced Standards for the South Carolina Physical Fitness Test

Test Item	Age											
	9	10	11	12	13	14	15	16–19	20–29	30–39	40–49	50–59
						Males						
1-mile run (min:sec)	10:00	9:45	9:10	8:30	8:00	8:00	8:00	8:00	8:00	8:30	9:00	9:30
9-minute run (yds)	1580	1620	1730	1860	1980	1980	1980	1980	1980	1860	1760	1670
Sit-ups	25	28	32	34	35	38	40	40	40	36	33	30
Sit and reach (cm)	23	23	23	23	23	23	23	23	23	23	23	23
ΣSkinfolds (mm)	25	25	28	29	30	34	34	34	34	34	34	34
						Females						
1-mile run (min:sec)	10:00	9:45	9:35	9:30	9:00	9:00	9:00	9:00	9:00	9:30	10:00	10:30
9-minute run (yds)	1580	1620	1650	1670	1760	1760	1760	1760	1760	1670	1580	1500
Sit-ups	25	28	30	30	30	32	33	34	34	30	27	24
Sit and reach (cm)	23	23	23	23	23	23	23	23	23	23	23	23
ΣSkinfolds (mm)	25	25	28	29	30	34	34	34	34	34	34	34

Source: R. Pate, ed., *South Carolina physical fitness test manual,* 2d ed., Columbia, S.C.: South Carolina Association for Health, Physical Education, Recreation, and Dance, 1983.

every child and adolescent can and should achieve, is endorsed by the American College of Sports Medicine. The FYT Program manual includes (1) a complete FYT curriculum; (2) a detailed FYT conditioning protocol; (3) a four-component FYT health awards program; (4) a three-level integrated FYT awards program; and (5) a comprehensive computer support program, available for Apple and IBM computers. The criterion-referenced standards are set at values that are reasonable for children and teenagers to achieve. Table 15.4 includes the criterion-referenced standards.

FYT awards include medals, patches, pins, and certificates that may be purchased by the school for presentation to students. FYT prizes may be purchased by any student qualifying for any of the FYT awards. The prizes include T-shirts, caps, sports bags, wristbands, backpacks, and other items. The FYT All Star Award recognizes the student who meets the criterion standard in all four FYT test categories. The FYT Star Award recognizes the student who meets the criterion standard in the Steady-State Jog and at least one other category of the test. The FYT Award recognizes the student who makes significant improvement in performance between the FYT pretest and posttest or in subsequent posttests, based on results, effort, and teacher discretion.
Age Level. Grades K through 12.

Equipment. Stopwatch, flat running surface, mat, sit and reach box, skinfold caliper.

Test Components
Note: Rather than body composition criterion standards, weight/height criterion standards are included for grades K–3.

1. Aerobic fitness and cardiorespiratory endurance: Steady-state jog or continuous movement. Before testing, students must be properly instructed and trained in a manner similar to that presented in the FYT conditioning protocol. Students in grades K–1 and 2–3 are instructed to jog or to move continuously for 12 minutes and 15 minutes, respectively. These times reflect the aerobic fitness criterion standards for K–3 students. Students in grades 4–12 are instructed to jog at a steady pace for 20 minutes. If the grade 4–12 student can attain the criterion reference standard by walking rapidly, or by a combination of walking and running, that is acceptable. The distance covered is recorded to the nearest $1/10$ mile.
2. Abdominal muscular strength and endurance: 2-minute bent-knee curl-up. Curl-ups are performed with arms crossed on chest and partner holding feet. Heels are placed 12 to 18 inches from the buttocks. The arms remain in contact with the chest while touching the thighs with the elbows. Lower shoulder blades must return to the testing

TABLE 15.4 Criterion-Referenced Standards for the FYT Test

Test Item	K–1	2–3	4	5	6	7	8	9	10	11	12
					Grade Level						
					Males						
Steady-state run (miles)	12 min jog or 12 min continuous activity	15 min jog or 15 min continuous activity	1.8	2.0	2.2	2.4	2.4	2.4	2.4	2.4	2.4
Curl-up	25	32	34	36	38	40	40	40	40	40	40
Sit and reach (in.)	9	9	9	9	9	9	9	9	9	9	9
Body composition ΣSkinfolds (mm)	Ht/wt standards used	Ht/wt standards used	23	26	29	29	29	27	25	23	23
% Fat			19	21	23	23	23	22	20	19	19
					Females						
Steady-state run (miles)	12 min jog or 12 min continuous activity	15 min jog or 15 min continuous activity	1.6	1.8	2.0	2.2	2.2	2.2	2.2	2.2	2.2
Curl-up	25	32	34	36	38	40	40	40	40	40	40
Sit and reach (in.)	9	9	9	9	9	9	9	9	9	9	9
Body composition ΣSkinfolds (mm)	Ht/wt standards used	Ht/wt standards used	32	32	33	34	34	34	34	34	34
% Fat			26	26	27	28	28	28	28	28	28

Source: Adapted from *FYT Program Manual,* Austin, TX: American Health and Fitness Foundation, 1986.

surface. This item is different from other sit-up tests in that the test is for a 2-minute period.

3. Trunk flexion: Sit and reach. This test is performed with the sit and reach box. The student is permitted four consecutive trials, and each trial must be held for at least 3 seconds.
4. Body composition: The sum of the triceps and medial-calf skinfold measurements.

■ YMCA Physical Fitness Test
(Golding, Myers, and Sinning 1989)

The YMCA Physical Fitness Test is administered as part of a health-related physical fitness program sponsored by the YMCA. A medical examination is required before the test is administered. An exercise program based on results of the test items is prescribed. Table 15.5 includes norms for the "Good" rating on the test items. The reference includes norms from the range of "Very Poor" to "Excellent."

Age Level. Eighteen through sixty-five-plus.

Equipment. Skinfold caliper; bicycle ergometer; 12-inch-high, sturdy bench; yardstick; barbell; weights; metronome; mat.

Test Components

1. Body composition: Both men and women use the sum of four skinfold sites—abdomen, ilium, triceps, and thigh. Three sites should be used only if the thigh skinfold cannot be measured accurately.
2. Cardiorespiratory endurance: The bicycle ergometer is used to measure this component. Maximal physical working capacity (PWC) and maximal oxygen uptake (VO_2max) are predicted from the performer's response to a submaximal workload.

The 3-minute step test may be used as a substitute for the bicycle ergometer test. The individual steps up and down on a 12-inch bench for 3 minutes at a rate of 24 steps per minute. The score is the total 1-minute postexercise heart rate (count must begin within 5 seconds after completion of the test).

TABLE 15.5 Standards for the Rating of "Good" for the YMCA Physical Fitness Test

Test Item	Age					
	18–25	26–35	36–45	46–55	56–65	65+
Males						
% Fat	8–10	13–15	16–18	18–20	19–21	19–21
3-min step test (heart rate)	82–88	83–88	86–94	89–96	89–97	89–95
PWC Max (kgm)	1705–1905	1665–1820	1565–1725	1385–1520	1240–1400	1045–1175
VO$_2$max (ml/kg)	53–59	50–54	44–49	40–43	37–39	33–36
Flexibility (in.)	18–20	18–19	17–19	16–17	15–17	13–15
Bench press (repetitions)	30–34	26–30	24–28	20–22	14–20	10–14
Sit-ups	45–48	41–45	36–40	29–33	26–29	22–26
Females						
% Fat	18–20	19–21	20–23	23–25	24–26	22–25
3-min step test (heart rate)	88–97	91–97	93–101	96–102	97–103	93–100
PWC Max (kgm)	1175–1320	1115–1245	1035–1135	930–1045	840–970	640–725
VO$_2$max (ml/kg)	48–54	46–51	39–44	35–39	32–36	28–31
Flexibility (in.)	21–23	20–22	19–21	18–20	18–19	18–19
Bench press (repetitions)	28–32	25–29	21–25	20–22	16–20	12–14
Sit-ups	37–41	33–37	27–30	22–25	18–21	18–22

Source: Adapted from L. A. Golding, C. R. Myers, and W. E. Sinning, eds., *The Y's way to physical fitness,* 3d ed., Champaign, Ill.: Human Kinetics, 1989.

3. Trunk flexion: Sit and reach. A yardstick is placed on the floor with tape across it at right angles to the 15-inch mark. The performer sits with the yardstick between the legs, with the zero (0) mark toward the body, and extends the legs with the feet approximately 12 inches apart. The heels of the feet should nearly touch the edge of the taped line. With one hand on top of the other, the individual reaches forward as far as possible and holds the position momentarily. The score (to the nearest ¼ inch) is the best of three trials.

4. Muscular strength and endurance.

Bench press. Metronome is set for 6 beats per minute (bpm), and individuals must repeat the up-and-down movement with each click. Males use an 80-pound barbell, and females use a 35-pound barbell. The score is the number of successful repetitions. The test is terminated when full extension cannot be completed or when the individual cannot keep up with the cadence. For safety, at least one spotter should be present during the test.

1-minute bent-knee sit-ups. Sit-ups are performed with fingers interlaced behind the neck and a partner holding the feet. The elbows should alternately touch the opposite knee as the performer comes into the up position; the performer must return to supine position until the shoulders touch the mat.

■ ACSM Fitness Test
(American College of Sports Medicine 1998)

The ACSM Fitness Test consists of four components. Table 15.6 includes the average standards for the push-up and sit and reach tests. Scores above and below these standards indicate above-average and below-average standards.

Age Level. Twenty through adulthood.

Equipment. Stopwatch; flat, measured surface; yardstick; adhesive tape.

Test Components
1. Aerobic fitness: Rockport 1-mile walk. This test and the performance standards are described on pages 120–121.
2. Muscular fitness: Push-ups. Males perform the push-up described on page 152 (legs straight and weight on feet

Test Item	Age				
	20–29	30–39	40–49	50–59	60+
	Males				
Push-up	35–44	25–34	20–29	15–24	10–19
Sit and reach (in.)	13–18	12–17	11–16	10–15	9–14
	Females				
Push-up	17–33	12–24	8–19	6–14	3–4
Sit and reach (in.)	16–21	15–20	14–19	13–18	12–17

Source: Adapted from American College of Sports Medicine, *ACSM fitness book,* Champaign, Ill.: Human Kinetics, 1998.

and hands); females perform the push-up described on page 152 (knees bent at right angles and weight on knees and hands); complete as many push-ups as possible.

3. Flexibility: Sit and reach. A yardstick is placed on the floor and taped in place at the 15-inch mark. The individual sits on the floor at the zero (0) end of the yardstick and with the yardstick between the legs. The feet should be 10 to 12 inches apart, and the heels even with the 15-inch mark. With one hand on top of the other, the individual slowly stretches forward and slides the hands along the yardstick. The score, recorded to the nearest inch, is the best reach in three attempts.

4. Body composition: Body mass index (BMI). The procedure for determining BMI is described on page 174. The desirable BMI is 19 to 25.

5. Waist-to-hip ratio (W/H). The procedure for determining the waist-to-hip ratio is described on page 174. Ratios below .80 for females and below .90 for males are desirable.

■ The Canadian Physical Activity, Fitness & Lifestyle Appraisal: CSEP's Guide to Healthy Living—Health Related Fitness Appraisal
(Canadian Society for Exercise Physiology 1998)

Note: Because several test items are unique, the Health Related Appraisal of the Canadian Physical Activity, Fitness & Lifestyle Appraisal is described in greater detail than the other tests presented in this chapter.

The Canadian Physical Activity, Fitness & Lifestyle Appraisal manual is a straightforward and systematic approach outlining the proper procedures for the appraisal and counseling of persons aged 15 to 69, emphasizing the health benefits of physical activity. The topics of understanding behavior change, helping people change, healthy physical activity participation, healthy lifestyle, basic exercise physiology, and health-related fitness are covered. The manual outlines the background material required for certification as a CSEP-certified fitness consultant (CFC) and includes appraisal tools, case studies, and references. Information about the manual may be found at the Web site of the Canadian Society for Exercise Physiology: www.csep.ca. You also may write to the Canadian Society for Exercise Physiology, 185 Somerset Street West, Suite 202, Ottawa, Ontario K2P 0J2, or you may call 613-234-3755.

The health-related fitness appraisal includes muscular power as a component of musculoskeletal fitness, and all appraisal measurements are reported in metric values. Preappraisal screening procedures described in the manual include measurement of resting heart rate, blood pressure, and utilization of the Physical Activity Readiness Questionnaire (PAR-Q) found in figure 10.2, page 127.

Age Level. Fifteen through sixty-nine.

Equipment. Tape measure, weight scale, skinfold caliper, stethoscope, ergometer steps, mCAFT CD or cassette player, stopwatch, masking tape, heart rate monitor, hand dynamometer, metric ruler, flexometer, gym mat, metronome, chalk.

Test Components

1. Body composition: Standing height (without shoes), weight (without shoes and in light clothing), and waist girth are measured. The test performer stands in a relaxed position, and the waist is measured at a level of noticeable

waist narrowing, at the end of a normal expiration. Skinfold measurements are made at the triceps, biceps, subscapular, iliac crest, and medial-calf sites. The indicators of body composition are:

body mass index (BMI): weight (kg)/height² (meters)
sum of five skinfolds (SO5S) (mm)
waist girth (WG) (cm)
sum of two trunk skinfolds—subscapular and iliac crest (SO2S) (mm)

Table 15.7 (reported in metric system) includes the healthy range for each indicator of the test performer's body composition. The body composition indicators are used to place performers in the appropriate health-benefit zone. The results for BMI and SO5S are combined for a point score, and the results of the WG and SO2S are combined for a second point score. Table 15.8 indicates how the two point scores are used to determine the health benefit zone. You should note two things about the points in Table 15.8.(1) The same 8-point score is awarded whether the individual has a healthy or an unhealthy BMI. It is possible for an individual to have a high BMI and not be overfat. The higher BMI is due to a greater than normal muscle mass, which is indicated by the SO5S falling within the healthy range. (2) A higher risk (fewer health-benefit points) is assigned to the combination of "WG

unhealthy and SO2S healthy" than to the combination of "WG unhealthy and SO2S unhealthy." Current research indicates that internal visceral fat is the greatest health risk. It is concluded that if two identical waist girths are assigned "WG unhealthy" but one has less subcutaneous fat (i.e., "SO2S healthy"), the waist girth with less subcutaneous fat must have more visceral fat. Therefore, the "WG unhealthy and SO2S healthy" represents a higher risk than "WG unhealthy and SO2S unhealthy."

2. Aerobic fitness: The Modified Canadian Aerobic Fitness Test (mCAFT), a step test, is used to measure this component. It is recommended that high-quality heart rate monitors be used, but the post-exercise heart rate can be determined with a stethoscope or by palpation at the radial artery. Figure 15.1 shows the ergometer steps that are used to administer the mCAFT. The manual provides guidelines for construction of the steps. For the test, performers complete one or more stepping sessions of 3 minutes at predetermined cadences based on their age and gender. All test performers begin the stepping sequence on double 20.3-cm steps and complete as many progressively more demanding 3-minute sessions as necessary to equal or exceed the ceiling postexercise heart rate. The ceiling is set at 85% of the predicted maximum heart rate for their age: $.85 \times (220 - age)$. Individuals with a high level of fitness may complete the test with a single-step sequence

TABLE 15.7 Healthy Ranges for Indicators of Body Composition (The Canadian Physical Activity, Fitness & Lifestyle Appraisal)

	Age					
	15–19	20–29	30–39	40–49	50–59	60–69
Males						
BMI (wt in kg/ht² in meters)	19–24	20–25	20–25	21–25	21–25	21–27
SO5S (mm)	31–47	32–58	32–63	37–63	31–62	33–63
WG (cm)	67–88	71–93	75–94	78–94	83–94	82–94
SO2S (mm)	11–24	13–32	14–33	15–34	17–33	17–34
Females						
BMI (wt in kg/ht² in meters)	19–24	20–25	20–25	20–25	20–25	21–27
SO5S (mm)	46–69	46–72	48–83	48–81	48–84	54–82
WG (cm)	61–81	61–81	63–83	65–85	67–85	66–85
SO2S (mm)	13–29	13–36	14–39	14–37	16–39	16–38

Source: Adapted from Canadian Society for Exercise Physiology, *The Canadian Physical Activity, Fitness & Lifestyle Appraisal,* 2d ed., Ottawa, Ontario: Canadian Society for Exercise Physiology, 1998.

TABLE 15.8 Determination of Health Benefit Zones for Body Composition (The Canadian Physical Activity, Fitness & Lifestyle Appraisal)

Scoring of Body Composition Assesssments

Indicators	Points	Indicators	Points
BMI healthy and SO5S healthy	8	WG healthy and SO2S healthy	8
BMI unhealthy and SO5S healthy	8	WG healthy and SO2S unhealthy	4
BMI healthy and SO5S unhealthy	3	WG unhealthy and SO2S unhealthy	2
BMI unhealthy and SO5S unhealthy	0	WG unhealthy and SO2S healthy	0

Health Benefit Zones for Healthy Body Composition

Zone	Points
Excellent	16
Very good	12
Good	7–11
Fair	4–5
Needs improvement	0–3

Interpretation of Health Benefit Zones

Zone	Description
Excellent	Body composition falls within a range that is generally associated with optimal health benefits.
Very good	Body composition falls within a range that is generally associated with considerable health benefits.
Good	Body composition falls within a range that is generally associated with many health benefits.
Fair	Body composition falls within a range that is generally associated with some health benefits but also some health risks; progressing from here into GOOD zone is a very significant step to increasing the health benefits associated with your body composition.
Needs improvement	Body composition falls within a range that is generally associated with considerable health risks; try to achieve and maintain a healthy body composition by enjoying regular physical activity and healthy eating.

Source: Adapted from Canadian Society for Exercise Physiology, *The Canadian Physical Activity, Fitness & Lifestyle Appraisal,* 2d ed., Ottawa, Ontario: Canadian Society for Exercise Physiology, 1998.

using a step 40.6 cm in height (stages 7 and 8 for males and stage 8 for females). The starting stages and the step cadences for each stage are found in table 15.9. The test is structured so that in the first 3 minutes most individuals step at an intensity equal to 65% to 70% of the average aerobic power of a person 10 years older. Instruction and time signals are given on the CD or cassette tape provided with the manual. These instructions tell when to start and stop exercising and how to count the 10-second measurement of the postexercise heart rate.

Before beginning the test, test performers should have completed all preappraisal screening items. The test performers also should perform mild calf stretches before and after the stair stepping. After a demonstration, the test performers are permitted to practice the stepping sequence.

At the conclusion of the initial 3-minute session, the test performers cease to step and remain motionless, while standing. The heart rate monitor is immediately read. If a heart rate monitor is not used, the postexercise heart rate is counted for 10 seconds with a stethoscope placed either on the sternum or over the second intercostal space on the left side. The heart rate also may be determined by palpation at the radial artery. The determination of an accurate

Physical Fitness   **199**

FIGURE 15.1 Ergometer steps for mCAFT.

TABLE 15.9 Starting Stages and Cadence for the Modified Canadian Aerobic Fitness Test (mCAFT)

Starting Stage		
Age	Males	Females
60–69	1	1
50–59	2	1
40–49	3	2
30–39	3	3
20–29	4	3
15–19	4	3

Cadence for Stages (footplants/min)		
Stage	Males	Females
1	66	66
2	84	84
3	102	102
4	114	114
5	132	120
6	144	132
7	118*	144
8	132*	118*

Source: Adapted from Canadian Society for Exercise Physiology, *The Canadian Physical Activity, Fitness & Lifestyle Appraisal,* 2d ed., Ottawa, Ontario: Canadian Society for Exercise Physiology, 1998.
*Single step (40.6 cm).

postexercise heart rate is the critical measurement for deciding if the performers should continue to the next 3-minute session of stepping. They *do not* continue if the heart rate is *equal to* or *above* the ceiling postexercise heart rate (85% of predicted maximum heart rate). If the heart rate is below the ceiling heart rate, the performers immediately begin the next 3-minute session. This process is continued until the ceiling heart rate is reached. After the performer has completed the test, the heart rate and blood pressure should be monitored for a specified period of time.

For both step sequences, the performer may start with either foot, but the instructions have the performer starting with the right foot. Test performers should feel free to stop stepping if they experience discomfort at any time.

Two-step sequence. Stand in front of the first step with feet together.

1. Place the right foot on the *first* step.
2. Place the left foot on the *second* step.
3. Place the right foot on the *second* step so the feet are together.
4. Start down with the left foot to the *first* step.
5. Place the right foot on the *ground* level.
6. Place the left foot on the *ground* level so that both feet are together.
7. Stop stepping at any time if you experience discomfort.

One-step sequence. Stand at the back or side of the top step with feet together.

1. Place the right foot on the *top* step.
2. Place the left foot on the *top* step so feet are together.
3. Place the right foot on *ground* level.
4. Place the left foot down on *ground* level so feet are together.

The aerobic fitness score is determined by using the oxygen cost of the step test and the performer's weight and age in the equation:

$$10[17.2 + (1.29 \times O_2 \text{ cost}) - (.09 \times \text{wt in kg}) - (.18 \times \text{age in years})]$$

Table 15.10 includes the oxygen cost of the test (reported in milliliters per kilogram body weight per minute), and Table 15.11 includes the health benefit zone for the score. The interpretation of the health benefit zones, included in the manual, is very similar to the interpretation of the zones for body composition.

3. Musculoskeletal fitness: Five components of musculoskeletal fitness are appraised. *Grip strength.* The grip strength of both hands is measured with a hand dynamometer. The grip is taken between the fingers and the palm at the base of the thumb, and the dynamometer is held in line with the forearm at the level of the thigh, away from the body. During the test neither hand nor the dynamometer should touch the body or any other object. Alternating hands, two trials per hand are administered. The grip score is recorded to the nearest kilogram, and the maximum score for each hand is combined for the test score.

Push-ups. Individuals who have lower back problems should not perform the push-up test. Males perform the push-up described on page 152, with the exception that the chin must touch the floor or the mat. Females perform the modified push-up (knees touch floor or mat) described on page 152, with the exception that the chin must touch the floor or the mat. For both males and females, the push-ups are performed consecutively and without a time limit. The test is stopped when the performer is seen to strain forcibly or is unable to maintain the proper push-up over two consecutive repetitions.

Trunk-forward flexion. The test procedure is very similar to the sit and reach test described on page 130. The Modified Wells and Dillon Flexometer is used, however, rather than the sit and reach box. Before performing this item, all individuals should be permitted to warm up. Without shoes, the test performer sits with the legs fully extended and the soles of the feet placed flat against the flexometer. The flexometer should be adjusted to a height that enables the balls of the feet to be against the upper crossboards. The inner edge of the soles are placed 2 cm from the edge of the scale. The test performer assumes a position with the knees fully extended, arms evenly stretched, and palms down. The performer bends, reaches forward, and pushes the sliding marker along the scale with the fingertips as far forward as possible. The position of maximum flexion must be held for approximately 2 seconds. The test is performed twice, and the maximum reach, recorded to the nearest 0.5 cm, is the score.

Partial curl-up. Tape is placed across a mat to mark an area that is 10 cm wide. One end of the area is designated as zero (0) and the other end as 10 cm. The test performer assumes a supine position, with the head resting on the mat, arms straight at the sides and parallel to the trunk, and palms in contact with the mat. The middle fingertip of

TABLE 15.10 Oxygen Cost and Stepping Cadence for Stages of the Modified Canadian Aerobic Fitness Test

Males								
Stage	1	2	3	4	5	6	7	8
Stepping cadence	66	84	102	114	132	144	118*	123*
O_2 cost (ml)	15.9	18.0	22.0	24.5	29.5	33.6	36.2	40.1
Females								
Stage	1	2	3	4	5	6	7	8
Stepping cadence	66	84	102	114	120	132	144	118*
O_2 cost (ml)	15.9	18.0	22.0	24.5	26.3	29.5	33.6	36.2

Source: Adapted from Canadian Society for Exercise Physiology, *The Canadian Physical Activity, Fitness & Lifestyle Appraisal,* 2d ed., Ottawa, Ontario: Canadian Society for Exercise Physiology, 1998.
*Single step (40.6 cm).

TABLE 15.11   Health Benefit Zones for Aerobic Fitness Scores (The Canadian Physical Activity, Fitness & Lifestyle Appraisal)

Zone	Age					
	15–19	20–29	30–39	40–49	50–59	60–69
	Males					
Excellent	574+	556+	488+	470+	418+	384+
Very good	524–573	506–555	454–487	427–469	365–417	328–383
Good	488–523	472–505	401–453	355–426	301–364	287–327
Fair	436–487	416–471	337–400	319–354	260–300	235–286
Needs improvement	<436	<416	<337	<319	<260	<235
	Females					
Excellent	490+	472+	454+	400+	366+	358+
Very good	437–489	420–471	401–453	351–399	340–365	328–357
Good	395–436	378–419	360–400	319–350	310–339	296–327
Fair	368–394	350–377	330–359	271–318	246–309	235–295
Needs improvement	<368	<350	<330	<271	<246	<235

Source: Adapted from Canadian Society for Exercise Physiology, *The Canadian Physical Activity, Fitness & Lifestyle Appraisal,* 2d ed., Ottawa, Ontario: Canadian Society for Exercise Physiology, 1998.

both hands should be at the 0 mark. The knees should be bent at a 90° angle. The performer slowly curls the upper spine up far enough so that the middle fingertips of both hands reach the 10 cm mark. The palms and heels must remain in contact with the mat, and anchoring of the feet is not permitted. The performer then returns to the starting position. The shoulderblades and the head must contact the floor, and the fingertips of both hands must touch the 0 mark. The curl-ups are performed slowly at a controlled rate of 25 curl-ups per minute. The score is the number of curl-ups performed, without pausing, to a maximum of 25 in the 1-minute time period. The test is terminated if the performer cannot maintain the required cadence or cannot execute the proper curl-up technique over two consecutive repetitions.

Vertical-jump. This test, described on page 153, is scored as a straight height jump and leg power. The highest jump of three trials, recorded to the nearest 0.5 cm, is the jump score. A rest period of 10 to 15 seconds is recommended between trials. Leg power, recorded as kilogram-meters per second is determined with the formula:

$$\text{leg power} = 2.21 \times \text{weight (kg)} \times \sqrt{\text{vertical jump (m)}}$$

Table 15.12 includes the "Good" health benefit zone for the grip strength, push-ups, trunk forward flexion, partial curl-up, vertical jump, and leg power. Scores above the "Good" zone are "Very Good" or "Excellent." Scores below are "Fair" or "Needs Improvement." The manual provides an interpretation of the zones.

Tests of Skill-Related Physical Fitness

Rarely does a single test battery include all components of skill-related physical fitness. If you prefer a certain test but would like to measure additional components, add those components to the test. However, remember to administer components that are appropriate for the group being tested.

■ AAU Physical Fitness Test
(Amateur Athletic Union 1994)

Because the Amateur Athletic Union (AAU) is responsible for the administration of the President's Challenge, the organization no longer promotes the AAU Physical Fitness

TABLE 15.12 "Good" Health Benefit Zones for Musculoskeletal Fitness (The Canadian Physical Activity, Fitness & Lifestyle Appraisal)

	Age					
	15–19	20–29	30–39	40–49	50–59	60–69
Males						
Grip strength* (kg)	95–102	106–112	105–112	102–109	96–101	86–92
Push-ups	23–28	22–28	17–21	13–16	10–12	8–10
Trunk Fwd Flexion (cm)	29–33	30–33	28–33	24–28	24–27	20–24
Partial Curl-Up	21–22	21–22	21–22	16–21	14–19	10–15
Vertical Jump (cm)	27–36	30–38	27–36	23–30	20–28	17–23
Leg Power (kg-m/sec)	73–87	89–101	87–101	81–95	76–92	75–83
Females						
Grip strength* (kg)	59–63	61–64	61–65	59–64	55–58	51–53
Push-ups	18–24	15–20	13–19	11–14	7–10	5–11
Trunk Fwd Flexion (cm)	34–37	33–36	32–35	30–33	30–32	27–30
Partial curl-up	21–22	19–22	16–21	13–20	9–15	6–10
Vertical Jump (cm)	22–28	20–27	16–23	15–18	13–16	10–13
Leg power (kg-m/sec)	58–66	56–64	54–63	56–59	57–62	53–55

Source: Adapted from Canadian Society for Exercise Physiology, *The Canadian Physical Activity, Fitness & Lifestyle Appraisal,* 2d ed., Ottawa, Ontario: Canadian Society for Exercise Physiology, 1998.

*Combined right and left hand.

Test. The test is presented, however, because of the uniqueness of some test items and the availability of test standards. Table 15.13 includes the criteria for Outstanding Achievement and Attainment certificates. The Outstanding Performance standard is at the eightieth percentile, and the Attainment standard is at the forty-fifth percentile.

Age Level. Six through seventeen.

Equipment. Stopwatch, flat running surface, mat, tape measure, yardstick, horizontal bar, fifteen objects (tennis balls, beanbags, blocks, etc.), two chairs or traffic cones, one collection box, one large object-supply box, and three blocks or erasers.

Test Components

1. Cardiorespiratory endurance: Two test options are provided.

   Distance run: ¼ mile for ages six and seven; ½ mile for ages eight and nine; ¾ mile for ages ten and eleven; and 1 mile for ages twelve through seventeen.

   Hoosier endurance shuttle run. Two chairs are placed 20 yards apart. The performer runs from chair 1 and picks up an object placed by the helper on the seat of chair 2; returns by running around chair 1 and dropping the object in the container behind the chair. This action is repeated for 6 minutes. Count each object placed in the container, including the last object picked up, even if the runner has not reached the container. No partial credit should be given to the runner if an object has not been picked up. The scorekeeper must keep count of the number of objects removed from the container. The score is the number of objects collected in 6 minutes.

2. Trunk strength and endurance: 1-minute bent-knee sit-ups. Sit-ups are performed with arms crossed on the chest and partner holding feet. The arms remain in contact with the chest while touching the thighs with the elbows. The performer must return to the starting position after each sit-up.

3. Flexibility of hamstrings and lower back: Sit and reach test. A yardstick or tape measure is placed on the floor. The test performer sits near the zero (0) end of the tape and straddles the measuring tape, with the heels 12 inches

TABLE 15.13 Awards Performance Criteria for AAU Physical Fitness Test

Event	Level of Performance	Age Level											
		6	7	8	9	10	11	12	13	14	15	16	17
							Girls						

Required:

Event	Level of Performance	6	7	8	9	10	11	12	13	14	15	16	17
1a. Endurance run (fractions of mile) (min:sec)	Attainment	¼ mi 2:30	¼ mi 2:24	½ mi 5:02	½ mi 4:57	¾ mi 7:30	¾ mi 7:25	1 mi 9:54	1 mi 9:50	1 mi 9:50	1 mi 9:50	1 mi 9:54	1 mi 9:51
	Outstanding Achievement	2:05	2:00	4:06	4:04	6:10	6:06	8:15	8:04	8:08	8:00	8:07	8:16
OR 1b. Hoosier endurance shuttle run (no. of objects)	Attainment	20	21	22	22	23	23	23	23	23	23	23	24
	Outstanding Achievement	23	24	25	25	26	26	26	26	26	26	27	27
2. Bent-knee sit-ups (1-minute time limit)	Attainment	22	25	29	31	32	33	35	35	36	35	35	36
	Outstanding Achievement	31	34	38	39	40	42	43	45	45	44	44	44
3. Sit and reach (in.)	Attainment	17	17	17	17	17	17	19	20	20	20	20	20
	Outstanding Achievement	19	20	20	21	21	21	21	23	23	23	23	24
4a. Pull-ups*	Attainment	1	1	1	1	1	1	1	1	1	1	1	1
	Outstanding Achievement	1	1	2	2	2	2	2	1	1	1	1	1
OR 4b. Flexed-arm hang (seconds & tenths)	Attainment	6.0	7.0	8.0	8.5	10.0	12.4	15.0	15.9	13.0	12.0	10.2	8.1

Optional:

Event	Level of Performance	6	7	8	9	10	11	12	13	14	15	16	17
1. Long jump (feet & inches)	Attainment	3'4"	3'8"	3'11"	4'2"	4'5"	4'9"	5'1"	5'3"	5'5"	5'4"	5'5"	5'6"
	Outstanding Achievement	4'0"	4'3"	4'6"	4'11"	5'1"	5'4"	5'9"	5'11"	6'0"	6'1"	6'1"	6'2"
2. Isometric push-up (seconds & tenths)	Attainment	11.0	15.0	15.0	17.0	18.0	18.0	19.0	19.0	20.0	21.0	19.0	19.0
	Outstanding Achievement	26.8	31.1	36.0	38.9	35.2	35.2	38.0	42.0	43.0	43.3	37.0	37.0
3. Push-ups (modified) (30-second time limit)	Attainment	14	15	17	21	21	21	21	22	22	21	21	23
	Outstanding Achievement	20	22	24	26	27	28	28	32	32	29	30	31
4. Phantom chair (isometric leg squat) (min:sec)	Attainment	:38	:50	1:02	1:02	1:03	1:03	1:04	1:05	1:09	1:02	1:02	1:05
	Outstanding Achievement	1:16	1:30	1:54	2:00	2:06	2:10	2:15	2:20	2:23	2:02	2:02	2:00
5. Shuttle run** (seconds & tenths)	Attainment	14.2	13.5	13.1	12.2	12.2	11.8	11.6	11.2	11.2	11.2	11.2	11.1
	Outstanding Achievement	12.9	12.5	12.0	11.5	11.3	10.9	10.5	10.3	10.4	10.4	10.4	10.2
6. Sprint (in yards) (seconds & tenths)	Attainment	50 yd 10.5	50 yd 10.0	50 yd 9.2	50 yd 9.1	50 yd 8.8	50 yd 8.5	50 yd 8.4	100 yd 15.8	100 yd 15.4	100 yd 15.5	100 yd 15.6	100 yd 15.7
	Outstanding Achievement	9.6	9.0	8.8	8.4	8.0	7.8	7.8	14.4	14.1	14.1	14.2	14.2

Source: The Amateur Physical Fitness Program, 1994.
*Standards for these items are based on data from the 1985 School Population Fitness Survey conducted by the University of Michigan Institute for Social Research.
**Should be conducted on gym floor or other clean, firm surface.

TABLE 15.13 *Continued*

Event	Level of Performance	Age Level											
		6	7	8	9	10	11	12	13	14	15	16	17
		Boys											

Required:

1a.	Endurance run (fractions of mile) (min:sec)	Attainment	¼ mi 2:23	¼ mi 2:13	½ mi 4:31	½ mi 4:20	¾ mi 6:35	¾ mi 6:27	1 mi 8:34	1 mi 7:54	1 mi 7:33	1 mi 7:27	1 mi 7:21	1 mi 7:08
		Outstanding Achievement	2:00	1:52	3:41	3:42	5:30	5:19	7:10	6:45	6:28	6:18	6:14	6:12
OR 1b.	Hoosier endurance shuttle run (no. of objects)	Attainment	21	23	23	24	25	25	25	25	26	26	26	26
		Outstanding Achievement	25	26	26	27	28	29	29	29	29	30	30	30
2.	Bent-knee sit-ups (one-minute time limit)	Attainment	22	27	31	34	36	38	40	41	44	44	44	46
		Outstanding Achievement	31	36	39	43	45	48	49	51	53	53	53	55
3.	Sit and reach (inches)	Attainment	15	15	15	15	15	15	15	15	16	17	17	17
		Outstanding Achievement	17	18	18	18	18	18	18	18	19	20	20	20
4a.	Pull-ups	Attainment	2	2	2	2	2	3	3	4	5	6	7	8
		Outstanding Achievement	4	4	4	4	4	5	7	8	9	10	10	11
OR 4b.	Flexed-arm hang* (seconds & tenths)	Attainment	5.0	7.0	9.0	8.0	10.0	10.0	10.0	12.0	17.0	28.0	25.0	29.0

Optional:

1.	Long jump (feet & inches)	Attainment	3'7"	4'0"	4'3"	4'7"	4'11"	5'1"	5'4"	5'10"	6'4"	6'7"	6'11"	7'3"
		Outstanding Achievement	4'2"	4'6"	4'10"	5'3"	5'6"	5'9"	6'1"	6'7"	7'3"	7'5"	7'8"	8'0"
2.	Isometric push-up (seconds & tenths)	Attainment	15.1	16.0	18.5	22.7	21.0	23.4	28.5	33.0	35.0	40.8	44.9	47.0
		Outstanding Achievement	32.4	35.5	38.0	45.5	47.0	50.5	53.0	55.0	58.3	60.0	68.0	70.0
3.	Push-ups (modified) (30-second time limit)	Attainment	:34	:53	1:02	1:06	1:06	1:16	1:20	1:22	1:24	1:25	1:30	1:30
		Outstanding Achievement	1:07	1:30	2:00	2:08	2:37	2:43	2:59	3:02	3:00	3:28	3:00	3:00
4.	Phantom chair (isometric leg squat) (min:sec)	Attainment	13.6	13.1	12.5	12.0	11.8	11.2	11.1	10.6	10.2	9.9	9.7	9.6
		Outstanding Achievement	12.6	12.0	11.6	11.4	10.8	10.4	10.2	9.8	9.5	9.1	9.1	8.7
5.	Shuttle run** (seconds & tenths)	Attainment	50 yd 10.3	50 yd 9.8	50 yd 9.4	50 yd 9.0	50 yd 8.5	50 yd 8.3	50 yd 8.2	100 yd 14.8	100 yd 13.9	100 yd 13.2	100 yd 13.1	100 yd 12.6
		Outstanding Achievement	9.3	8.9	8.5	8.4	7.6	7.5	7.4	13.4	12.6	12.2	12.2	11.9

*Standards for these items are based on data from the 1985 School Population Fitness Survey conducted by the University of Michigan Institute for Social Research.
**Should be conducted on gym floor or other clean, firm surface.

apart, even with the 15-inch mark of the tape. With the legs straight and flat on the floor, and hands overlapped and facing the floor, the performer slides the hands as far as possible along the tape without bending the knees. Another person should hold the ankles for stability. The score is the farthest point touched by the tip of the fingers in the best of three trials.

4. Upper-body strength and endurance: Pull-ups (palms may face toward or away from body). The performer pulls the body up until the chin is raised above the bar. The body then is lowered until the arms are fully extended. Swinging, kicking, and resting are not permitted. The score is the number of complete pull-ups. Both males and females must do pull-ups to qualify for the Outstanding award. Participants who are unable to perform one pull-up are permitted to substitute the flexed-arm hang for this event but do not qualify for the Outstanding award. Such participants, however, are eligible for the Attainment or Participation award.

The following are optional test items:

1. Explosive leg strength and efficiency of control of body mass in space: Standing long jump. Three trials.
2. Upper-body static endurance (males): Isometric push-ups. The test performer takes the resting push-up position. On the command to begin, the body is pushed up until the elbows are bent at a 90° angle. The score is the time this position can be held.
3. Upper-body strength and endurance (females): Modified push-ups with 30-second time limit.
4. Static leg endurance: Isometric leg squat (phantom chair). With back flat against wall, the performer slides down the wall until the knees form a 90° angle. The feet should point directly forward and must be flat on the floor, and the arms should hang at the sides. The score is the length of time this position can be held.
5. Agility and quickness: Shuttle run. Two lines are placed 30 feet apart with masking tape. One block is placed at the starting line and two blocks at the parallel line. On the command to begin, the test performer runs to the line with two blocks; picks up a block; runs back to the starting line and places the block on the starting line; picks up the block originally placed on the starting line; runs back to the parallel line and places the block on the line; picks up the third block; and returns as rapidly as possible across the starting line. The score is in seconds and tenths.
6. Speed, quickness, and anaerobic capacity: Sprint. 50 yards for ages nine through twelve; 100 yards for ages thirteen through seventeen.

■ The President's Challenge
(President's Council on Physical Fitness and Sports 2000)

Participants in the President's Challenge can strive for one of three awards. Males and females who score at or above the eighty-fifth percentile on all five items of the test are eligible to receive the Presidential Physical Fitness Award. Participants scoring at or above the fiftieth percentile, but less than the eighty-fifth percentile, are eligible to receive the National Physical Fitness Award. The Participant Physical Fitness Award is given to individuals who attempt all five items on the test but whose scores fall below the fiftieth percentile on one or more of them. The performance standards for the Presidential Physical Fitness Award and the National Physical Fitness Award are included in table 15.14.

The President's Challenge also provides a health-criterion–referenced award as an alternative to the traditional physical fitness awards. The Health Fitness Award (HFA) can be earned by students whose test scores meet or exceed the specified health criteria on each of the five items constituting the President's Challenge Health Test. The five items are partial curl-ups, 1-mile run or distance option, V-sit reach or sit and reach, right-angle push-ups or pull-ups, and body mass index (BMI).

Emblems and certificates are available for individuals who complete the requirements for each award. The State Champion Award is presented to the top schools in each state, one in each of three enrollment categories (50–100, 101–500, 501-plus) that qualify the highest percentage of students for the Presidential Physical Fitness Award. The President's Challenge also includes modifications for students with special needs. The modifications are described in chapter 17.

Information about the President's Challenge may be found at the Web site www.indiana.edu/~preschal. You also may write to the President's Challenge, 400 East 7th Street, Bloomington, IN 47405-3085, or you may call at 800-258-8146.

Age Level. Six through seventeen.

Equipment. Mat, flat running surface, two blocks of wood or similar object (2" × 2" × 4"), horizontal bar, yardstick or tape measure.

Test Components

1. Abdominal strength/endurance: Curl-ups. For the 1-minute bent-knee curl-ups the performer does sit-ups with arms crossed on chest; the arms remain in contact with the chest while touching the thighs with the elbows. A partner holds the feet. The scapulas must touch the mat when the back is lowered to the mat. Partial curl-ups may be used as an option to curl-ups. The test performer assumes a supine position on a mat, with the knees flexed, feet flat on the mat, and the heels about 12 inches from buttocks. The feet

TABLE 15.14 Performance Standards for the President's Challenge (Continued on page 208)

The Presidential Physical Fitness Award (Qualifying Standards; Eighty-fifth Percentile)

Age	Curl-Ups (Timed One Min)	Or	Partial Curl-Ups (Number)	Shuttle Run (Sec)	V-Sit Reach (Inches)	Or	Sit and Reach (Centimeters)	One-Mile Run (Min/Sec)	Or	Distance Option (Min/Sec) ¼ Mile	½ Mile	Pull-Ups	Or	Rt. Angle Push-Ups (Number)
Boys
6	33		22	12.1	+3.5		31	10:15		1:55		2		9
7	36		24	11.5	+3.5		30	9:22		1:48		4		14
8	40		30	11.1	+3.0		31	8:48			3:30	5		17
9	41		37	10.9	+3.0		31	8:31			3:30	5		18
10	45		35	10.3	+4.0		30	7:57				6		22
11	47		43	10.0	+4.0		31	7:32				6		27
12	50		64	9.8	+4.0		31	7:11				7		31
13	53		59	9.5	+3.5		33	6:50				7		39
14	56		62	9.1	+4.5		36	6:26				10		40
15	57		75	9.0	+5.0		37	6:20				11		42
16	56		73	8.7	+6.0		38	6:08				11		44
17	55		66	8.7	+7.0		41	6:06				13		53
Girls
6	32		22	12.4	+5.5		32	11:20		2:00		2		9
7	34		24	12.1	+5.0		32	10:36		1:55		2		14
8	38		30	11.8	+4.5		33	10:02			3:58	2		17
9	39		37	11.1	+5.5		33	9:30			3:53	2		18
10	40		33	10.8	+6.0		33	9:19				3		20
11	42		43	10.5	+6.5		34	9:02				3		19
12	45		50	10.4	+7.0		36	8:23				2		20
13	46		59	10.2	+7.0		38	8:13				2		21
14	47		48	10.1	+8.0		40	7:59				2		20
15	48		38	10.0	+8.0		43	8:08				2		20
16	45		49	10.1	+9.0		42	8:23				1		24
17	44		58	10.0	+8.0		42	8:15				1		25

TABLE 15.14 Continued

The Presidential Physical Fitness Award (Qualifying Standards; Fiftieth Percentile)

Age	Curl-Ups (Timed One Min)	Or	Partial Curl-Ups (Number One Min)	Shuttle Run (Sec)	V-Sit Reach (Inches)	Or	Sit and Reach (Centimeters)	One-Mile Run (Min/Sec)	Or	Distance Option (Min/Sec) 1/4 Mile	Distance Option (Min/Sec) 1/2 Mile	Pull-Ups or Flexed-Arm Hang Number (Sec)		Or	Rt. Angle Push-Ups (Number)
							Boys								
6	22		10	13.3	+1.0		26	12:36		2:21		1	6		7
7	28		13	12.8	+1.0		25	11:40		2:10		1	8		8
8	31		17	12.2	+0.5		25	11:05			4:22	1	10		9
9	32		20	11.9	+1.0		25	10:30			4:14	2	10		12
10	35		24	11.5	+1.0		25	9:48				2	12		14
11	37		26	11.1	+1.0		25	9:20				2	11		15
12	40		32	10.6	+1.0		26	8:40				2	12		18
13	42		39	10.2	+0.5		26	8:06				3	14		24
14	45		40	9.9	+1.0		28	7:44				5	20		24
15	45		45	9.7	+2.0		30	7:30				6	30		30
16	45		37	9.4	+3.0		30	7:10				7	28		30
17	44		42	9.4	+3.0		34	7:04				8	30		37
							Girls								
6	23		10	13.8	+2.5		27	13:12		2:26		1	5		6
7	25		13	13.2	+2.0		27	12:56		2:21		1	6		8
8	29		17	12.9	+2.0		28	12:30			4:56	1	8		9
9	30		20	12.5	+2.0		28	11:52			4:50	1	8		12
10	30		24	12.1	+3.0		28	11:22				1	8		13
11	32		27	11.5	+3.0		29	11:17				1	7		11
12	35		30	11.3	+3.5		30	11:05				1	7		10
13	37		40	11.1	+3.5		31	10:23				1	8		11
14	37		30	11.2	+4.5		33	10:06				1	9		10
15	36		26	11.0	+5.0		36	9:58				1	7		15
16	35		26	10.9	+5.5		34	10:31				1	7		12
17	34		40	11.0	+4.5		35	10:22				1	7		16

Source: From the President's Challenge Physical Fitness Program. Reprinted by the permission of The President's Council on Physical Fitness and Sports, 2000.

are not held or anchored. The arms are extended forward with the fingers resting on the thighs and pointing toward the knees. A test partner is behind the performer's head with the hands cupped under the head. The performer curls up slowly, sliding the fingers up the legs until the fingertips touch the knees, then back down until the head touches the partner's hands. The curl-ups are done to a metronome, with one complete curl-up every 3 seconds, and are continued until the test performer can do no more in rhythm (has not done the last three in rhythm) or has reached the target number for the Presidential Physical Fitness Award.

2. Speed and agility: Shuttle run. Two parallel lines are placed 30 feet apart with marking tape. Two blocks of wood or similar objects (with an approximate size of 2" × 2" × 4") are placed behind one of the lines. On the signal "Ready? Go!" the test performer runs to the blocks, picks one up, runs back to the starting line, places the block behind the line, runs back and picks up the second block, and runs back across the starting line. Blocks should not be thrown across the line. The score is recorded to the nearest tenth of a second.

3. Heart/lung endurance: 1-mile run/walk. The ¼ mile run is an option for six to seven years old, and the ½ mile run is an option for eight to nine years old.

4. Upper body strength/endurance: Maximum number of pull-ups with palms facing away from body. Right-angle push-ups may be used as an option to pull-ups. This component is similar to the push-up described in chapter 12. The difference is that the performer lowers the body only until there is a 90° angle at the elbows. A test partner holds her or his hands at the point of the 90° angle so that the test performer goes down only until the shoulders touch the partner's hands. The push-ups are done to a metronome, with one complete push-up every 3 seconds, and are continued until the performer can do no more in rhythm (has not done the last three in rhythm) or has reached the target number for the Presidential Physical Fitness Award. The flexed-arm hang, described in chapter 12, may be used as an alternative to pull-ups for the National and Participant Physical Fitness Awards.

5. Flexibility of lower back and hamstrings: V-sit reach. A straight line 2 feet long is marked on the floor as the baseline. A measuring line is drawn perpendicular to the midpoint of the baseline extending 2 feet on each side and is marked off in inches. The point where the baseline and the measuring line intersect is the zero (0) point. The test participant sits on the floor, without shoes, with the measuring line between the legs and the soles of the feet immediately behind the baseline. The heels should be 8 to 12 inches apart. With palms down and thumbs clasped so that the hands are together, the participant places his or her hands on the measuring line. With the legs

held flat by a partner, the test participant slowly reaches forward as far as possible. After three practice trials, the fourth reach is held for 3 seconds while distance is recorded.

The sit and reach test on page 130 may be used as an option to the V-sit reach.

■ AAHPERD Youth Fitness Test
(AAHPERD 1976)

Although the AAHPERD Youth Fitness Test was last published in 1976, it is included as a fitness test because norms are included for all test items.

Age Level. Nine through seventeen-plus.

Equipment. Horizontal bar, mat, stopwatch, flat running surface, measuring tape.

Test Components

1. Arm and shoulder girdle strength and endurance: Pull test (palms forward) for males and flexed-arm hang for females. Administration of these test items and norms for them are provided in chapter 12.

2. Abdominal strength and endurance: 1-minute bent-knee sit-ups. The hands are placed at the back of the neck; the feet are held by a partner; the elbows must touch the knees; and the performer must return to the starting position with elbows on the surface. Table 15.15 reports percentile norms.

3. Agility in running and changing direction: AAHPERD shuttle run. Administration of this item and norms are included in chapter 8.

4. Leg power: Standing long jump. Administration of this item and norms are provided in chapter 12.

5. Speed: 50-yard dash. Two runners should run at the same time (for competition), and all runners should be instructed not to slow down before crossing the finish line. Table 15.16 reports norms.

6. Cardiorespiratory function: 600-yard run. Table 15.17 provides percentile norms. Optional long-distance runs include the 1-mile or 9-minute run for ages ten through twelve, and the 1.5-mile or 12-minute run for ages thirteen or older. Descriptions and norms for these runs are provided in chapter 10.

Development of Health-Related and Skill-Related Physical Fitness

If either health-related or skill-related physical fitness is to be developed, a program must consist of different activities and exercises. One particular type of activity or

TABLE 15.15 Norms for AAHPERD Youth Fitness Sit-Ups Test for Ages Nine Through Seventeen+

	Age							
Percentile	9–10	11	12	13	14	15	16	17+
Males								
95	47	48	50	53	55	57	55	54
75	38	40	42	45	47	48	47	46
50	31	34	35	38	41	42	41	41
25	25	26	30	30	34	37	35	35
5	13	15	18	20	24	28	28	26
Females								
95	45	43	44	45	45	45	43	45
75	34	35	36	36	37	36	35	35
50	27	29	29	30	30	31	30	30
25	21	22	24	23	24	25	24	25
5	10	9	13	15	16	15	15	14

Source: Adapted from AAHPERD, *Youth fitness test manual,* Reston, Va.: American Alliance for Health, Physical Education, Recreation, and Dance, 1976.

TABLE 15.16 Norms in Seconds and Tenths of Second for AAHPERD 50-Yard Dash for Ages Nine Through Seventeen+

	Age							
Percentile	9–10	11	12	13	14	15	16	17+
Males								
95	7.3	7.1	6.8	6.5	6.2	6.0	6.0	5.9
75	7.8	7.6	7.4	7.0	6.8	6.5	6.5	6.3
50	8.2	8.0	7.8	7.5	7.2	6.9	6.7	6.6
25	8.9	8.6	8.3	8.0	7.7	7.3	7.0	7.0
5	9.9	9.5	9.5	9.0	8.8	8.0	7.7	7.9
Females								
95	7.4	7.3	7.0	6.9	6.8	6.9	7.0	6.8
75	8.0	7.9	7.6	7.4	7.3	7.4	7.5	7.4
50	8.6	8.3	8.1	8.0	7.8	7.8	7.9	7.9
25	9.1	9.0	8.7	8.5	8.3	8.2	8.3	8.4
5	10.3	10.0	10.0	10.0	9.6	9.2	9.3	9.5

Source: Adapted from AAHPERD, *Youth fitness test manual,* Reston, Va.: American Alliance for Health, Physical Education, Recreation, and Dance, 1976.

TABLE 15.17 Norms in Minutes and Seconds for AAHPERD 600-Yard Run Test for Ages Nine Through Seventeen+

	Age							
Percentile	9–10	11	12	13	14	15	16	17+
				Males				
95	2:05	2:02	1:52	1:45	1:39	1:36	1:34	1:32
75	2:17	2:15	2:06	1:59	1:52	1:46	1:44	1:43
50	2:33	2:27	2:19	2:10	2:03	1:56	1:52	1:52
25	2:53	2:47	2:37	2:27	2:16	2:08	2:01	2:02
5	3:22	3:29	3:06	3:00	2:51	2:30	2:31	2:38
				Females				
95	2:20	2:14	2:06	2:04	2:02	2:00	2:08	2:02
75	2:39	2:35	2:26	2:23	2:19	2:22	2:26	2:24
50	2:56	2:53	2:47	2:41	2:40	2:37	2:43	2:41
25	3:15	3:16	3:13	3:06	3:01	3:00	3:03	3:02
5	4:00	4:15	3:59	3:49	3:49	3:28	3:49	3:45

Source: Adapted from AAHPERD, *Youth fitness test manual,* Reston, Va.: American Alliance for Health, Physical Education, Recreation, and Dance, 1976.

exercise usually will not develop all components. For example, though running is an excellent activity for the development of cardiorespiratory fitness, other activities must be performed for the development of arm and shoulder strength and flexibility. The same is true of many cardiorespiratory fitness programs. Also, weight-lifting programs are excellent for muscular strength and endurance, but other types of programs are better for cardiorespiratory fitness. Activities and exercises that may be used to develop the components of health-related and skill-related physical fitness have been described in previous chapters. Through selection of the appropriate activities for different ages, you should be able to design sound programs.

textbook? If they do, do you consider them as components of health-related or skill-related physical fitness?

2. Interview several teachers in the local school system about their use of health-related and skill-related physical fitness tests. Ask which tests they prefer, and why.

3. Administer the President's Challenge test to several of your classmates. Ask them to provide constructive criticism of your test administration.

4. Design a program to develop health-related physical fitness for the age group sixteen through eighteen.

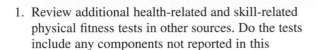

REVIEW PROBLEMS

1. Review additional health-related and skill-related physical fitness tests in other sources. Do the tests include any components not reported in this

16 Older Adult

Upon completion of this chapter, you should be able to

1. Define functional fitness;

2. State why the functional fitness of older adults should be measured;

3. Measure the functional fitness of older adults;

4. Prescribe activities and exercise for the development of functional fitness for the older adult.

Functional fitness is the physical capacity of the individual to perform ordinary daily activities safely and independently without undue fatigue (Osness et al. 1996; Rikli and Jones 1999a). In the United States, more of us are living longer, and as we age we hope to maintain a high level of functional fitness. At the beginning of the twentieth century, approximately 4% of the U.S. population were individuals over 65 years of age. By the year 2020, nearly 20% of the U.S. population will be 65 or older (U.S. Bureau of the Census 1996). As the number of individuals over the age of 65 increases, so will the number of the oldest old (85 and older); in this latter group, we can expect an increase in the number of individuals who are unable to function effectively in society.

Why Measure Functional Fitness?

Although a sedentary lifestyle is often directly related to chronic diseases associated with aging, the activity level of many individuals declines with age even if they have no chronic disease. Regrettably, largely because of a sedentary lifestyle, many older individuals must exert maximum effort just to perform daily physical activities. Research indicates that much of the age-related physical decline in our older years may be prevented through an active lifestyle. Research also indicates that older individuals can experience health benefits when changing from a sedentary lifestyle to an active lifestyle. To ensure the quality of life they desire, we must encourage the older population to be physically active. Before older individuals initiate such a program, however, it is important to identify any physical limitations (cardiorespiratory fitness, muscular strength and endurance, flexibility, and so on) that could place them at risk of bodily harm. In addition to identifying at-risk individuals, proper measurement and assessment can serve to:

- identify physical weaknesses or deficiencies that will limit success with the initiation of an active lifestyle
- identify physical abilities in which further decline may be prevented or reduced
- provide a baseline for evaluating improvement in physical performance

213

- provide feedback to individuals about their limitations and motivate them to initiate an active lifestyle
- provide data for evaluation of program effectiveness

?ARE YOU ABLE TO DO THE FOLLOWING:

‣ define functional fitness and state why the functional fitness of older adults should be measured?

Tests of Functional Fitness

Many older individuals are capable of completing some of the physical performance test items presented in previous chapters. Some individuals will be better served, however, by attempting the items presented in this chapter. These test items can be administered without costly laboratory equipment and are related to the daily functions of life.

■ Functional Fitness Assessment for Adults Over 60 Years
(Osness et al. 1996)

Test Objective. To evaluate the ability of adults to carry on certain daily activities.

Age Level. Over sixty.

Equipment. Weight scale, tape measure, chair with arms (16-inch seat height), masking or duct tape, two cones, stopwatch, three unopened 12-ounce soda pop cans, a table, four 8-pound weights (or a half-gallon plastic milk bottle with handle), one-gallon plastic milk bottle with handle, sand, water, normal chair with arms.

Validity. Assumed for ponderal index, sit and reach, and agility course; soda pop was validated using typical laboratory procedures for reaction time (r = .59), hand steadiness (r = .399), and hand-eye coordination (.349); arm-curl was validated using a cybex protocol elbow curl (r = .82); and 880-yard walk was validated by measurement of maximal oxygen intake per minute (r = .615)

Reliability. Test-retest studies were done in multiple laboratories; only one correlation value for each item is included in this test description.

Pondral index: men and women (r = .994)

Sit and reach: men (r = 0.988); women (r = .978)

Agility course: men and women (r = .995)

Soda pop: men (r = .911); women (r = .853)

Arm-curl: men and women (r = .833)

880-yard walk: men (r = .82)

Norms. Table 16.1 reports average standards for ages sixty through ninety.

Test Components

1. Ponderal index. Body weight is recorded to the closest pound and height is recorded in feet and inches to the nearest ½ inch; shoes and heavy garments should be removed. The measured weight in pounds is marked on the right scale of figure 16.1, and the measured height is marked on the left scale of figure 16.1. A straight edge is used to connect these two points. The point of intersection on the center scale is the ponderal index. The higher the ponderal index, the greater the degree of leanness. Record the ponderal index to the nearest .1 of one unit.

2. Trunk/leg flexibility: Sit and reach. This test procedure is similar to the sit and reach test item included in the YMCA Physical Fitness Test. A yardstick is taped to the floor with a perpendicular line over the 25-inch mark. The test performer, with shoes removed, sits with the legs extended flat on the floor and the heels at the 25-inch mark. The yardstick should be between the legs, with the zero (0) point toward the performer. With the feet spread about 12 inches apart and one hand placed directly on top of the other, the performer slowly reaches forward, sliding the hands along the yardstick as far as possible. The performer must hold the final position for at least 2 seconds. The test administrator should place a hand on top of one of the performer's knees to ensure that the knees are not raised during the test. Two practice trials are permitted, and the best of two test trials is recorded. The score is recorded to the nearest ½ inch.

3. Agility/dynamic balance. The agility course is marked as illustrated in figure 16.2. The test performer sits in the chair, with heels on the floor. On the signal "Ready, go," the performer stands up, moves to the right, goes to the inside and around the cone (counterclockwise), returns to the chair, sits down, and raises the feet from the floor. Without hesitating, the test performer immediately stands up, moves to the left, again going to the inside and around the cone (clockwise), returns to the chair, and sits down, completing one circuit. The performer immediately stands up and completes the circuit a second time. The two

TABLE 16.1 Average Standards for Functional Fitness Assessment for Adults over 60

	Age					
	60–64	65–69	70–74	75–79	80–84	85–90
	Men					
Ponderal index (P.I. units)	12.36–11.48	12.37–11.41	12.67–11.39	12.57–11.29	12.16–11.06	12.56–11.20
Flexibility (inches and tenths of inches)	24.90–14.90	24.88–14.80	23.97–11.75	24.12–12.94	22.32–14.42	19.02–13.38
Agility/balance (seconds and tenths of seconds)	19.22–31.50	18.46–35.52	15.11–41.31	23.42–40.08	23.35–41.85	17.07–50.05
Coordination (seconds and tenths of seconds)	8.98–14.34	10.13–14.83	9.51–16.57	11.08–15.82	11.09–17.35	10.17–16.97
Strength/endurance (repetitions)	29.15–18.23	28.38–14.56	26.90–15.38	24.24–16.06	23.14–17.92	22.92–12.72
Aerobic fitness (minutes and hundreths of minutes)	5.84–8.40	6.30–9.34	7.07–9.61	5.99–13.47	6.69–9.49	8.15–10.89
	Women					
Ponderal index (P.I. units)	12.49–10.89	12.63–11.01	12.60–11.06	12.61–11.23	12.89–10.99	12.81–12.01
Flexibility (inches and tenths of inches)	28.25–18.21	29.72–17.43	28.35–16.85	29.23–16.59	26.77–14.99	25.74–13.32
Agility/balance (seconds and tenths of seconds)	19.54–30.40	21.13–33.61	21.99–36.09	23.40–44.64	21.99–52.19	29.59–57.91
Coordination (seconds and tenths of seconds)	8.92–15.31	9.18–16.04	9.20–16.66	8.99–18.13	10.74–18.34	12.41–18.95
Strength/endurance (repetitions)	27.98–15.58	27.94–14.48	26.85–14.73	22.87–12.53	22.48–12.70	20.97–11.43
Aerobic fitness (minutes and hundreths of minutes)	6.88–10.00	6.69–10.83	6.72–11.46	8.10–11.84	8.36–13.06	8.28–12.48

Source: Adapted from W. H. Osness, et al., *Functional Fitness for Adults over 60 Years*, 2d ed., Dubuque, Iowa: Kendall/Hunt Publishing, 1996.

circuits complete one trial. After a 30-second rest, a second trial is administered. A practice trial is administered to acquaint the performer with the test. Each trial is scored to the nearest 0.1 second. The score is the time for the best trial.

4. Coordination: Soda pop test. Place a 30-inch strip of ¾-inch masking tape on a table. The tape should be about 5 inches from the edge of the table. Starting at 2½ inches from either end of the tape, place a strip of tape (approximately 3 inches long) across the 30-inch strip of tape. Now place a second 3-inch strip exactly 5 inches from the first strip. Place additional strips until six 3-inch strips are placed across the 30-inch tape, 5 inches apart. For the purpose of the test, the 3-inch strips of tape are numbered 1 to 6. The preferred hand is used for the test. If the right hand is preferred, an unopened (12-ounce) soda can is placed on tapes 1, 3, and 5. To start the test, the performer places the right hand, with the thumb up, on can number 1. On the starting command, the test performer lifts the first can, turns it over and places it on tape number 2, then turns can 2 and places it on tape 4, and places can 3 on tape 6. The test performer immediately returns all three cans to their original places, beginning with can 1. On the "return trip," the cans are grasped with

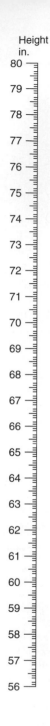

Height
in.

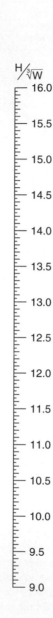

$H/\sqrt[3]{W}$

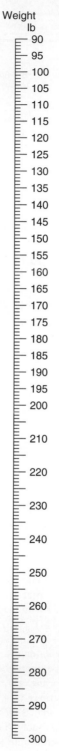

Weight
lb

FIGURE 16.1 Nomogram for ponderal index.

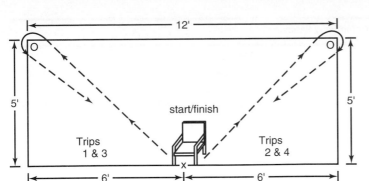

FIGURE 16.2 Agility course.

the hand in a thumb-down position. Upon completion of the return trip, without hesitation, the performer completes the entire process again. The trial consists of lifting, turning, and moving the cans a total of 12 times. After two practice trials, two test trials are performed. Each test trial is scored to the nearest 0.1 second; the best time is recorded as the score.

5. Strength/endurance. A 4-pound weight is used for women, and an 8-pound weight is used for men. As an alternative to weights, a ½-gallon plastic milk bottle filled with sand or water to the proper weight may be used. The test performer sits in a chair with the back straight against the chair and the nondominant hand at rest in the lap. The dominant arm hangs to the side. The weight is held in the dominant hand in a thumb-up position. The test administrator places a hand on the biceps of the test performer's dominant arm. On the signal to start, the test performer lifts the weight through the biceps' full range of motion until the lower arm touches the hand of the test administrator. The score is the number of repetitions that can be completed in 30 seconds.

6. Aerobic fitness: 880-yard walk. The test performer walks 880 yards as fast as possible. A measured, suitable test area is needed. One trial is administered, with the time recorded in minutes and seconds. The score is recorded to the nearest second. Individuals should be screened for cardiovascular or orthopedic problems. Individuals with the following conditions should consult their physician before attempting this test item:

- significant orthopedic problems that may be aggravated by prolonged continuous walking
- history of cardiac problems that can be negatively influenced by physical exertion
- lightheadedness while physically active or history of uncontrolled hypertension

■ Functional Fitness Test for Community-Residing Older Adults
(Rikli and Jones 1999a; Rikli and Jones 1999b)

Test Objective. To assess the major underlying physical parameters associated with functional mobility in independent older adults.

Age Level. Sixty to ninety-plus.

Equipment. Straightback or folding chair (without arms and seat height approximately 17 inches), stopwatch, 5- and 8-pound weights, long measuring tape, cones, Popsicle sticks, chalk, masking tape, tape measure or 30-inch piece of cord, and 18-inch ruler.

Validity. Criterion validity was estimated for the 30-second chair stand (.77), arm-curl (men = .81; women = .78); 6-minute walk (.78); 2-minute step (.73); and chair sit and reach (.83). The back scratch was considered to be the best measure of overall shoulder flexibility, and the 8-foot up-and-go was considered to be a good measure of combined physiological attributes.

Reliability. Reliability values were as follows: 30-second chair stand (.89), arm-curl (.81), 6-minute walk (.94), 2-minute step test (.90), chair sit and reach (.95), back scratch (.96), and 8-foot up-and-go (.95).

Norms. Table 16.2 reports percentile norms for ages sixty through ninety-four.

Test Components

1. Lower body strength: 30-second chair stand. The test performer sits in the middle of the chair, with back straight, feet flat on the floor, and arms crossed at the wrists and held against the chest. The chair should be placed against a wall or in some other way stabilized so that it does not move during the testing. On the signal "Go," the performer rises to a full stand and then returns to a fully seated position. The test performer is to stand up

TABLE 16.2 Percentile Norms for Functional Fitness Test for Community-Residing Older Adults

Percentile	Men						
	Age						
	60–64	65–69	70–74	75–79	80–84	85–89	90–94
Chair stand (no. of stands)							
25	14	12	12	11	10	8	7
50	16	15	15	14	12	11	10
75	19	18	17	17	15	14	12
90	22	21	20	19	18	17	15
Arm-curl (repetitions)							
25	16	15	14	13	13	11	10
50	19	18	17	16	16	14	12
75	22	21	21	19	19	17	14
90	25	25	24	22	21	19	17
6-minute walk (yards)							
25	610	560	545	470	445	380	305
50	675	630	610	555	525	475	405
75	735	700	680	640	605	570	500
90	790	765	745	715	680	660	590
2-minute step (no. of steps)							
25	87	86	80	73	71	59	52
50	101	101	95	91	87	75	69
75	115	116	110	109	103	91	86
90	128	130	125	125	118	106	102
Chair sit and reach (inches)							
25	−2.5	−3.0	−3.5	−4.0	−5.5	−5.5	−6.5
50	0.5	0.0	−0.5	−1.0	−2.0	−2.5	−3.5
75	4.0	3.0	2.5	2.0	1.5	0.5	0.5
90	6.5	6.0	5.5	5.0	4.5	3.0	2.0
Back scratch (inches)							
25	−6.5	−7.5	−8.0	−9.0	−9.5	−10.0	−10.5
50	−3.5	−4.0	−4.5	−5.5	−5.5	−6.0	−7.0
75	0.0	−1.0	−1.0	−2.0	−2.0	−3.0	−4.0
90	2.5	2.0	2.0	1.0	1.0	0.0	−1.0
8-foot up-and-go (seconds)							
25	5.6	5.7	6.0	7.2	7.6	8.9	10.0
50	4.7	5.1	5.3	5.9	6.4	7.2	8.1
75	3.8	4.3	4.2	4.6	5.2	5.3	6.2
90	3.0	3.8	3.6	3.5	4.1	3.9	4.4
BMI (kg/m²)							
25	24.6	24.7	24.0	23.8	23.8	23.3	22.4
50	27.4	27.5	26.6	26.4	26.1	24.9	24.9
75	30.2	30.3	29.2	29.0	28.4	26.5	27.4
90	32.8	32.9	31.6	31.4	30.5	28	29.6

TABLE 16.2 *Continued*

	Women						
Percentile	Age						
	60–64	65–69	70–74	75–79	80–84	85–89	90–94
Chair stand (no. of stands)							
25	12	11	10	10	9	8	4
50	15	14	13	12	11	10	8
75	17	16	15	15	14	13	11
90	20	18	18	17	16	15	14
Arm-curl (repetitions)							
25	13	12	12	11	10	10	8
50	16	15	15	14	13	12	11
75	19	18	17	17	16	15	13
90	22	21	20	20	18	17	16
6-minute walk (yards)							
25	545	500	480	430	385	340	275
50	605	570	550	510	460	425	350
75	660	635	615	585	540	510	440
90	710	695	675	655	610	595	520
2-minute step (no. of steps)							
25	75	73	68	68	60	55	44
50	91	90	84	84	75	70	58
75	107	107	101	100	91	85	72
90	122	123	116	115	104	98	85
Chair sit and reach (inches)							
25	−0.5	−0.5	−1.0	−1.5	−2.0	−2.5	−4.5
50	2.0	2.0	1.5	1.0	0.5	−0.5	−2.0
75	5.0	4.5	4.0	3.5	3.0	2.5	1.0
90	7.0	6.5	6.0	5.5	5.0	4.5	3.5
Back scratch (inches)							
25	−3.0	−3.5	−4.0	−5.0	−5.5	−7.0	−8.0
50	−0.5	−1.0	−1.5	−2.0	−2.5	−4.0	−4.5
75	1.5	1.5	1.0	0.5	0.0	−1.0	−1.0
90	4.0	3.5	3.0	3.0	2.5	2.0	2.0
8-foot up-and-go (seconds)							
25	6.0	6.4	7.1	7.4	8.7	9.6	11.5
50	5.2	5.6	6.0	6.3	7.2	7.9	9.4
75	4.4	4.8	4.9	5.2	5.7	6.2	7.3
90	3.7	4.1	4.0	4.3	4.4	5.1	5.3
BMI (kg/m^2)							
25	22.8	23.0	23.1	22.5	22.0	19.5	21.1
50	26.3	26.5	26.1	25.4	24.7	21.8	24.1
75	29.8	30.0	29.1	28.3	27.4	24.3	27.1
90	33.0	33.2	31.9	31.0	30.0	26.8	29.5

Source: Adapted from R. E. Rikli and C. J. Jones, Functional fitness normative scores for community-residing older adults, ages 60–94, *Journal of Aging and Physical Activity* 7:162–182, 1999.

and sit down as many times as possible in 30 seconds. After a demonstration by the test administrator, a practice trial of one to three repetitions should be done. The score is the total number of stands performed correctly in 30 seconds. If the test performer is more than halfway up at the end of 30 seconds, it counts as a full stand.

2. Upper body strength: Arm-curl. A 5-pound dumbbell is used for women, and an 8-pound dumbbell is used for men. The test performer sits in a chair, with back straight, feet flat on the floor, and the dominant side of the body close to the edge of the chair. The weight is held in the dominant hand (handshake grip), with the arm down beside the chair, perpendicular to the floor. On the signal "Go," the test performer turns the palm up while curling the arm through a full range of motion and then returns to the starting position (arm fully extended). At the down position, the weight again should be in the handshake position. The test administrator's fingers should be on the performer's mid-biceps to prevent upper arm movement and to ensure that a full curl is made. After a demonstration by the test administrator, a practice trial of one or two repetitions is given to check for proper form. The score is the number of curls made in 30 seconds. If the arm is more than halfway up at the end of 30 seconds, it counts as a curl.

3. Aerobic endurance. There are two options for the aerobic endurance item.

6-minute walk. The test area consists of a rectangle 20 yards long and 5 yards wide. The inside perimeter of the rectangle should be marked with cones, and the 20-yard sides should be marked into 5-yard segments. A complete trip around the rectangle is 50 yards. The test involves walking as fast as possible for 6 minutes. A Popsicle stick can be given to the test performer each time the start cone is passed, to keep track of the distance walked. The score is the total number of yards walked in 6 minutes, to the nearest 5 yards. The test should be discontinued if at any time the test performer shows signs of dizziness, pain, nausea, or undue fatigue.

2-minute step-in-place (an alternative to the 6-minute walk). The proper (minimum) knee-stepping height for each test performer is at a level even with the midway point between the middle of the kneecap and the top of the iliac crest. This point can be determined with a tape measure. To monitor the correct knee-stepping height, stack books on an adjacent table or attach a ruler to a chair or wall with masking tape to mark the proper knee height. On the signal "Go," the test performer begins stepping in place, starting with the right leg. Although both knees

must be raised to the correct height to be counted, only the number of times the right knee reaches the correct height is counted. A practice test should be administered before the test day so that the test performer is aware of the proper pace. The score is the number of times the right knee reaches the minimum height. To assist with the pacing, tell the test performer when 1 minute has passed and when there are 30 seconds to go.

4. Lower body flexibility (hamstrings): Chair sit and reach. The test performer sits on the front edge of a straightback or folding chair. The crease between the top of the leg and the buttocks should be even with the edge of the chair. One leg is bent, with the foot placed flat on the floor; the other leg (the preferred leg) is extended straight in front of the hip, with the heel on the floor and the foot flexed approximately 90°. With the extended leg as straight as possible (but not hyperextended), the performer slowly bends forward at the hip joint, sliding the hands (one on top of the other, with the tips of the middle fingers even) down the extended leg in an attempt to touch the toes. The spine should remain as straight as possible, with the head in line with the spine, not tucked. The reach must be held for 2 seconds. Performers should exhale as they bend forward, should avoid bouncing or rapid forceful movements, and should never stretch to the point of pain. After a demonstration by the test administrator, the test performer is asked to determine the preferred leg (the one that results in a better score). After two practice trials, two test trials are administered. With an 18-inch ruler, the number of inches by which the performer is short of reaching the toe (minus score) or reaches beyond the toe (plus score) is recorded. The middle of the toe at the end of the shoe represents a zero (0) score. The score, recorded to the nearest ½ inch, is the best score of the two trials.

5. Upper body (shoulder) flexibility: Back scratch. In a standing position, the test performer places the preferred hand over the same shoulder and reaches down the middle of the back as far as possible (palm toward the back, fingers extended, and elbow pointed up). The hand of the other arm is placed behind the back (palm up), reaching up as far as possible in an attempt to touch or overlap the extended middle finger of both hands. Without moving the performer's hands, the test administrator helps to see that the middle finger of each hand is directed toward the other middle finger. After a demonstration by the test administrator, the test performer is asked to determine which is the preferred hand (the one that results in a better score). Two practice trials are followed by two test trials. The score, measured with a ruler to the nearest ½ inch, is the distance of overlap (plus score) or the distance

between the tips of the middle fingers (negative score). The best score of the two trials is recorded.

6. Agility/dynamic balance: 8-foot up-and-go. A straightback or folding chair (seat height approximately 17 inches) is positioned against a wall or in some other way secured so that it does not move during testing. A cone is placed in front of the chair, with the back of the cone 8 feet from the front edge of the chair. The test begins with the test performer fully seated in the chair (erect posture), hands on thighs, and feet flat on the floor (one foot slightly in front of the other). On the signal "Go," the test performer gets up from the chair (pushing off of thighs is permitted), walks as quickly as possible around the cone, and returns to the seated position in the chair. After a demonstration, the performer should walk through the test one time for practice. Two test trials then are administered; the score is the elapsed time (nearest 0.1 second) from the signal "Go" until the performer returns to the seated position in the chair. The best score of the two trials is recorded.

7. Body composition: Body mass index. The body mass index (BMI) is a weight:height ratio that is correlated with body fat. It is determined by dividing weight (in kilograms) by height (in meters) squared: $BMI = kg/m^2$. An alternative formula consists of multiplying the weight (in pounds) by 703 and dividing by height (in inches) squared: $BMI = (pounds \times 703)/inches^2$. The following BMI ratings are generally used:

below 20: may indicate loss of muscle mass and bone tissue, especially in older adults

20–25: normal range

above 25: overweight; higher risk of health problems

Physical Activity for the Older Adult

The term *physical activity* may be defined in many different ways. In this discussion of the older adult, physical activity includes all movements associated with everyday life (e.g., work, routine activities, exercise activities, and recreational activities). Usually, older adults are retired or their work responsibilities require little physical activity. For this reason, it is important that the lifestyle of these individuals includes recreational activities, exercise, or other activities that require physical exertion.

The older adult can experience the benefits of physical activity in much the same way as younger individuals. It is the immediate benefits that encourage most individuals to maintain an active lifestyle. With an active lifestyle, older adults:

- have a better self-image
- sleep better
- maintain appropriate body composition
- have better muscle tone and strength
- better manage stress
- are more likely to have a positive attitude
- experience fewer minor infectious ailments
- have more frequent bowel movements (less constipation)

These benefits can be experienced shortly after changing to an active lifestyle. Over the long term, the benefits include:

- continuation of immediate benefits
- increased cardiorespiratory endurance
- increased muscle strength and endurance
- increased flexibility
- prevention of bone loss, decreased risk of osteoporosis
- prevention and/or postponement of declines in balance and coordination
- postponement of decline in speed of movement and reaction time
- improved mental health

It is now accepted that regular physical activity can provide benefits for all older individuals regardless of their physical health. It is not advisable, however, to prepare exercise or activity guidelines that can be applied to all older adults. In the preparation of such guidelines, individual differences in health status, physical fitness, and previous lifestyle must be considered. For most individuals, physical activity of mild to moderate intensity is not dangerous. Some individuals, however, should consult a physician before increasing their physical activity. The *ACSM Fitness Book* (1998) and PAR-Q & YOU in figure 10.2 provide a list of questions that will help individuals determine whether medical clearance should be obtained.

Even though individual differences should be considered, general exercise guidelines for older adults are as follows.

Activity

Large-muscle, rhythmic activities provide cardiorespiratory benefits. Examples of such aerobic activities are bicycling, jogging, swimming, and walking.

Frequency

The activities should be performed a minimum of two or three times a week. After a period of adjustment to the activity, most individuals are able to exercise 4 to 6 days a week without any negative consequences.

Duration

Although a sedentary individual can benefit from any activity increase, the typical exercise session would be:

warm-up and stretching: 10 to 20 minutes

aerobic activity: 20 to 30 minutes

cool down: 5 to 10 minutes

Intensity

The program should be one of low to moderate intensity and related to the functional capacity of the individual.

These guidelines are primarily for aerobic activities. Flexibility and muscular fitness (strength and endurance) exercises also should be included in an exercise program for the older adult. Upper and lower body muscle groups can benefit through the use of hand and leg weights. As are aerobic activities, muscle fitness exercises should be related to the functional capacity of the individual. Also, it is often best to avoid the use of rigid guidelines when prescribing any exercise for the older adult. Many sedentary individuals can experience health benefits through 10- to 15-minute segments of mild activity.

17 Special Populations

Upon completion of this chapter, you should be able to

1. Define the term *special populations,* and state what must be done in public physical education programs to meet the needs of special populations;

2. Describe the role of physical performance measurement in special physical education programs;

3. Justify the use of norm-referenced and criterion-referenced tests with special populations; and

4. Select appropriate perceptual-motor performance, motor performance, and physical fitness tests, and administer them to special populations.

The term **special populations** is used when referring to disabled, handicapped, or impaired individuals. Federal laws require all public agencies to ensure a continuum of alternative placements to meet children's needs for special education and related services; the children are to be educated in the least restrictive environment in which their educational needs can be provided. Therefore, when disabled individuals cannot benefit from placement in a regular physical education program, federal laws dictate that the program be adapted or modified to meet their needs. As a physical educator, you should seek approaches to these adaptations that will emphasize what the individuals can do; accentuate the positive. However, the adaptations will not be the same for everyone. Special needs vary for persons with different disabilities and with different degrees of the same disability. Your professional preparation should include one or two courses that promote a better understanding of the needs of disabled individuals and the means by which physical educators can provide appropriate and worthwhile programs for all disabled students. This chapter emphasizes the place of measurement and assessment in physical education programs for special populations and provides examples of perceptual-motor performance, motor performance, and physical fitness tests that may be used for screening and diagnostic purposes. Many tests are available. Though a few tests are described in this chapter, you should review other available tests and select the one that best meets your needs.

No activities for development of perceptual-motor abilities, motor abilities, and physical fitness will be described in this chapter. However, many activities or modifications of activities described in previous chapters can be used for such purposes. In addition, there are many types and degrees of disability, and the activities for development of perceptual-motor abilities, motor abilities, and physical fitness may vary with the type of disability.

Why Measure Special Populations?

Several public laws have had instrumental influence on educational programs for individuals with disabilities, but the Individuals with Disabilities Education Act of

1990 (Public Law 101–476 and subsequent amendments) includes the most recent version and amendments of these laws. This act expanded upon the previous Education for the Handicapped Act and amendments, including PL 91–230 in 1970, PL 94–142 in 1975, PL 98–199 in 1983, and PL 99–457 in 1986. The Individuals with Disabilities Education Act (IDEA) states that disabled students have a right to the following:

- A free and appropriate education
- Physical education
- Equal opportunity in athletics and intramurals
- An individualized education program (IEP) designed to meet unique needs
- Programs conducted in the least restrictive environment
- Nondiscriminatory testing and objective criteria for placement
- Due process
- Related services to assist in special education

Although all of the public laws listed above have implications for the role of physical education, the Education for All Handicapped Children Act of 1975, PL 94–142, emphasizes the importance of evaluation in the education of disabled and handicapped children. Through the law, a framework has been established in which evaluation is the key to the type of program provided. Not all aspects of the law pertaining to evaluation will be described here, but the major points are as follows:

1. Every state is required to develop a plan for identifying, locating, and evaluating all disabled and handicapped students.
2. All disabled and handicapped children and their parents are guaranteed procedural safeguards. Known as due process, this requirement means that parents and their children must be informed of their rights, and they may challenge educational decisions they feel are unfair. The law also includes the following requirements: the parents must give written permission for their child to be evaluated; the results of the evaluation must be explained to the parents; the parents may request that an independent evaluation be conducted outside the school; and if the parents and the school cannot agree on the evaluation findings, a special hearing

must be held. All evaluation results must be kept confidential.
3. Standards for evaluation must be followed. Tests must be used that measure achievement level rather than impaired sensory, manual, or speaking skills, and more than one test procedure must be used to determine the student's educational status. Since many disabled and handicapped students have communication problems, tests must be administered to test ability rather than communication skills. Finally, a multidisciplinary team of qualified professionals must administer the test and interpret the results.

If you assume a professional position that includes responsibilities with special populations, you should be familiar with all aspects of IDEA and PL 94–142, as well as with all other public laws for disabled individuals.

Regardless of federal laws, individuals with disabilities should have the opportunity to participate in physical activity. For the most part, they can gain very similar benefits from physical activity as individuals without disabilities. Through physical activity, they can enhance the functioning and health of their heart, lungs, muscles, and bones; improve their flexibility, mobility, and coordination; and lessen the negative effects of some conditions or slow the progression of others. In addition, physical activity can develop stamina to make the demands of their daily living easier.

Norm-Referenced or Criterion-Referenced Tests?

Should norm-referenced or criterion-referenced tests be used with special populations? Really, it is not a choice of using only one or the other, for both norm-referenced and criterion-referenced tests are needed when working with handicapped students. Norm-referenced tests serve the same purposes as they do for other populations: standardized norms are useful in screening for motor problems, in comparing students with similar handicaps, in program evaluation, and in the placement of students. Criterion-referenced tests are especially useful in measuring student progress and for making instructional decisions about individual students. These tests also can be used for screening purposes when students are asked to perform certain basic skills.

- define the term *special populations,* and state what must be done in public physical education programs to meet the needs of special populations?
- describe the role of physical performance measurement in special physical education programs?
- state why norm-referenced and criterion-referenced measurement should be used in physical education programs for special populations?

Perceptual-Motor Performance Tests

Perceptual-motor performance tests sample the ability of children to integrate sensory information with past experience to make decisions about movement. There is little doubt that perception is an important aspect of successful movement, so perceptual-motor performance tests can be valuable educational tools. However, they should not be interpreted as providing an overall measurement of motor ability. Rather, each item of the test battery should be used to measure a separate, specific factor. Components of perceptual-motor efficiency include balance, postural and locomotor awareness, visual perception, auditory perception, kinesthetic perception, tactile perception, body awareness, and laterality and directionality. Perceptual-motor programs for the handicapped are important, but they should not be used in place of physical education programs. A strong physical education program is essential to every child's motor development. Some handicapped children may need both programs.

Before any formal testing of disabled students, familiarize yourself with their basic motor behavioral patterns. You may obtain much information through the informal techniques of observation, self-testing, discussion with others, and rating scales and checklists. The preferred hand and foot should be determined, as well as any movement patterns that can be used in a positive way. Preliminary measurement of such skills as running, skipping, balancing, catching, throwing, striking an object, and kicking may be conducted with a rating scale by ask-ing the students to perform these skills while you observe. This type of preliminary testing may prevent problems during the formal testing.

Many perceptual-motor tests are available, but only three are presented as examples to illustrate the types of test components that may be included in perceptual-motor tests. You should refer to other sources before selecting a test. The test you choose to administer will depend on your needs and the age group you wish to test.

■ Purdue Perceptual Motor Survey
(Roach and Kephart 1966)

Though referred to as a test, the Purdue Perceptual Motor Survey is a survey. The survey manual includes clear and precise instructions for scoring and administering each item as well as illustrations clarifying exactly what the child is expected to do. Forms for recording each child's performance are provided. The survey may be purchased from Merrill Publishing Co., Inc., P.O. Box 508, Columbus, OH 43216.
Age Level. Six through ten.
Equipment. Visual achievement forms, chalkboard, chalk, yardstick, penlight.

Test Components
1. Balance and posture. Walking forward, backward, and sideward on a walking board and performing a series of jumping, hopping, and skipping tasks while maintaining balance.
2. Body image and differentiation. Identification of body parts, imitation of movement, and participation in various obstacle-course activities.
3. Perceptual-motor match. Drawing circles and lines on a chalkboard and performing eight rhythmic writing tasks.
4. Ocular control. Ocular-pursuit tasks involving individual eye movement and simultaneous eye movement.
5. Form-perception. Drawing various geometric shapes on a sheet of paper.

■ Ayres Southern California Perceptual-Motor Tests
(Miller and Sullivan 1982)

To perform this test, the child must understand simple verbal directions. In addition, because five of the six items call for adequate motor responses, caution must be taken in testing children with neuromuscular impairment. The test battery can be administered in approximately 20 minutes. The test may be purchased from Western Psychological Services, Los Angeles, California.

Age Level. Four through eight.

Equipment. Watch, table, chairs.

Test Components

1. Imitation of postures. Imitate twelve postures demonstrated by the instructor.
2. Crossing midline of body. Point at, or touch, the designated ear or eye, using the left or the right hand.
3. Bilateral motor coordination. Use the palms of the hands to gently slap or touch the thighs with a rhythmical motion.
4. Right-left discrimination. Identify own left and right sides, those of another pupil, or of various objects.
5. Standing balance, eyes open. Maintain balance while standing on one foot, then change to the other foot. Balance is timed for each foot.
6. Standing balance, eyes closed. Same as component 5, except the eyes are kept closed throughout.

■ Andover Perceptual-Motor Test
(Nichols, Arsenault, and Giuffre 1980)

The Andover Perceptual-Motor Test measures the basic perceptual-motor areas necessary for normal development and motor learning. The test should be used as a quick screening device, not as a diagnostic tool. It can be administered to a group of twenty-five children in two 30-minute class sessions.

Age Level. Four through seven.

Equipment. Primary balance beam, two 8-inch balls, marking tape, dowel or stick.

Test Components

1. Balance. The ability to maintain static and dynamic balance.
2. Eye-hand coordination. The ability to coordinate the eyes and hands to accomplish a task.
3. Locomotion. The ability to ambulate the body through space; a combination of strength, coordination, and balance is needed to perform this item.
4. Spatial awareness. The ability to make spatial judgments and perceive the body in relation to other objects in space.
5. Rhythm. The ability to hear, interpret the sounds heard, and respond to what is interpreted.

Motor Performance Tests

For many years, educators have been interested in the relationship of age and motor performance. Because of this interest, many tests have been established for measurement of motor skills and to compare an individual's motor performance with that of other individuals of similar age. (Many of these tests have been described in previous chapters.) Motor performance tests also have been established to serve as screening instruments, to help identify individuals with motor deficiencies and those in need of special education.

However, these tests often are incorrectly used to measure individual growth and progress over a period of time. Some teachers mistakenly believe that test scores will improve if students participate in a variety of movement experiences. But you should not expect changes in test scores unless the students practice items or skills that are very similar to the test items. Because many motor performance skills are highly specific, transfer of learning does not always occur because of participation in general movement experiences. On the other hand, assuming that no improvement in motor performance has taken place if test scores do not change is also incorrect. The students may have improved in skills that are not measured by the test. In addition, a general background in motor performance serves as a foundation for the development of specific motor skills. There are many motor performance tests, but only four are presented as examples.

■ The Bruininks-Oseretsky Test of Motor Proficiency
(Arnheim and Sinclair 1985; Safrit 1986)

The Bruininks-Oseretsky Test of Motor Proficiency can be administered in two forms: as a complete form or as a short form. The complete form consists of eight subtests composed of forty-six separate items. Four subtests measure gross motor skills, three measure fine motor skills, and one measures both fine and gross motor skills. The complete test requires 45 to 60 minutes to administer. The short form also consists of eight subtests, but only fourteen items. The short form can be administered in 15 to 20 minutes. The division of the test into eight basic areas permits the teacher to be specific in determining where to place the emphasis in remedying the children's movement problems. No special training is required of test administrators. The test kit may be purchased from the American Guidance Service, Inc., 4201 Woodland Road, Circle Pines, MN 55014–1796.

Age Level. 4¼ through 14¼.

Equipment. Balance beam, ball, mazes, scissors, balance rod, matchbook, coins, small boxes, thread, playing cards, matchsticks, ballpoint pen, paper.

Test Components

Long Form
Subtest 1: Running speed and agility (one item).
Subtest 2: Balance (eight items).
Subtest 3: Bilateral coordination (eight items).
Subtest 4: Strength (three items).
Subtest 5: Upper-limb coordination (nine items).
Subtest 6: Response speed (one item).
Subtest 7: Visual-motor control (eight items).
Subtest 8: Upper-limb speed and dexterity (eight items).

Short Form
Subtest 1: Running speed and agility.
Subtest 2: Standing on preferred leg while making circles with fingers.
Walking forward heel-to-toe on balance beam.
Subtest 3: Tapping feet alternately while making circles with feet. Jumping up and clapping hands.
Subtest 4: Standing broad jump.
Subtest 5: Catching a ball with both hands. Throwing a ball at a target with preferred hand.
Subtest 6: Response speed.
Subtest 7: Drawing a line through a straight path with preferred hand.
Copying a circle on paper with preferred hand.
Copying overlapping pencils with preferred hand.
Subtest 8: Sorting shape cards with preferred hand. Drawing dots in circles with preferred hand.

■ The Basic Motor Ability Tests
(Arnheim and Sinclair 1979)

The Basic Motor Ability Tests (BMATs) are a battery of eleven tests designed to evaluate the selected motor responses of small- and large-muscle control, static and dynamic balance, eye-hand coordination, and flexibility. Each of the eleven subtests requires little training to administer. One child can be tested in approximately 12 to 15 minutes, and a group of five children can be tested in about 25 minutes, by one test administrator.

Age Level. Four through twelve.

Equipment. ½-inch beads; 18-inch round shoelace with ¾-inch plastic tip; 4" × 5" beanbags; wastepaper basket, 14 inches high; table; chair; transfer board consisting of two 8-ounce margarine containers, 4 inches in diameter, attached to and positioned on the board 12 inches apart; 30 regular-sized

marbles; yardstick; 4' × 6' mat; blindfold; stopwatch; balance board with width of 1¾ inches; basketball; 50-foot tape measure; two Nerf balls (3-inch diameter ball and 10-inch diameter ball); target consisting of four vertical lines, 1-inch wide and 8 feet high, which are connected at the top by a horizontal line 1-inch wide (vertical lines are 2 feet apart); playground ball, 10 inches in diameter; four cones.

Test Components
Subtest 1: Bilateral eye-hand coordination and dexterity. Bead stringing with 40-second time limit.
Subtest 2: Eye-hand coordination. Target throwing with beanbags and wastepaper basket.
Subtest 3: Speed of hand movement, crossing from one side of the body to the other. Transfer of marbles from one container to another; both hands are tested, with 20-second time limit for each hand.
Subtest 4: Flexibility of back and hamstring muscles. Sit and reach.
Subtest 5: Strength and power in the thigh and lower-leg muscles. Standing long jump.
Subtest 6: Speed and agility in changing from a prone to a standing position. Move from face-down to standing position and touch mark on wall; repeat cycle as many times as possible in 20 seconds.
Subtest 7: Static balance. Static balance on 1¾-inch balance board; performed with eyes open and blindfolded on preferred foot and other foot; maximum of 10 seconds per trial.
Subtest 8: Arm and shoulder girdle explosive strength. Two-hand chest pass with basketball; three trials.
Subtest 9: Coordination associated with striking. Ability to strike Nerf ball with hand and hit target drawn on wall; five swings with each arm.
Subtest 10: Eye-foot coordination. Ability to kick ball at target; five kicks with each foot.
Subtest 11: Agility. Rapidly move the body and alter direction; zigzag pattern around cones.

■ The Stott, Moyes, and Henderson Test of Motor Impairment
(Miller and Sullivan 1982)

The objective of the Stott, Moyes, and Henderson Test of Motor Impairment is to ascertain and assess motor impairment of functional or presumed neurological origin. The test was

derived from the original Oseretsky test and the revised
Lincoln-Oseretsky test. The revised form contains sets of five
test items each, one set for each year, ages five through
fourteen. It can be administered to most pupils in
approximately 20 minutes. Test procedures are available from
Brook Educational Publishing Ltd., P.O. Box 1171, Guelph,
Ontario NIH6N3.

Age Level. Five through fourteen.

Equipment. See test items (equipment varies for each age).

Test Components

1. Control and balance of the body while immobile.
2. Control and coordination of the upper limbs.
3. Control and coordination of the body while in motion.
4. Manual dexterity with emphasis on speed.
5. Simultaneous movement and precision.

Age Five

1. Balancing on tiptoes; feet together, eyes open.
2. Bouncing a ball and catching it in two hands.
3. Jumping over a cord at knee height.
4. Posting coins into a bank box.
5. Placing counters simultaneously into a box.

Age Six

1. Balancing on one leg; eyes open.
2. Bouncing a ball and catching it in one hand.
3. Hopping forward for 5 yards, between two lines.
4. Threading beads onto a lace.
5. Tracing a circular track with a pencil.

Age Seven

1. Balancing on one foot with arms raised; eyes open.
2. Following a track of holes in a wooden board with a
   pencil.
3. Walking heel-to-toe along a line.
4. Placing pegs on a board, one by one.
5. Touching tips of the fingers in order.

Age Eight

1. Balancing on one foot with other foot placed on the knee;
   eyes open.
2. Throwing a ball at a wall and catching the rebound.
3. Jumping sideward, three jumps, with feet together.
4. Threading a lace through a series of holes in a wooden
   board.
5. Walking while balancing a bead on a board.

Age Nine

1. Balancing on a wide board; eyes open.
2. Catching a ball in one hand.
3. Jumping and clapping twice before landing.
4. Placing a wooden pin through a series of holes.
5. Placing pegs simultaneously into a board.

Age Ten

1. Balancing on a narrow board; eyes open.
2. Guiding a ball round an obstacle course on a table.
3. Jumping over a knee-height cord; taking off with two feet
   together and landing on one foot.
4. Placing matchsticks in four small boxes.
5. Placing holed-squares simultaneously on two rods.

Ages Eleven and Twelve

1. Balancing heel-to-toe on two narrow boards; eyes open.
2. Hitting a target with a ball.
3. Hopping sideward into two squares.
4. Piercing holes in paper track.
5. Placing pegs on a board and squares on pins,
   simultaneously.

Ages Thirteen and Fourteen

1. Balancing on the toes of one foot.
2. Moving a ring along a rod.
3. Jumping backward and forward inside large circles.
4. Moving a pen around a track.
5. Piercing holes simultaneously with two styluses.

■ Test of Gross Motor Development
(Ulrich 1986)

The Test of Gross Motor Development consists of two
subtests. Subtest one includes seven items that measure
locomotor skills. Subtest two includes five items that measure
object control skills. The test provides standards for successful
performance of each item; the tester rates the performer as
successful or unsuccessful.

Age Level. Three to ten.

Equipment. Flat running surface, masking tape, 4- to 6-inch
lightweight ball, plastic bat, 8- to 10-inch playground ball, flat
hard surface, 6- to 8-inch sponge ball, 6- to 10-inch plastic or
slightly deflated playground ball, tennis ball, wall.

Test Components
Locomotor Skills

1. Speed run 50 feet.
2. Gallop 30 feet.
3. Hop three times.
4. Leap from one foot to the other.
5. Horizontal jump (standing broad jump).
6. Skip 30 feet.
7. Slide 30 feet.

Object Control Skills

1. Two-hand strike (baseball swing).
2. Stationary bounce. Bounce ball with one hand three times.
3. Catch ball with hands.

4. Kick stationary ball.
5. Overhand throw.

Physical Fitness Tests

The development of physical fitness is important for special populations for the same reasons it is important for other individuals. All children should be instructed in the why and how of a healthy lifestyle, and they should be provided the opportunity for development of health-related and skill-related physical fitness.

There is another important reason why special populations need to develop and maintain physical fitness: poor physical fitness can limit a child's performance and slow the rate of improvement in motor performance. For example, scores on balance and agility tests may be influenced by a child's poor muscular endurance and cardiorespiratory fitness. Any individual whose fitness limitations restrict progress in motor development should be involved in a program to strengthen those weaknesses.

The health-related and skill-related physical fitness of many handicapped individuals may be measured with the same tests or test items presented in chapter 15. Adjustments in the items may be necessary, depending on the type and degree of handicap. For example, distance runs may be reduced in distance. If it is necessary to reduce the distance to the point that it is no longer a valid measure of cardiorespiratory fitness, the run may be used as a motivational item. (When it is necessary to adjust a test item for an individual, it is important to not compare the resulting score with scores achieved by individuals who can perform the item without adjustments.)

■ The Brockport Physical Fitness Test
(Winnick and Short 1999)

In 1993, the U.S. Department of Education funded Project Target, a research study designed primarily to develop a health-related, criterion-referenced physical fitness test for persons with disabilities, age 10 to 17. The Brockport Physical Fitness Test (BPFT), the test developed through Project Target, is designed primarily for individuals with mental retardation, spinal cord injury, cerebral palsy, blindness, congenital anomalies, and amputations. The test, however, can be used for young people with other disabilities and in the general population. There are twenty-seven test items in the

BPFT, but generally four to six items can be used to assess the health-related physical fitness of an individual. Guidelines are provided in the test manual as to which items should be administered to the different populations and how the items may be modified. The manual also includes standards for each age, gender, and population.

Age Level. Ten to seventeen.

Equipment. Audio cassette player, PACER audio cassette, measuring tape, marker cones, electronic heart monitor (recommended), stopwatch, skinfold caliper, barbells and weights, gym mat, chair, adjustable horizontal bar, grip dynamometer, sturdy armchair, yardstick, standard wheelchair ramp, sit and reach box, sturdy table.

Test Components

1. Aerobic functioning: Four test options are provided.

   20-meter PACER. The procedure and scoring are the same as those for the PACER (included in the FITNESSGRAM) on page 190.

   16-meter PACER. The test procedure is the same as that of the 20-meter PACER. The shorter version is recommended particularly for individuals with mental retardation and mild limitations in physical fitness.

   Target aerobic movement test. This item measures the ability of the performer to exercise at or above a recommended target heart rate for 15 minutes. Test performers can engage in virtually any physical activity as long as the activity is of sufficient intensity to reach a minimal target heart rate and to sustain the heart rate in a target heart rate zone. One test trial is given; the score is pass/fail.

   1-mile run or walk. The test performers run or walk 1 mile in the shortest time possible. One test trial is administered, and the score is recorded in minutes and seconds.

2. Body Composition: Two items are included.

   Skinfolds. Skinfold measurements are used to estimate body fat. The measurements may be taken at three sites: triceps, subscapular, or calf. With one exception, the directions for skinfold testing described in chapter 13 should be followed. Rather than always performing the measurements on the right side, however, the measurements should be taken on the individual's dominant or preferred side. Three measurements should be taken at each skinfold site used. The middle measurement value is recorded as the criterion score. If a skinfold reading at the same site differs from other readings by 2 mm or more, an additional measurement should be taken, and the measurement that is substantially different should be deleted.

Body mass index. The body mass index (BMI) provides an indication of the appropriateness of an individual's weight for the individual's height. The BMI can be determined by using a chart in the test manual or by using the following equations: BMI = body weight (kg)/height^2 (m)

$$BMI = [body\ weight\ (lb) \times 704.5]/height^2\ (in.)$$

3. Musculoskeletal Functioning—Muscular Strength and Endurance: Sixteen items are provided.

Bench press. A 35-pound barbell is used to measure upper extremity strength and endurance. The test performer lies supine on a bench, with knees bent and feet flat on the floor or on rolled mats placed on each side of the bench. The performer grasps the bar, with the hands directly above the shoulders and the elbows flexed. On the start command, the performer raises the barbell to a straight-arm position and then returns to the ready position. This procedure is repeated without rest until the barbell cannot be raised or until fifty repetitions for males or thirty repetitions for females are completed. One repetition should be completed every 3 to 4 seconds. One trial is administered, and the score is the number of repetitions performed correctly, up to 50 for males and 30 for females.

Curl-up. This test measures abdominal strength and endurance. The procedure and scoring are the same as those for the FITNESSGRAM curl-up described on page 192. One trial is administered.

Modified curl-up. This test is similar to the curl-up with the following exceptions:

- The hands are placed on the front of the thighs.
- As the test performer curls up, the hands slide along the thighs until the fingertips contact the patellae. The hands should slide approximately 4 inches to the patellae or beyond, if necessary.
- If necessary, the test administrators can place their hands on the performer's kneecaps to provide a reach target.

Dumbbell press. A 15-pound dumbbell is used to measure arm and shoulder strength and endurance. While seated in a wheelchair or a sturdy chair, the performer grasps the dumbbell with the dominant hand. The elbow should be flexed so that the weight is close to and in front of the dominant shoulder. On the start command, the performer extends the elbow and flexes the shoulder so that the weight is lifted straight up and above the shoulder. When the elbow is completely extended, the weight is returned to the starting position. One repetition should be performed every 3 to 4 seconds until the performer is no

longer able to completely extend the elbow or until 50 repetitions are completed. One trial is administered, and the score is the number of presses performed correctly, up to 50.

Extended-arm hang. This test measures hand, arm, and shoulder strength and endurance. Using an overhand or pronated grip, the performer hangs from a bar or similar hanging apparatus for as long as possible, up to 40 seconds. The performer may jump to the hanging position, be lifted to it, or move to it from a chair. A fully extended position, with the feet clear off the floor, must be maintained throughout the test. The performer can be steadied to prevent swaying. One trial is administered, and the score is the elapsed time to the nearest second, up to 40 seconds.

Flexed-arm hang. This test measures hand, arm, and shoulder strength and endurance. Using an overhand grip, the performer maintains a flexed arm position while hanging from a bar for as long as possible. The performer is assisted to a position where the body is close to the bar and the chin is clearly over, but not touching, the bar. The body must not swing, the knees must not be bent, and the legs must not kick. One trial is administered, and the score is the time to the nearest second that the flexed-arm position can be maintained.

Dominant grip-strength. A grip dynamometer is used to measure hand and arm strength. The test performer is seated on a straightback, armless chair, with the feet flat on the floor. The dynamometer is squeezed with the second finger on the adjustable handle. After the handle is adjusted to the correct position, the performer squeezes the handle as hard as possible. The hand grasping the dynamometer should be held away from the body and the chair during the test. Three trials are administered with at least 30 seconds allowed between trials. The middle score, recorded to the nearest kilogram, serves as the criterion score.

Isometric push-up. This test measures strength and endurance of the upper body. The test performer assumes a front-leaning rest position with the hands directly below the shoulders, arms extended, the whole body in a straight line, and toes touching the floor. The test is ended when the correct push-up position can no longer be held. One trial is administered, and the score, recorded to the nearest second, is the length of time the proper position is maintained.

Pull-up. This test measures upper-body strength and endurance. Using an overhand (pronated) grip, the performer completes as many pull-ups as possible. The body must not swing, the knees must not be bent, and the legs must not kick during the pull-up. One trial is administered, and the score is the number of pull-ups completed.

Modified pull-up. This test measures upper-body strength and endurance. The test performer completes as many pull-ups as possible using the apparatus illustrated in figure 12.6, page 151. There is no time limit, but the pull-ups should be continuous. One trial is administered, and the score is the number of correct pull-ups completed.

Push-up. This test measures upper-body strength and endurance. The test performer completes as many push-ups as possible at a cadence of one push-up every 3 seconds. One trial is administered, and the score is the number of correct push-ups completed.

40-meter push or walk. This test measures whether the individual has the strength and endurance to traverse a distance of 40 meters without reaching a moderate level of exertion. The test performers walk or push their wheelchair a distance of 40 meters with a 5-meter start zone at a speed that is comfortable for them. The test performers are encouraged to travel at the speed that they usually use to move around the community. To pass the test, performers must be able to cover the 40 meters in 60 seconds or less while keeping the heart rate below the criterion for moderate exercise intensity. The test is timed to the nearest second. As soon as a test performer crosses the finish line, the test administrator counts the performer's radial pulse for 10 seconds. For the correct level of exercise intensity, test performers who walk or push a wheelchair with their legs must have a posttest 10-second pulse rate of 20 beats or less. Individuals who push a wheelchair with their arms must have a posttest 10-second pulse of 19 beats or less. Two trials can be administered. If two trials are used, the performer's pulse must be at or near resting level before the second trial is administered. The test is scored on a pass/fail basis. Performers pass when they can cover the distance within 60 seconds at the acceptable pulse rate.

Reverse curl. This test measures hand, wrist, and arm strength. The test performer lifts a 1-pound dumbbell with the preferred arm while seated in a chair or wheelchair. The movement starts with the weight resting on the midpoint of the thigh while the performer is in a normal seated position. The fingers are wrapped around the weight, and the forearm is pronated. With the wrist extended, the individual flexes the elbow and lifts the

weight until the elbow is flexed to at least 45° (the arm remains pronated throughout the movement). The weight is held in this position for 2 seconds and then returned to the starting position. The movement must be controlled and the downward movement must be slower than the gravitational pull. One trial is administered, and the test is passed if the performer can complete one correct reverse curl.

Seated push-up. This test measures upper-body strength and endurance. With the hands placed on the handles of push-up blocks, on the armrests of a wheelchair, or on the armrests of a chair, the performer attempts a seated push-up and holds it for 20 seconds. The buttocks are raised from the supporting surface by extension of the elbows. The extension position is maintained for as long as possible. One trial is administered, and the score is the time that the position is held, up to 20 seconds.

Trunk lift. This test measures trunk extension, strength, and flexibility. The procedure and scoring are the same as those for the FITNESSGRAM trunk lift described on page 192.

Wheelchair ramp test. This test measures upper-body strength and endurance. The test performers push their chairs up a standard wheelchair ramp. The test is not timed, and multiple trials are permissible. Going beyond the 8-foot line meets the minimal standard; the preferred standard is met when the performer either goes beyond the 15-foot line or makes it to the top of a longer ramp that the individual frequently encounters.

4. Musculoskeletal Functioning—Flexibility or Range of Motion: Five items are provided.

Modified Apley test. This test measures upper-body flexibility. The test performer attempts to reach back and touch with one hand the superior medial angle of the opposite scapula. One trial is administered for each arm. Scoring for this test is:

3—touch the superior medial angle of opposite scapula
2—touch the top of the head
1—touch the mouth
0—unable to touch the mouth

Back-Saver sit and reach. This test measures the flexibility of the hamstring muscles. The procedure and scoring are the same as those for the FITNESSGRAM back-saver sit and reach described on page 192.

Shoulder stretch. This test measures upper-body flexibility. The procedure and scoring are the same as those for the FITNESSGRAM shoulder stretch described on page 192.

Modified Thomas test. This test measures the length of the performer's hip flexor muscles. A thin strip of masking tape is placed on a sturdy table 11 inches from one of the short edges. The test performer lies in a supine position on the table so that the head of the femur is level with the strip of the tape (i.e., the hip joint is 11 inches from the edge of the table). The lower legs are relaxed as they hang off the table. To test the right hip, the performer lifts the left knee toward the chest and, with the hands, pulls the knee toward the chest until the back is flat against the table. At that point, the test administrator observes the position of the performer's right thigh. A maximum score is earned if the performer can keep the thigh in contact with the table surface while the back is flat. The procedure is repeated on the opposite side of the body. One trial is administered for each leg. The test is scored from 0 to 3 points as follows:

3—The tested leg remains in contact with the surface of the table when the opposite knee is pulled toward the chest, and the back is flat.

2—The tested leg does not remain in contact with the surface of the table, but the height of the performer's leg above the edge of the table is less than 3 inches.

1—The tested leg lifts more than 3 inches but less than 6 inches above the edge of the table.

0—The tested leg lifts more than 6 inches above the edge of the table.

Target stretch test. This test is a screening instrument used to estimate the extent of movement in various joints. For each movement, the performer is asked to achieve the maximum movement extent, and the test administrator evaluates the movement limit against sketches included in the manual. The eight movements are wrist extension, elbow extension, shoulder extension, shoulder abduction, shoulder external rotation, forearm supination, forearm pronation, and knee extension.

■ Kansas Adapted/Special Physical Education Test
(Johnson and Lavay 1988)

The Kansas Adapted/Special Physical Education Test Manual was developed primarily to address the need for health-related physical fitness testing of children with special needs in the state of Kansas. It is based on the rationale that all children can benefit from a structured program of physical activity and no child should be excluded, regardless of his or her handicapping condition. After proper testing, the test results should be used to develop individualized physical activity programs.

Age Level. Five through twenty-one.

Equipment. Mat, tape measure or yardstick, 12-inch ruler, 12-inch-high solid bench or box, masking tape, stopwatch, bar and weights (35 pounds), large enough area for adequate aerobic movement.

Test Components

1. Abdominal strength and endurance: Bent-knee sit-ups. Arms are crossed on the chest; individual may grasp the shirt. Feet are held by partner; elbows touch the thighs, and shoulder blades must touch the flat surface with each return to the start position. The exercise is continued until the performer stops for 4 seconds, quits, or completes fifty correctly executed repetitions. The test performer is encouraged by the tester and class through cheers, praise, and the act of rhythmically counting repetitions. Three tape reference lines can be placed on the mat or floor to help the teacher keep the performer's heels within 12 to 18 inches from the buttocks. Line one is for placement of the buttocks, line two is 12 inches from line one, and line three is 18 inches from line one.

2. Flexibility of lower back and posterior thighs: Sit and reach. Tape a 12-inch ruler to the front edge of a 12-inch bench or box where the 6-inch mark is at the front edge and the ruler is at a right angle to the edge. The front edge of the bench or box (6-inch mark) is considered the zero (0) position. The test is administered in the same way as the standard sit and reach test. If the test performer has an impairment in the limbs, the best functioning limb should be used. The position must be held for 1 second, and the score is the best of five trials. If the performer is unable to reach the 6-inch mark, the score is recorded as a negative score.

3. Upper-body strength and endurance: Isometric push-up and bench press. The isometric push-up score is the length of time (nearest tenth of a second) that the correct up position of a push-up can be held. The bench press is recommended for individuals thirteen years of age or older. The test performer assumes a supine position on the bench, with the knees bent and the feet placed on the floor on each side of the bench. The performer grasps a 35-pound barbell with both hands directly above the shoulders and raises the barbell to a straight-arm "ready" position. On command, the barbell is lowered until it touches the chest; it then is raised to the straight-arm position at a 90° angle to the body. This action is repeated until either the barbell cannot be raised any longer or fifty repetitions for males and thirty repetitions for females have been completed correctly. The flexed-arm hang and pull-ups are tests that may be used also.

4. Cardiovascular endurance: Run, walk, propelling in wheelchair, stationary bicycle, or propelling on scooter

board. Performer may use any fashion to elevate heart rate above the resting heart rate. The major objective is for the test performer to reach and maintain a heart rate between 140 and 180 beats per minute for 12 minutes after a 6-minute warm-up. The tester monitors the performer's heart rate every 3 minutes by counting the pulse rate at the carotid artery for 6 seconds. If the pulse rate is above 18 beats, the performer is asked to slow down and is closely monitored for stress. If the performer's pulse rate is above 20 beats for two consecutive checkpoints, the performer is stopped and the test is terminated. All test performers should be allowed 6 minutes of warm-up activity before starting this test item. The performer's score is the number of minutes he or she performs the test, as indicated in table 17.1.

■ FITNESSGRAM Modifications for Special Populations
(Cooper Institute for Aerobics Research 1999)

This test is a modification of the FITNESSGRAM test described in chapter 15. General and specific suggestions are provided for modifying testing procedures, the FITNESSGRAM report, and the recognition program so that the physical fitness of special populations can be addressed. Criterion standards for special populations are not available. The test activities may be used to establish an individual baseline for each student, and performances on subsequent tests can be compared with the baseline performance. Before the assessment, students should practice the items. If the teacher suspects that the disabled student does not understand the test administration, instruction and practice should be provided.

The recognition system used by FITNESSGRAM is *You Stay Active!* Exercise behaviors are emphasized rather than fitness performance. The program places its highest priority on the development and reinforcement of health-related behaviors, which are attainable by all students. It is intended that recognition be available to all children and teenagers. The criteria for earning recognition may be adapted to meet individual needs of students as necessary.

Age Level. Five through high school.

Equipment. Flat surface (e.g., parking area), swimming facility, skinfold caliper, mats.

Test Components

1. Aerobic capacity: Swimming, stationary bicycle, propelling a wheelchair, or walking. The following recommendations are for disabled students whose condition allows for maximal or near maximal estimates of aerobic capacity. The distances are arbitrary selections and may be modified on the basis of individual capabilities. Aerobic assessment is important to the disabled student because when it is repeated, performance improvement is probably due to an improvement in aerobic capacity.

   Swimming. If swimming is used as testing event, the student must be able to swim or to use a flotation device. The distance of the swim is 300 yards (younger elementary); 400 yards (upper elementary); 500 yards (junior high); or 700 yards (high school). The score is the time taken to complete the distance.

TABLE 17.1 Scoring for the Cardiovascular Endurance Event of the Kansas Adapted/Special Physical Endurance Test

Time Interval	Heart Rate		
	Below 14	Between 14 and 18	Above 18
First 3 min	Allow to continue, but give no credit	Credit for 3 minutes	Ask to slow down; monitor closely; credit for 3 minutes
Second 3 min	Allow to continue, but give no credit; encourage to speed up	Credit for 3 minutes	Ask to slow down; monitor closely; credit for 3 minutes
Third 3 min	Allow to continue, but give no credit; encourage to speed up	Credit for 3 minutes	Ask to slow down; monitor closely; credit for 3 minutes
Fourth 3 min	Give no credit	Credit for 3 minutes	Credit for 3 minutes

Source: R. E. Johnson and B. Lavay, *Kansas adapted/special physical education test manual,* Topeka, Kans.: Kansas State Department of Education, 1988.
Note. The test performer is stopped when the pulse rate is above 20 beats per minute for two consecutive checkpoints.

Stationary bicycle. Pedaling may be done with the arms or the legs. With the resistance set at a moderate level, the student makes as many revolutions as possible in 5 minutes. The score is the number of revolutions or the distance covered during the 5 minutes.

Propelling a wheelchair. The goal is to cover a specified distance in the minimal amount of time. The distance is 600 yards (younger elementary); 800 yards (upper elementary); 1,200 yards (junior high); or 1 mile (high school). The score is the time required to cover the distance.

Walking. The goal is to cover a specified distance in the minimal amount of time. The distances are the same as those for the wheelchair event.

2. Body composition: Triceps and calf skinfold thickness. If problems prevent measurement of skinfold thickness on the right side of the body, the left side may be used. The mixing of measurements from both sides is preferable to no measurements at all. If necessary, only one site may be used, or measurement may be made at the abdominal site. The measurements are used as reference points to indicate an increase or decrease in total body fat.
3. Muscular strength, endurance, and flexibility: Many mat movements may be used to test these fitness components. Students may be asked to do the movement as many times as they can with or without a time limit or to do a certain number of repetitions. Students with motor control problems probably will need to have timing factors removed from the testing as long as the movement is rhythmic and there is no pause longer than 2 seconds between repetitions. The important consideration is to establish a baseline performance that can be used as a basis of comparison to determine progress.

■ The President's Challenge for Students with Special Needs
(PCPFS 1999)

The President's Challenge as a measure of skill-related physical fitness is described in chapter 15. The test may be modified for students with special needs who meet the following criteria:

1. The individual has medical, orthopedic, or other health problems that should be considered before participation in physical activities, including physical fitness testing.
2. The individual has been participating in an appropriate physical fitness program that develops and maintains cardiorespiratory endurance; muscle strength, endurance, and power; and flexibility.

3. The individual has a disability or other problem that adversely affects performance on one or more test items.
4. The individual has engaged in all five test items, modified or substituted as necessary to accommodate the individual's condition.
5. The individual has performed all five test items in each of the five fitness categories and has performed at a level equivalent to a Presidential, National, or Participant Physical Fitness Award.

■ AAHPERD Motor Fitness Test for the Moderately Mentally Retarded
(Johnson and Londeree 1976)

The AAHPERD Motor Fitness Test for the Moderately Mentally Retarded is a modification of the AAHPERD Youth Test. It is intended to be used when testing mentally retarded children who are capable of learning (IQs ranging from 50 to 70). The test may include thirteen items, but six items are recommended as sufficient for testing the motor fitness of the moderately retarded. The remaining items of height, weight, sitting bob and reach, hopping, skipping, tumbling progression, and target throw may or may not be included depending on the testing situation.

Age Level. Norms are published for boys and girls, ages six through twenty.

Equipment. Metal or wooden bar 1½ inches in diameter, tumbling mat, stopwatch, tape measure, softballs, flat running surface.

Test Components
1. Arm-and-shoulder strength and endurance: Flexed-arm hang.
2. Abdominal strength and endurance: 30-second sit-ups.
3. Explosive leg power: Standing long jump.
4. Coordination: Softball throw for distance.
5. Speed: 50-yard dash.
6. Cardiorespiratory fitness: 300-yard run or walk.

■ Special Fitness Test for Mildly Mentally Retarded Persons
(AAHPERD 1976b)

The Special Fitness Test for Mildly Mentally Retarded Persons is a modification of the AAHPERD Youth Fitness Test. The norms are different, but the components are similar to those of the Motor Fitness Test for the Moderately Mentally Retarded.

Age Level. Eight through eighteen.

Equipment. Metal or wooden bar 1½ inches in diameter, tumbling mat, stopwatch, tape measure, softballs, flat running surface.

Test Components

1. Arm-and-shoulder strength and endurance: Flexed-arm hang.
2. Abdominal strength and endurance: 1-minute straight-leg sit-ups.
3. Agility: Shuttle run.
4. Explosive leg power: Standing long jump.
5. Speed: 50-yard dash.
6. Coordination: Softball throw for distance.
7. Cardiorespiratory fitness: 300-yard run.

■ Fait Physical Fitness Test for Mildly and Moderately Mentally Retarded Students
(Fait and Dunn 1984)

The Fait Physical Fitness Test is suitable for use with the educable and a majority of the medium and high trainables, if they do not have other handicaps that prevent safe performance of the test.

Age Level. Nine through twenty.

Equipment. Horizontal bar or doorway bar, mat, flat running surface.

Test Components

1. Speed: 25-yard run.
2. Static muscular endurance of the arm-and-shoulder girdle: Bent-arm hang.
3. Dynamic muscular endurance of the flexor muscles of the leg and of the abdominal muscles: Leg lift.
4. Static balance: Balance on one leg with eyes closed.
5. Agility: 20-second squat thrust.
6. Cardiorespiratory endurance: 300-yard run or walk.

■ Buell AAHPERD Youth Fitness Adaptation for the Blind
(Buell 1982)

This test for the blind is an adaptation from the AAHPERD Youth Fitness Test.

Age Level. Ten through seventeen.

Equipment. Horizontal bar or doorway bar, mat, stopwatch, tape measure, basketball, flat running surface.

Test Components

1. Arm-and-shoulder girdle strength and endurance: Pull-ups (boys) and flexed-arm hang (girls).
2. Abdominal strength and endurance: 1-minute bent-knee sit-ups.
3. Leg power: Standing long jump.
4. Speed: 50-yard dash.
5. Cardiorespiratory function: 600-yard run or walk.
6. Upper-body power: Basketball throw.

The norms for pull-ups (boys), flexed-arm hang (girls), sit-ups, and standing long jump are the same as in the revised AAHPERD Youth Fitness Test (1976a). Separate norms were developed for the 50-yard dash and for the 600-yard run or walk. The shuttle run test was eliminated, and a basketball throw was added to measure upper-body power.

 REVIEW PROBLEMS

1. Ask physical education teachers in local schools to describe the tests they are using to screen special populations.
2. Review in other sources additional perceptual-motor performance, motor performance, and physical fitness tests for special populations.

18 Sports Skills

Upon completion of this chapter, you should be able to

1. Measure sports skills;

2. State how sports skills tests may be used in physical education; and

3. Locate and select individual, dual, and team sports skills tests.

Many sports skills tests are described in the professional literature you will read. Some of these tests are valid and reliable; others are not. No attempt is made in this chapter to describe all good sports skills tests, but a very adequate sampling is provided. Unless indicated otherwise, the described tests may be administered to males and females. Collins and Hodges (1978), describe 103 tests for twenty-six sports. Their comprehensive guide is an excellent source for skills tests.

Selection of any sports skills test should be based on the criteria described in chapter 4. In addition to selecting a good test, you should recognize that some tests measure only one aspect of a sport. When such a test is administered, no generalization should be made about an individual's overall skill in a particular sport.

Norms are available for many sports skills tests, but unless you want to make national comparisons, it may be more appropriate to develop local norms. Often local norms are more meaningful, owing to differences in movement experiences, the socioeconomic environment of the group being tested, and the group used to develop the test norms.

Why Measure Sports Skills?

Perhaps the most popular purpose of sports skills measurement is to determine an individual's progress or level of achievement in a particular sport. Other important purposes for the measurement of sports skills follow.

Classification. A skills test can be administered early in the instruction in a sport to classify all participants. This early test eliminates the need to observe the individuals for several group meetings before attempting to classify them.

Diagnosis. Determining the strengths and weaknesses of the students can aid in the planning of unit objectives and can help identify students who may need special attention.

Motivation. Used correctly, a skills test can motivate individuals to improve their abilities in a sport. The challenge of competing against one's own scores often is more motivating than the challenge of competing against others.

Practice. While performing the test items, the students are actually practicing the skills of the sport.

Program Accountability. Test scores, as well as other information, can be used to demonstrate to the administration, parents, and the public the objectives and values of physical education. When no such information is available, the perception of physical education as a "play period" is reaffirmed.

?ARE YOU ABLE TO DO THE FOLLOWING:

- state how sports skills tests may be used in physical education?

Individual and Dual Sports

Archery

■ AAHPER Archery Test
(AAHPER 1967)

Test Objective. To measure archery skill.
Age Level. Twelve through eighteen.
Equipment. Standard 48-inch target faces, bows ranging from 15 to 40 pounds in pull, matched arrows (eight to ten per person) 24 to 28 inches in length, archery accessories (arm guards and finger tabs).
Validity. Face validity.
Reliability. No reliability estimate is provided, but the test manual states that no test item in the battery has a reliability less than .70.
Administration and Directions. No more than four archers should shoot at one target. Two ends of six arrows (total of twelve) are shot at distances of 10, 20, and 30 yards for boys and 10 and 20 yards for girls. All archers begin at the 10-yard distance and move to the 20-yard line when the two ends have been completed. This process is repeated for each line. However, individuals who do not score at least 10 points at one distance may not advance to the next distance. Each archer is given four practice shots at each distance.
Scoring. Standard target scoring is used, with the point values 9, 7, 5, 3, and 1 for the respective circles from the center outward. Arrows falling outside the outer circle or missing the target are scored 0. Arrows passing completely through or rebounding off the target are awarded 7 points.

Badminton

■ French Short-Serve Test
(Scott et al. 1941)

Test Objective. To measure the ability to serve accurately with a low and short placement (degree of serving skill should be developed before the test is administered).
Age Level. Junior high through college-age.
Equipment. Badminton racket, shuttles, rope to stretch above net, floor marking tape.
Validity. When tournament rankings were used as a criterion, a coefficient of .66 was reported.
Reliability. For college women, coefficients of .51 to .89 were reported.
Administration and Directions. A rope is stretched 20 inches directly above and parallel to the net. A series of 2-inch lines in the form of arcs are placed at distances of 22, 30, 38, and 46 inches from the midpoint of the intersection of the center line and the short-service line of the right service court. Each measurement includes the width of the 2-inch lines. The test performer may stand anywhere in the right service area, diagonally opposite the target. Twenty legal serves (may be two groups of ten) are attempted at the target (see figure 18.1). To earn points, the serve must pass between the rope and net and land somewhere in the proper service court area for doubles play.
Scoring. The scorer stands in a position (center of left service court, facing the target) to determine if the shuttle passes between the rope and net and to determine the point value of each serve. A score is awarded to any legal serve that passes between the rope and net and lands in the proper service court for doubles play. A score of 0 is recorded for any shuttle that does not pass between the rope and the net. The awarded points (5, 4, 3, 2, and 1) are based on the placement of the shuttle. Shuttles that land on a target line are awarded the point value of the higher area. If a shuttle hits the rope, the trial is not counted. Illegal serves may be repeated. The test score is the sum of the twenty serves.
Comment. The test performer should have the opportunity to practice this skill before attempting the test, because the reliability of the test is not as high for unskilled players. Drawing the target on the corner of a sheet or canvas for placement on the court will prevent the need of placing tape on the floor each time the test is administered.

■ Scott and French Long-Serve Test
(Scott and French 1959)

Test Objective. To measure the accuracy of the long serve.
Age Level. High school through college-age.

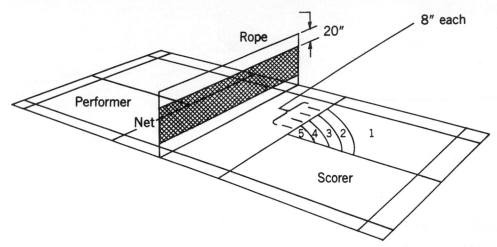

FIGURE 18.1 French short-serve test.

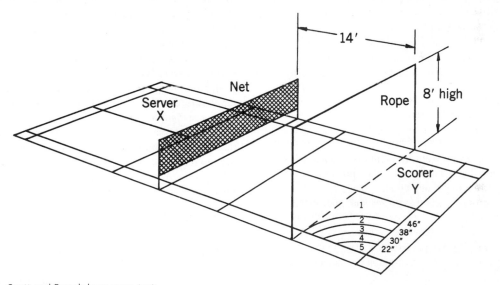

FIGURE 18.2 Scott and French long-serve test.

Equipment. Badminton racket, shuttles, and floor marking tape.

Validity. A coefficient of .54 was found by correlating the scores of college women with the subjective rating of judges.

Reliability. The internal consistencies of reliability estimates for college women were .77 and .68.

Administration and Directions. With the use of additional standards, a rope is stretched across the court 14 feet from and parallel to the net at a height of 8 feet. Floor markings are identical to those described for the French Short-Serve Test,

except for their location. The intersection of the long service line and the left side boundary line for singles is used for placement of the target (see figure 18.2). Standing anywhere in the service court diagonally across from the target, the performer attempts twenty legal serves over the net and rope to the target area.

Scoring. A score (5, 4, 3, 2, or 1) is awarded to any legal serve that passes over the net and rope and lands in the target area. Serves that hit the rope are taken over, and shuttles that land on a target line are awarded the point value of the higher

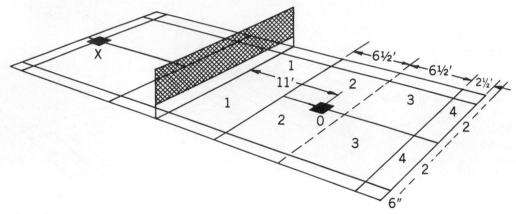

FIGURE 18.3 Poole forehand clear test.

target. Illegal serves may be repeated. The test score is the sum of the twenty serves.

Comments. Any serve that lands beyond the back line receives 0 points. Because most opponents play serves that would land close to the back line, the test administrator may choose to develop a point system that includes an area 2 to 3 inches beyond the back line.

■ **Poole Forehand Clear Test**
(Poole and Nelson 1970)

Test Objective. To measure ability to hit the forehand clear from the backcourt, high and deep into the opponent's court.
Age Level. High school through college-age.
Equipment. Badminton rackets, shuttles, and floor marking tape.
Validity. When tournament play was used as a criterion measure, a coefficient of .70 was found.
Reliability. With the test-retest method, a coefficient of .90 was found.
Administration and Directions. The scoring zones are marked as shown in figure 18.3. A 15" × 15" square is drawn 11 feet from the net astride the center line (0 in figure 18.3). Another square of equal size is drawn on the other side of the court at the intersection of the doubles long-service line and the center line (X in figure 18.3). If right-handed, the test performer stands with the right foot on the X square (left-handed, left foot) and a player stands at point 0 with a racket extended overhead. The performer places a shuttle, with the feather end down, on the forehand side of the racket, tosses the shuttle into the air, and hits it with an overhead forehand clear over the player's extended racket. The player calls out, "Low," if the shuttle fails to pass over the racket.

Scoring. The point value of the zone in which the shuttle lands is recorded, and the best ten of twelve shots are totaled for the test score. Shuttles landing on a target line are given the higher point value, and one point is deducted for any shuttle that fails to clear the extended racket of the player. The maximum score is 40.
Comments. The test performer should practice the tossing of the shuttle. The test also can be used to measure the backhand clear: The right-handed performer stands with the left foot in the X square, places the shuttle on the forehand side of the racket, tosses it into the air, and executes a backhand clear deep into the opponent's court.

Golf

Outdoor golf tests are preferable to indoor golf tests, and many such tests are available. In addition, it would not be difficult for you to devise accuracy tests for various clubs. Because of time and space limitations, however, it is sometimes necessary to administer indoor tests.

■ **Clevett's Putting Test**
(Clevett 1931)

Test Objective. To measure general golf putting ability.
Age Level. Junior high through college-age.
Equipment. Putters, golf balls and smooth carpet, 20 feet long and 27 inches wide (marked as shown in figure 18.4).
Validity and Reliability. Not reported.
Administration and Directions. The carpet is placed on a level, smooth surface. It is divided into three equal 9-inch sections running the full length of the putting surface. Beginning 8 feet from the starting point, 48 scoring areas, each 9 inches

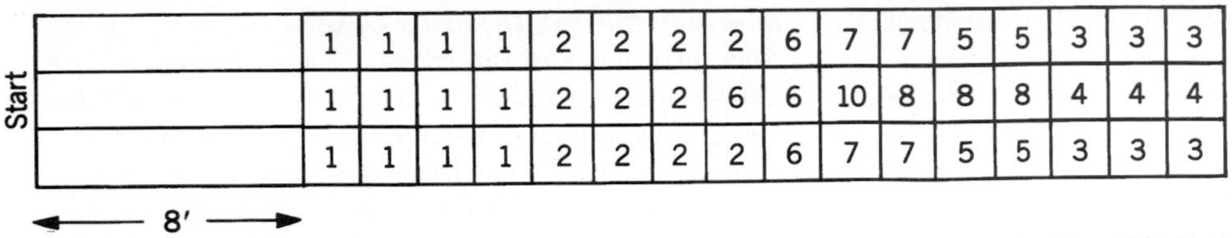

FIGURE 18.4 Clevett's putting test.

square, are marked off. The square 10, or the imaginary hole, is located 15 feet from the starting line. Ten putts are attempted.

Scoring. Each putt receives a numerical score based on the square on which the ball stops. The final score is the total points for the ten putts. Balls that stop on a line are given the higher point value. The test performer should be advised to putt too long rather than too short.

Comments. Cutting a hole in the 10 square makes the test more realistic. Also, with additional carpet, the distances can be varied.

■ Indoor Golf Skill Test for Junior High School Boys
(Shick and Berg 1983)

Test Objective. To measure golf skill with the 5-iron.

Equipment. Two 5-iron clubs (one right-handed and one left-handed), plastic golf balls, an orange cone, floor tape, tape measure, driving mat, floor mat.

Validity. A coefficient of .84 was found using a criterion measure of the best of three scores on a par-3, nine-hole golf course.

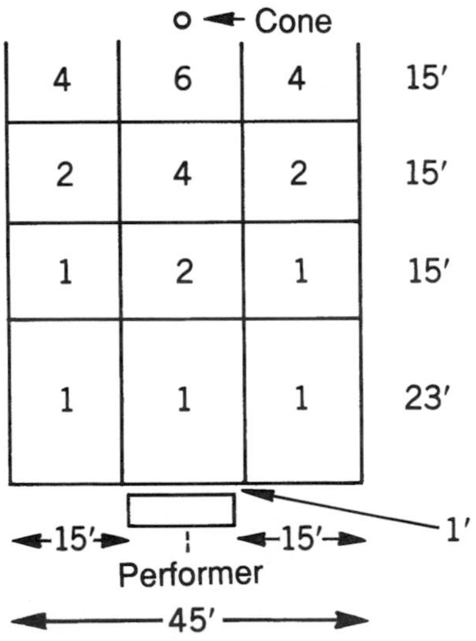

FIGURE 18.5 Indoor golf skill test.

Reliability. Coefficients of .97 and .91 were found for single test and test-retest administrations, respectively.

Administration and Directions. A target is placed on the floor of the testing area (see figure 18.5). Identifying the scoring areas with different colors will facilitate the scoring process. A mat is placed at the front edge of the target, and a driving mat is placed on the mat one foot from the target line. The test performer stands on the mat and hits the plastic ball as far as possible off the driving mat with a 5-iron, aiming for the orange cone. After two practice trials, twenty test trials are completed.

Scoring. Each trial score is the landing point of the ball on the target. Balls landing beyond the target but in line with the 4, 6, 4 target areas are given the point value of the closest target area. A topped ball that rolls through the scoring area is given one point. A ball landing on a target line is given the value of the highest adjacent target area. The test score is the sum of the twenty trial scores.

Handball

■ Tyson Handball Test
(Tyson 1970)

Test Objective. To measure essential handball skills.

Age Level. Originally designed for college males but also may be administered to males and females in high school through college.

Equipment. Handballs, gloves, stopwatch.

Validity. The coefficient of .92 was found for the three-item battery. Coefficients of .87, .84, and .76 were found for the 30-second volley, front-wall kill with the dominant hand, and back-wall kill with the dominant hand, respectively.

Reliability. Coefficients of .82, .82, and .81 were found for the items in their order of previous presentation.

30-Second Volley

Administration and Directions. Standing behind the short line holding a handball, the test performer puts the ball into play with a toss to the front wall, then volleys the ball against the front wall as many times as possible within the 30-second time period. Each return must be hit from behind the short line. Returns do not count when the short line is violated or the ball has bounced more than once. If the performer loses control of the ball, the test administrator quickly tosses him or her another ball. Either hand may be used.

Scoring. The item score is the total number of legal hits made in 30 seconds.

Front-Wall Kill with Dominant Hand

Administration and Directions. If right-handed, the test performer assumes a position in the doubles service box against the left sidewall, or if left-handed, the right sidewall. The test administrator stands in the middle of the service zone and begins the trial by tossing the ball against the front wall so that it rebounds to the right of the right-handed performer or to the left of the left-handed performer. As soon as the test administrator releases the ball, the performer is free to move, being sure to cross behind the test administrator to get into a better position for hitting the ball. Five trials to place the ball in the target area on the front wall and floor are attempted (see figure 18.6).

Scoring. The item score is the total number of points accumulated on the five trials, with 25 points being the maximum.

Back-Wall Kill with Dominant Hand

Administration and Directions. The initial position of the test performer is the same as that for the front-wall kill item. The test administrator, however, is now positioned in the center of the court, 6 feet behind the short line. The test administrator tosses the ball to the front wall so that it rebounds and bounces 8 to 12 feet behind the short line and approximately 10 feet from the right sidewall for a right-handed performer, or 10 feet from the left sidewall for a left-handed person. For best results, the toss should be aimed for a spot between 15 and 18 feet high on the front wall. (A bad toss does not have to be played.) As the toss is made, the test performer may leave the starting position and move into a position that allows him or her to hit the ball with his or her dominant hand as the ball rebounds off the back wall. Five trials to place the ball in the target area on the front wall and floor are attempted (see figure 18.7).

Scoring. The item score is the points accumulated on the five trials, with 25 being the maximum.

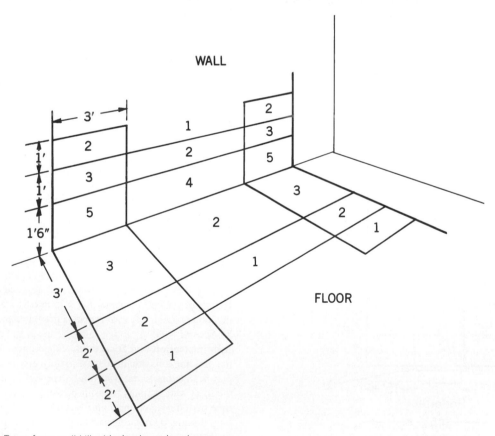

FIGURE 18.6 Tyson front-wall kill with dominant hand test.

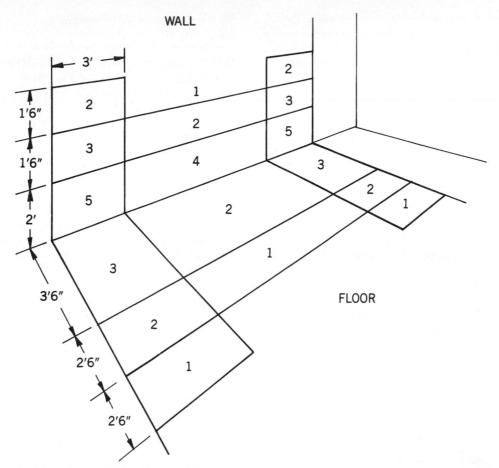

WALL

FLOOR

FIGURE 18.7 Tyson back-wall kit with dominant hand test.

Comments. The test administrator should practice the different tosses before administering the test items. Test performers should be aware that they do not have to return bad tosses.

Racquetball

■ Racquetball Skills Test
(Hensley, East, and Stillwell 1979)

Test Objective. To measure basic racquetball skills.
Age Level. High school through college-age.
Equipment. Rackets, four new racquetballs, colored floor marking tape, stopwatch.
Validity. With instructor ratings as the criterion, concurrent coefficients of .79 and .86 were found for the short wall volley and the long wall volley, respectively.

Reliability. Test-retest coefficients ranging from .76 to .86 for the short wall volley and the long wall volley for college men and women were found.
Short Wall Volley Test
Administration and Directions. The test consists of two 30-second trials, preceded by a 30-second practice period. Holding two racquetballs, the test performer stands behind the short service line, drops a ball, and volleys it against the front wall for 30 seconds. All strokes must be made from behind the short line. The ball may be hit in the air or after bouncing one or more times, and any stroke may be used to keep the ball in play. If the ball does not return past the short line or if the performer misses it, the ball may be retrieved or a new ball may be put into play. The test administrator should be standing near the back wall with two additional racquetballs in the event they are needed. Each time a new volley is started,

the ball must be put into play by being bounced behind the short line. The stopwatch is started when the performer drops the ball to begin the volley.

Scoring. The item score is the sum of the legal hits against the front wall for the two trials.

Long Wall Volley Test

Administration and Directions. The testing procedures for this item are the same as for the short wall volley test item, except the ball must be volleyed from behind a restraining line drawn 12 feet behind the short line. Two extra balls are placed in the crease of the back wall because the test administrator should not be in the court during this test.

Scoring. The scoring is the same as for the short wall test.

Tennis

■ Hewitt's Revision of the Dyer Backboard Tennis Test
(Hewitt 1965)

Test Objectives. To classify beginning and advanced tennis players by measuring rallying ability.

Age Level. High school through college-age.

Equipment. A smooth wall 20-feet high and 20-feet wide, tennis racket, at least one dozen new tennis balls, a basket, tape measure, stopwatch, floor and wall marking tape.

Validity. Coefficients ranging from .68 to .73 for beginner classes and from .84 to .89 for advanced classes were found.

Reliability. With the test-retest method, coefficients of .82 and .93 were found for beginner and advanced classes, respectively.

Administration and Directions. A line 1-inch wide, 20 feet long, and at a height of 3 feet is placed on the wall. A restraining line 1-inch wide, 20-feet long, and 20 feet from the wall is placed on the floor. A basket of tennis balls is placed at one end of the restraining line. The test performer, standing behind the restraining line with two tennis balls and a racket, serves the ball against the wall. (Any type of serve is allowed.) The stopwatch is started when the ball hits above the net line on the wall. On the rebound, the performer begins a rally from behind the restraining line and attempts to hit the ball continuously against the wall so it hits on or above the line on the wall. If the ball gets away, the test performer may take another ball from the basket. Each time a new rally is started, the ball must be served. Three trials of 30 seconds each are given.

Scoring. One point is scored each time the ball hits on or above the wall line. If the test performer steps on or in front of the restraining line to hit a ball, the rally is continued but no point is scored. No points are scored on the serve. The test score is the average of the three trials.

■ Hewitt Tennis Achievement Test
(Hewitt 1966)

Test Objective. To measure the basic tennis skills of the service, forehand drive, and backhand drive.

Age Level. High school through college-age.

Equipment. Tennis rackets, thirty-six new tennis balls, court markings, poles or standards, rope longer than width of court.

Validity. Coefficients ranging from .52 to .93 were found.

Reliability. Coefficients ranging from .75 to .94 were found.

Service Placement

Administration and Directions. A rope is placed 7 feet above the ground and parallel to the net. The right service court is marked as shown in figure 18.8. A 10-minute warm-up is permitted. The test performer stands to the right of the center line behind the baseline and serves ten balls into the marked service court. The ball must be served between the rope and the net. Net balls and balls that hit the rope are repeated.

Scoring. The point value for the zone in which each ball lands is totaled for the ten trials. Balls going over the rope are given a score of 0.

Speed of Service

Administration and Directions. The court is divided into zones as shown in figure 18.8. The distance the ball bounces after it hits in the service area gives an indication of the speed the ball travels. The score is based on the zone in which second bounce lands. Ten trials are given. This test can be conducted at the same time as the service placement test.

Scoring. The point value for the zone in which each ball bounces is totaled for the ten trials.

Forehand and Backhand Drive Tests

Administration and Directions. A rope is placed 7 feet above the ground and parallel to the net. The court is marked as shown in figure 18.9. The test performer stands at the center of the baseline. The test administrator is positioned, with a basket of balls, on the other side of the net at the intersection of the center line and the service line. The administrator hits five practice balls to the performer, who uses either the forehand or the backhand to return the balls. The balls hit by the administrator should land just beyond the service line. Twenty test trials are then administered the same way, the performer choosing which ten balls to hit with the forehand and which ten balls to hit with the backhand. If the drive goes between the net and the rope, points are scored, as indicated in figure 18.9. All net balls and those that hit the rope are repeated.

Scoring. The point value for the zone in which each ball lands is totaled for the twenty trials. Balls hit over the rope

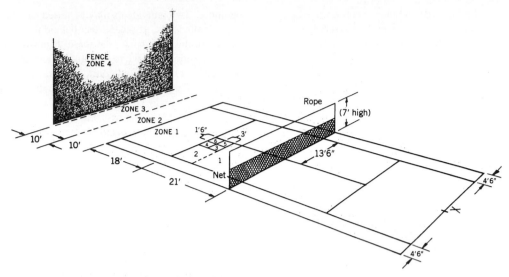

FIGURE 18.8 Hewitt service placement and speed of service tests.

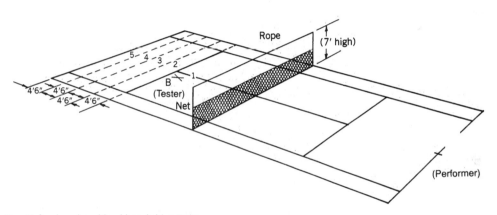

FIGURE 18.9 Hewitt forehand and backhand drive tests.

and landing in the scoring zones score one-half the regular value.

■ AAHPERD Tennis Skills Test
(AAHPERD 1989)

Test Objective. To measure the basic tennis skills of ground strokes (forehand and backhand) and the serve. A volley test is included as an optional item.

Age Level. Grade 9 through college.

Equipment. Tennis court, racket, twenty tennis balls, tape or chalk.

Validity. Concurrent coefficients ranging from .65 to .91 were found for the three items.

Reliability. Coefficients ranging from .69 to .95 were found for the three items.

Ground Strokes

Administration and Directions. Lines are placed on the court as shown in figure 18.10. A 5-minute warm-up period is permitted. The test performer takes a position behind and at the center mark of the baseline. The test administrator is stationed with ten to twelve balls on the other side of the net, within approximately 3 feet of the net and along the center line. Using an overhand motion, the tester tosses twelve consecutive balls to the forehand and twelve consecutive balls to the backhand. The first two tosses to each side serve as practice. The ball should be tossed so that it lands beyond the service line on the desired side and within 6 feet of the test performer. The test performer may elect *not* to swing at no more than two tosses for each side. This decision must be made before attempting to stroke the ball. The performer should attempt to hit the ball over the net into the designated scoring area within the singles court.

Scoring. Each of the ten trials for both the forehand and backhand is scored for placement and power. The placement score is determined according to the target area in which the ball lands. The power score is determined according to the power zone in which the ball lands on the second bounce. Balls that are wide, long, or hit into the net receive a score of 0 for both placement and power. The total score is the sum of the placement and power scores for each of the scored trials.

Serve

Administration and Directions. Lines are placed on the court as shown in figure 18.11. A 5-minute warm-up is permitted. Two individuals may be tested simultaneously. A box of balls is placed several feet behind the center mark on the end of the court where the server is positioned. One server takes a position to serve to the deuce court; the other takes a position to serve to the ad court. Two practice serves are permitted. Four trials are attempted into the designated scoring area; each trial may consist of a second service attempt if the first serve is a fault. The first four trials are directed to the outside half of the designated service court, and the next four are directed toward the inside half. After each server has attempted eight scored trials to the designated service court, the servers trade positions and repeat the procedure (no additional warm-up serves are permitted). Let serves are reserved.

Scoring. Each of the sixteen service attempts is scored for both placement and power. The placement score is determined according to the target area within the service court in which the ball lands. Serves landing in the designated half of the court are awarded 2 points; serves landing elsewhere in the service court are awarded 1 point; and those landing outside of

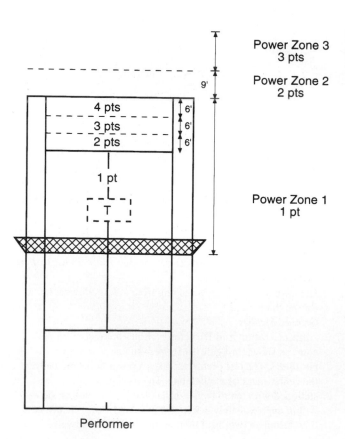

FIGURE 18.10 AAHPERD tennis ground stroke test—forehand and backhand drive.

Power Zone 3
3 pts

Power Zone 2
2 pts

Power Zone 1
1 pt

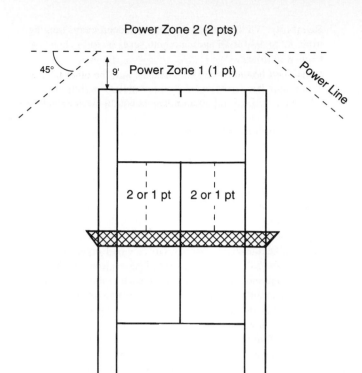

Power Zone 2 (2 pts)

45°   9'   Power Zone 1 (1 pt)

Power Line

2 or 1 pt | 2 or 1 pt

S   S

FIGURE 18.11   AAHPERD tennis serve test.

the service court are awarded 0 points. The power score is determined according to the power zone in which the ball lands on the second bounce. Serve balls that land outside the appropriate service court are scored 0 for power.

Volley (Optional Item)

Administration and Directions.   Lines are placed on the court as shown in figure 18.12. A 5-minute warm-up period is permitted. The test performer takes a position 3 to 6 feet from the net in the center of the court. The tester is stationed with a box of tennis balls near the center of the baseline. Using a forehand stroke, the tester hits ten balls to the forehand side and ten balls to the backhand side of the performer. The first four balls to each side are for practice. The tester should hit the balls at a consistent, moderate speed, approximately 1 to 3 feet above the net (waist high to head high of the test performer). The performer may elect not to attempt to volley a total of two trials for each side. This decision must be made before attempting to return the ball. If the tester judges that an improper setup ball was responsible for a low score on a performer's attempt, the trial may be repeated.

Scoring.   Each of the six designated trials for both the forehand and backhand are scored for placement. The placement score is determined according to the target area in which the ball lands. Balls that are wide, long, or hit into the net receive a score of 0. The score is the sum of the scores for all twelve trials.

Team Sports

Basketball

■ **AAHPERD Basketball Skills Test**
(Hopkins, Shick, and Plack 1984)

Age Level.   Ten through college-age.
Equipment.   Basketballs, stopwatch, floor and wall marking tape, tape measure, six cones.
Validity.   Coefficients ranging from .37 to .91 for all ages and both sexes on individual test items and from .65 to .95 for test battery as a whole were found.

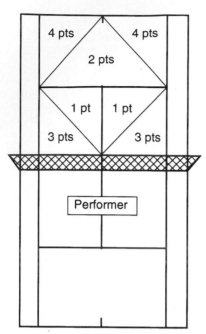

FIGURE 18.12   AAHPERD tennis volley test.

Reliability. With the test-retest method, coefficients ranging from .82 to .97 for all ages and both sexes on individual test items were found.

Speed Spot Shooting

Test Objective. To measure skill in rapidly shooting from different positions and, to a limited extent, to measure agility and ball handling.

Administration and Directions. Floor markers are placed on the floor as shown in figure 18.13. The distances for spots B, C, and D are measured from the center of the backboard; those for spots A and E are measured from the center of the basket. For fifth and sixth graders, the shooting distance is 9 feet; for grades 7, 8, and 9, it is 12 feet; and for grades 10 through college, it is 15 feet. Holding a basketball, the test performer begins the test with one foot behind any one of the five markers. On the signal, "Ready, Go," the performer shoots, retrieves the ball, and dribbles to and shoots from another spot. At least one shot must be taken from each of the five markers. A maximum of four lay-up shots may be attempted, but no two may be taken in succession. Three 60-second trials are administered, with the first being a practice trial.

Scoring. Two points are given for each shot made, and 1 point is given for each unsuccessful shot that hits the rim (from above). The item score is the sum of the scores for

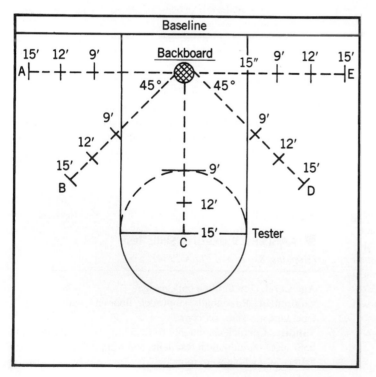

FIGURE 18.13   AAHPERD speed spot shooting test.

the two trials. The test administrator must record the number of lay-ups attempted, the point value of the attempted shots, and if the performer attempts at least one shot from each of the five markers. No score is given for shots that follow ball-handling infractions such as traveling and double dribbling or for more than four lay-up attempts. If the performer fails to shoot from each of the five markers, the trial is repeated.

Passing

Test Objective. To measure skill in chest passing and recovering the ball while moving.

Administration and Directions. A restraining line is drawn on the floor 8 feet from the wall and parallel to it, and squares are marked on the wall (as shown in figure 18.14). Only chest passes are permitted. Holding a basketball, the test performer stands behind the restraining line facing target A. On the signal, "Ready, Go," the ball is passed to target A. The rebound is recovered while moving to be in line with target B. The ball is then passed to target B. This sequence is continued until target F is reached, where two passes are attempted. The performer then moves back toward the target A. Three 30-second trials are taken, with the first being a practice trial.

Scoring. Each pass that lands in the target or on the target line earns 2 points. Passes hitting the wall between the targets earn 1 point. The item score is the sum of the two trials. No points are given if the performer's foot is on or over the line; if a second pass is made at targets B, C, D, or E; or if a pass other than a chest pass is used.

Control Dribble

Test Objective. To measure ball-handling skill (dribbling) while moving.

Administration and Directions. Six cones are placed as shown in figure 18.15. On the signal, "Ready, Go," the test performer begins dribbling with the nondominant hand from the nondominant side of cone A to the nondominant side of cone B. For the remainder of the course the performer may use the dominant hand, and hands may be changed when appropriate. Three timed trials are given, with the first being a practice trial.

Scoring. The trial score is recorded to the nearest one-tenth of a second. The item score is the sum of the two trials. The trial is retaken for ball-handling infractions, failure of the performer or ball to remain outside any cone, and failure to continue the test from the spot where loss of ball control occurred.

Defensive Movement

Test Objective. To measure basic defensive-movement skills.

Administration and Directions. The court is marked as shown in figure 18.16. The boundaries are the free-throw line, the end line behind the basket, and the free-throw lane lines. The middle lines on the free-throw lane serve as markers for C and F. Marks A, B, D, and E must be made with floor tape. The test performer stands at point A, facing away from the basket. On the signal, "Ready, Go," the performer slides to the left, without crossing the feet, to point B and touches the floor outside the lane with the left hand. Then, executing a drop step (changing defensive direction by moving the trailing foot

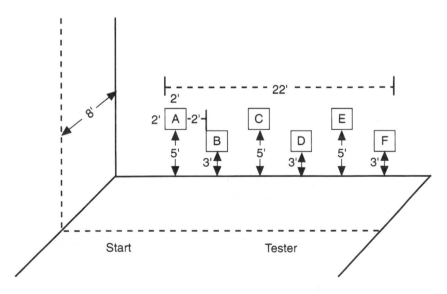

FIGURE 18.14 AAHPERD basketball passing test.

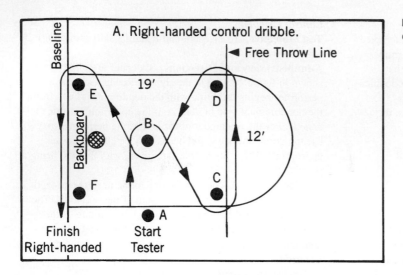

FIGURE 18.15 AAHPERD control dribble test.

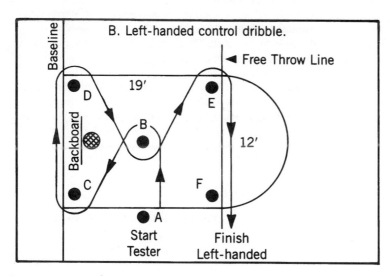

in a sliding motion in the direction of the next move), the performer slides to point C and touches the floor outside the lane with the right hand, performs a drop step, and slides to point D. The test is continued (as shown in figure 18.16) until both feet cross the finish line. Three timed trials are given, with the first being a practice trial.

Scoring. The trial score is recorded to the nearest one-tenth of a second. The item score is the sum of the two trials. The trial is repeated for crossing the feet during the slide or turn, running, failing to touch the hand to the floor outside the lane, and performing the drop step before the hand touches the floor.

Field Hockey

■ Chapman Ball Control Test
(Chapman 1982)

Test Objective. To measure the ability to combine quickness in stick movement with ability to control the force that is necessary to move the ball.

Age Level. High school through college-age.

Equipment. Hockey sticks, hockey balls, floor marking tape, stopwatch.

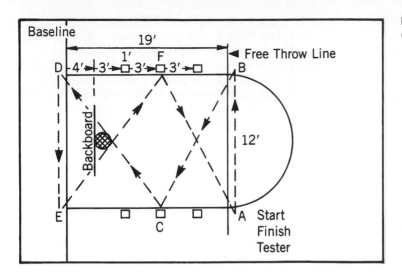

FIGURE 18.16 AAHPERD defensive-movement test.

Validity. Logical validity and, with a criterion measure of ratings of stickwork skills, concurrent validity coefficients of .63 and .64 were found.

Reliability. With single test administration, the coefficient of .89 was found.

Administration and Directions. A pattern is placed on the gymnasium floor (as shown in figure 18.17). The lines that divide the outer circle into three equal segments are ⅛-inch wide. (It is recommended that these segments be of a color that contrasts with both the hockey ball and the gymnasium floor.) The ball is placed just outside the outer circle, and on the signal, "Ready, Go," the performer taps the ball through or into and out of the center circle with a hockey stick. Each time the ball is tapped through or out of the center circle, it must roll outside the outer circle. Three 15-second trials are given. It is recommended the test administrator be assisted by a separate time keeper who can start and stop the trials at the end of 15 seconds. An alternate administration method is to tape record the "go" and "stop" commands at 15-second intervals, so the test administrator does not have to observe the stopwatch and the test performer simultaneously. Test administration should include a demonstration of the scoring techniques, a brief practice period, and rest between all test trials. Providing two practice targets enables two performers to practice while a third is tested.

Scoring. One point is scored each time the ball is tapped (not pushed) through or into the center circle. A point also may be scored when the ball is tapped from the center circle to outside of the outer circle and if it passes through a different segment from the one it entered. Points can be scored only when the ball is tapped outside of the outer circle or from

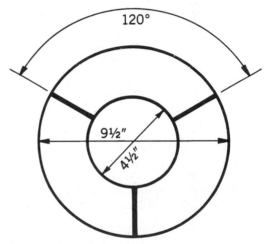

FIGURE 18.17 Chapman ball control test.

within the center circle. No points are scored when the ball is tapped while inside the outer circle or when it is tapped with the rounded side of the stick.

Football

■ AAHPER Football Skills Test
(AAHPER 1965)

The AAHPER Football Skills Test includes ten items that measure different football skills. Eight items, which measure skills also used in touch or flag football, are described in this chapter. No validity or reliability coefficients were reported.

Test Objective. Each item measures a single basic skill.

Age Level. Ten through eighteen; although designed for males, some of the items may be administered to females.

Equipment. Footballs, 8' × 11' canvas, five chairs, kicking tee, tape measure.

Forward Pass for Distance

Administration and Directions. The pass is made from within a 6-foot restraining area. The contact point of the performer's first pass is marked with a metal or wooden stake. Three trials are given, and the stake is moved if the second or third pass is longer. If the test item is administered on a football field, the restraining area should be placed parallel to the yard lines. (Administration of the test on a football field facilitates the measurement process because it is necessary to measure only the distance from the stake to the yard line immediately behind the stake.) The distance is measured to the last foot passed and at a right angle to the throwing line.

Scoring. The item score is the best pass of the three trials.

50-Yard Dash with Football

Administration and Directions. While carrying the football, the performer runs as fast as possible for 50 yards. The starter shouts, "Go," and simultaneously swings a white cloth down. The timer starts the watch with the downward arm movement of the starter and stops it when the runner crosses the finish line. Two trials are administered, with a rest period in between.

Scoring. The score is the better time of the two trials to the nearest one-tenth second.

Forward Pass for Accuracy

Administration and Directions. A target is painted on an 8' × 11' canvas. The diameter is 2 feet for the center circle; 4 feet for the middle circle; and 6 feet for the outer circle. The bottom of the circle is 3 feet from the ground. The target is hung from the crossbar of the goalposts and tied to the goalposts so that it remains taut. A restraining line is placed 15 yards from the target. The test performer runs two or three small steps along the line in the direction of the dominant arm, turns, and throws the football at the target. The pass should be made with good speed. Ten trials are administered.

Scoring. The target values are three (inner circle), two (middle circle), and one (outer circle). Passes striking a line are given the higher value. The score is the point total for the ten trials.

Punt for Distance

Administration and Directions. The performer takes one or two steps within a 6-foot kicking zone and punts the ball as far as possible. The test is administered the same as the forward pass for distance.

Scoring. Same as forward pass for distance.

Ball-Changing Zigzag Run

Administration and Directions. Five chairs are placed in a line, with the first chair 10 yards from the starting line and the others 10 yards apart. The test performer stands behind the starting line, holding a football under the right arm. On the signal, "Go," the performer runs to the right of the first chair, shifts the ball to the left arm, and runs to the left of the second chair. The run is continued in and out of the chairs (as shown in figure 18.18). The ball must be under the outside arm, and the inside arm must be extended (as in stiff-arming an opponent) each time a chair is passed. The runner is not permitted to touch the chairs. Two trials are administered.

Scoring. Each trial is timed to the nearest one-tenth of a second from the signal, "Go," until the performer passes back over the starting line. The score is the better time of the two trials.

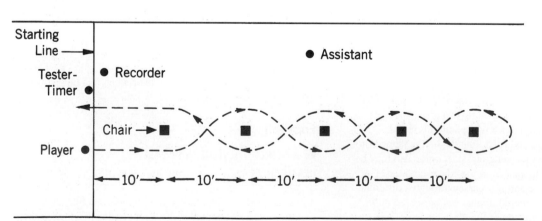

FIGURE 18.18 AAHPER ball-changing zigzag run test.

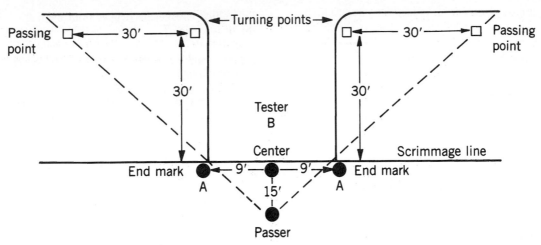

FIGURE 18.19 AAHPERD catching forward pass test.

Catching the Forward Pass

Administration and Directions. Two end marks, located 9 feet to the right and left of the center, are placed on the scrimmage line. Turning points are placed 30 feet in front of the end marks (see figure 18.19). The test performer stands on the right end mark and faces straight ahead. On the signal, "Go," the performer runs toward the turning point directly in front of him or her, makes a 90° right turn behind the turning point, and while continuing to run parallel to the scrimmage line prepares to receive a pass at the passing point. On the "Go" signal the center snaps the ball to the passer. The passer then takes one backward step to be in position to pass the ball directly over the passing point, slightly above the head of the receiver. The same pattern is run from the left end mark, except the performer makes a left turn at the turning point. Ten trials are run around each turning point. Poorly thrown passes are repeated.

Scoring. One point is awarded for each pass caught. The score is the sum of the passes caught from both sides.

Pullout

Administration and Directions. The test performer assumes a 3-point stance midway between two goalposts. On the signal, "Go," the performer turns to the right and runs parallel to the imaginary scrimmage line, makes a 90° turn around the goalpost, and races straight ahead across a finish line 30 feet away. Two time trials are administered, with the time starting on "go" and stopping when the performer crosses the finish line.

Scoring. The score is the better time of the two trials, measured to the nearest one-tenth second.

Kickoff

Administration and Directions. A kicking tee is placed in the center of a yard line on the field. The football is placed on the tee so that it tilts slightly back toward the kicker. Taking as long a run as needed, the kicker attempts to kick the ball as far as possible. Three trials are administered.

Scoring. The score is determined in the same way as the forward pass and punt for distance tests.

Soccer

■ McDonald Soccer Test

(McDonald 1951)

Test Objective. To measure general soccer ability.

Age Level. High school through college-age.

Equipment. Three soccer balls and stopwatch.

Validity. A coefficient of .85 was found by correlating the test scores of fifty-three college soccer players from three varsity levels, with the subjective ratings of three coaches.

Reliability. Not reported.

Administration and Directions. A restraining line is marked 9 feet from a wall, 30 feet wide and 11½ feet high. A soccer ball is placed on the restraining line. On the signal, "Go," the test performer kicks the ball against the wall as many times as possible in 30 seconds. Two soccer balls are placed 9 feet behind the restraining line in the center of the test area. In the event of a wild kick, the test performer may retrieve the original ball or use one of the two additional balls. The hands may be used to retrieve a ball. Any type of kick may be used, but all kicks must be kicked from the ground behind the restraining line. Four trials are administered.

Scoring. The number of legal kicks in each 30-second period is recorded. The test score is the highest total of any three trials.

Mitchell Soccer Test
(Mitchell 1963)

Test Objective. To measure general soccer ability.

Age Level. Originally designed for fifth- and sixth-grade boys but may be administered to girls and boys in grades 5 through junior high.

Equipment. Soccer balls and stopwatch.

Validity. With fifth- and sixth-grade boys serving as subjects, coefficients of .84 and .76 were found.

Reliability. With the test-retest method, correlations of .93 and .89 were found.

Administration and Directions. A target 4 feet high from the base of the wall and 8 feet long is marked on a smooth, unobstructed wall. The total width of the kicking area on the wall should be at least 14 feet (3 feet on each side of the target). A restraining line is marked 6 feet from the wall, and a boundary line is marked 12 feet from the wall (6 feet behind the restraining line). A soccer ball is placed on the restraining line, and individuals who serve as ball retrievers are positioned around and behind the boundary line. On the signal, "Go," the test performer kicks the ball against the wall target as many times as possible in 20 seconds. Any kicking technique may be used with either foot or leg, but the hands or arms may not be used. If the test performer miskicks or fails to block a kick, the retrievers stop the ball and place it back on the boundary line at the point where it rolled out. The performer retrieves the ball from that point (may not use hands), repositions it, and continues the test. The trial is given again for any action by the retrievers that causes an unnecessary time delay. The performer may go anywhere to retrieve the ball, but all legal kicks must be made from behind the restraining line. Three consecutive trials are administered.

Scoring. The test score is the total number of legal kicks made in the three trials. Use of the hands or arms at any time results in a 1-point reduction.

Softball

AAHPERD Softball Skills Test
(AAHPERD 1991)

Test Objective. To measure the basic softball skills of batting, fielding, throwing, and baserunning.

Age Level. Grade 5 through college.

Equipment. Standard softball field, adjustable batting tee, bats, eight marking cones, lime, softballs, measuring tape, gloves, stopwatch.

Validity. Concurrent coefficients ranging from .54 to .94 were found for the four items. The majority of the coefficients were above .70.

Reliability. Coefficients ranging from .69 to .97 were found for the four items.

Batting

Administration and Directions. Lines are placed on the field as shown in figure 18.20. Eight cones are used to mark the boundary areas. Two cones are placed at points 120 feet (grades 5–8) or 150 feet (grades 9–college) on diagonal lines drawn from home plate through points on the baseline 20 feet on each side of second base. Cones are also placed on these diagonal lines at points 180 feet (grades 5–8) or 240 feet (grades 9–college) from home plate. Four other cones are placed at the respective distances on the outside fair-ball boundary lines. The cones and the chalked lines separate the field into three power zones and three placement areas. The batter assumes a batting stance at home plate and attempts to hit the ball off the batting tee as far as possible within the center field boundaries. The batting tee should be adjusted to approximately waist height and placed in the center of the strike zone, opposite the front hip of the batter. Two practice trials and six test trials are permitted.

Scoring. The batter's score is the sum of the values of the zone in which the ball stops rolling for the six test trials. A missed swing, balls hit into foul territory, and balls stopping within the infield score no points.

Fielding Ground Balls

Administration and Directions. A 20' × 60' area is marked off as shown in figure 18.21. The player being tested stands in ready position behind the restraining line (point A). A thrower (point B) stands behind the throwing line and throws two practice and six test balls to each player. Each throw must strike the ground before the 30-foot line and must stay within the sideline boundaries of the marked area. The throws should be sidearm, with sufficient velocity to carry an untouched ball a prescribed, age-adjusted distance beyond the end line: 65 feet (grades 5–6), 75 feet (grades 7–8), 90 feet (grades 9–12), and 100 feet (college). The prescribed distance beyond the end line is marked by a cone or similar object (point C). Of the six test trials, two balls (in varying order) should be thrown directly to the player, two to the right (between the player and the sideline), and two to the left side of the player. The player attempts to field the ball cleanly and toss it back to the thrower. On each trial, the player starts behind the 5-foot restraining line but must move forward of the 60-foot line toward the approaching ground ball to obtain maximum points. Any throw not made as specified should be repeated. The thrower should periodically check the velocity of the throw by occasionally instructing the player to let the ball go by untouched. Throws should be within 5 to 8 feet of the velocity marker.

Scoring. Each ball cleanly fielded in front of the 60-foot line counts 4 points. A ball that is stopped, but bobbled, counts

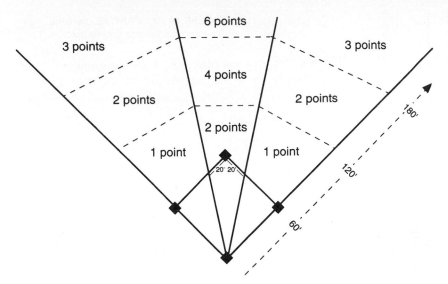

FIGURE 18.20 AAHPERD batting test for grades 5 through 8. Distance for grades 9 through college are 60 feet, 150 feet, and 240 feet.

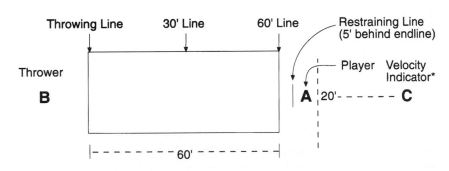

FIGURE 18.21 AAPHERD fielding ground balls test.

*Velocity indicator distances (past the 60' end line) are as follows:

65' - grades 5&6
75' - grades 7&8
90' - grades 9-12
100' - college

2 points. Only the player's glove and the ball must be in front of the line. Balls fielded behind the 60-foot line receive one-half the points normally earned, that is, 2 points for cleanly fielded balls and 1 point for bobbled balls. Balls that get past the player score no points. The score is the sum of the six trials.

Overhand Throwing for Distance and Accuracy
Administration and Directions. A throwing line is marked off in feet down the center of a large open field area, with a restraining line marked at one end perpendicular to the throwing line as shown in figure 18.22. A back boundary line is marked off 10 feet behind the restraining line. After the

proper warm-up, the player stands between the restraining line and the back boundary line, takes one or more steps, and throws as straight as possible down the throwing line. If a player steps over the restraining line before releasing the ball, the throw must be repeated. Two throws are attempted.
Scoring. The better of two throws is measured and recorded as the score. The score equals the throwing distance, measured at a point on the throwing line straight across from (perpendicular to) the spot where the ball landed, minus the number of feet the ball landed off target. Both error scores and distance scores are measured to the nearest foot. Figure 18.22 includes an example of scoring.

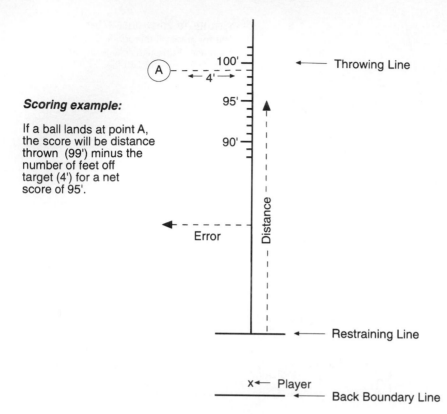

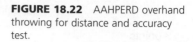

FIGURE 18.22 AAHPERD overhand throwing for distance and accuracy test.

Throwing Line

100'

4'

A

95'

Scoring example:

If a ball lands at point A, the score will be distance thrown (99') minus the number of feet off target (4') for a net score of 95'.

90'

Distance

Error

Restraining Line

x ← Player

Back Boundary Line

Baserunning

Administration and Directions. After a proper warm-up, the player takes a lead-off position in front of home plate with the back foot in contact with the front edge of the base. On the signal, "Ready, Go," the player runs around first base to second base. The player is to run through second base, rather than slide into it or stop on it. Two trials, with a rest between, are attempted.

Scoring. Trials are timed to the nearest tenth of a second from the signal "go" to the touching of second base. The score is the better of the two trials.

■ Fielding Grounders—Agility, Speed, and Accuracy Test
(Fringer 1961)

Test Objective. To measure the ability to field grounders, to run to a base, and to throw quickly and accurately to a target.

Age Level. Originally designed for high school girls but also may be administered to high school boys.

Equipment. Softball glove, several quality softballs, floor marking tape, stopwatch.

Validity. For high school girls, a coefficient of .70 was found.

Reliability. A test-retest coefficient of .72 was found.

Administration and Directions. A floor space of 30' × 40' with a 20' × 20' wall is needed. A target is placed on the wall, and markings are placed on the floor (as indicated in figure 18.23). Dimensions for the base markings are the same as for a softball base. The test performer stands with a foot on the start mark with a softball and glove. On the signal, "Go," the performer runs to either base, throws the ball at the target, rushes to field the ball, and quickly runs to the other base to make another throw at the target. The bases must be alternated for the throws, and a foot must be in contact with the base on each throw. Two 45-second trials are administered, with rest permitted between trials.

Scoring. Balls hitting on or in the target circle count. The test score is the sum of the target hits made in two trials.

■ Shick Softball Test Battery
(Shick 1970)

Test Objective. To measure defensive softball skills.

Age Level. Originally designed for college women, but the test also may be administered to males and females in high school through college.

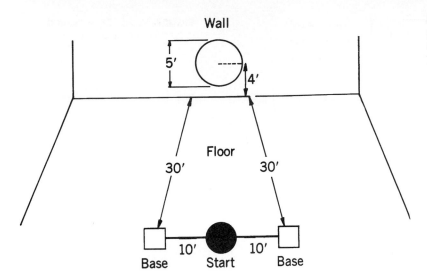

Equipment. Several softballs and stopwatch.

Validity. For two general softball classes of fifty-nine college females, a coefficient of .75 was found by correlating expert ratings with the test battery.

Reliability. A coefficient of .88 was found for the test battery.

Repeated Throws

Administration and Directions. A line is drawn on the wall 10 feet from and parallel to the floor. A restraining line is drawn on the floor 23 feet from and parallel to the wall. The test performer stands behind the restraining line, holding a softball. On the signal, "Go," the student throws the ball against the wall above the 10-foot line (overhand or sidearm throw is required) and attempts to catch the rebound in the air or field it from the floor. This action is repeated as many times as possible in 30 seconds. If fielding errors occur, the performer must recover the ball. However, there is no penalty other than the loss of time. The test consists of four 30-second trials, and the performer is given one practice throw before each trial.

Scoring. A ball thrown with the test performer's stepping on or across the restraining line or a ball hitting below the wall line does not count. The test score is the sum of the legal hits for the four trials.

Fielding Test

Administration and Directions. A line is drawn on the wall 4 feet from and parallel to the floor. A line also is drawn on the floor 15 feet from and parallel to the wall. The procedures are the same as those for the repeated throws test, except any type throw may be used, and all throws are to hit below the wall line.

Scoring. The scoring method is identical to the repeated throws scoring, except no ball that hits above the wall line is counted.

Target Test

Administration and Directions. The dimensions of the wall and floor targets are shown in figure 18.24. The wall target is 66 inches square, and its center is 36 inches from the floor. The target value areas are color coded as follows: five = red, four = medium blue, three = bright yellow, two = pale aqua, and one = black. A restraining line is marked on the floor 40 feet from and parallel to the wall. The test performer stands behind the restraining line for all throws. Two trials of ten throws each are administered. Two practice throws are permitted.

Scoring. Each throw is given two scores: one for the wall hit and one for the hit of the first bounce on the floor. Any hit outside the scoring areas of the wall and floor is recorded as 0. The test score is the sum of the two trials. The highest possible test score is 200 (50 per trial for the wall, and 50 per trial for the floor).

Volleyball

■ Brady Volley Test
(Brady 1945)

Test Objective. To measure general volleyball playing ability.

Age Level. College, but the test may also be appropriate for some high school groups. If administered to younger groups, it is suggested that the height of the target be lowered.

Equipment. Volleyballs, wall tape, tape measure, stopwatch.

Validity. For college males, a coefficient of .86 was found for the correlation between test scores and the subjective ratings of four qualified judges.

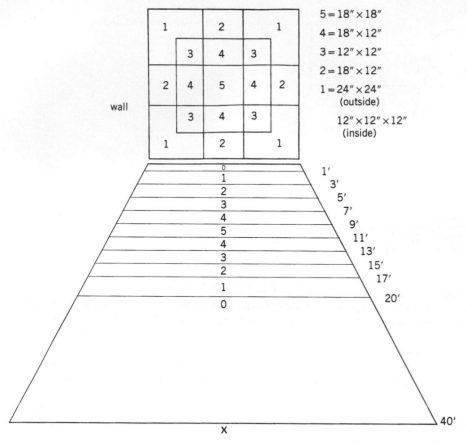

FIGURE 18.24 Shick target test.

$5 = 18'' \times 18''$

$4 = 18'' \times 12''$

$3 = 12'' \times 12''$

$2 = 18'' \times 12''$

$1 = 24'' \times 24''$
(outside)

$12'' \times 12'' \times 12''$
(inside)

Reliability. A test-retest coefficient of .93 was found.

Administration and Directions. A target consisting of a horizontal line 5 feet in length and 11½ feet from the floor is marked on a smooth wall. Vertical lines at the end of the horizontal line are extended toward the ceiling. The wall should be at least 15 feet high and 15 feet wide. No restraining line is used. The test performer begins the test by throwing the volleyball against the wall. On the rebound, and on all subsequent rebounds, the performer attempts to volley the ball within the boundaries of the target (balls landing on the target lines are counted). One 60-second trial is administered. Catching or losing control of the ball requires that the test performer rethrow the ball against the wall to continue the test.

Scoring. The test score is the number of legal hits in 60 seconds. Thrown balls do not count.

■ **Brumbach Volleyball Service Test**
(Brumbach 1967)

Test Objective. To measure the ability to serve the volleyball low and deep into the opponent's court.

Age Level. Junior high through college-age.

Equipment. Volleyballs, volleyball net, rope, tall standards, floor tape, and tape measure.

Validity and Reliability. Not reported.

Administration and Directions. A rope is placed 4 feet above and parallel to the net, and markings are placed on the floor (as shown in figure 18.25). The test performer stands behind the rear end line and attempts to serve the ball between the net and the rope so that it lands deep into the backcourt on the opposite side. Two sets of six trials are administered (total of twelve).

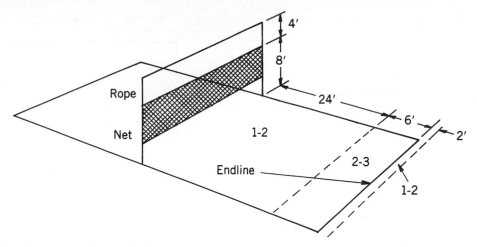

FIGURE 18.25 Brumbach volleyball service test.

Scoring. A serve that passes between the net and the rope receives the higher value for the target area in which it lands. Serves going over the rope receive the lesser value for the target areas. Serves that hit the rope are repeated. Foot faults, serves hitting the net, and serves landing outside the target area are given a 0 score. The test score is the sum of the ten best trials.

■ North Carolina State University Volleyball Skills Test Battery
(Bartlett et al. 1991)

Test Objective. To measure and evaluate the three basic volleyball skills: serve, forearm pass, and set.
Age Level. High school through college-age.
Equipment. Volleyballs, volleyball net, floor tape, two 8-foot poles or standards, two 10-foot poles or standards, 30-foot rope, 11-foot rope.
Validity. Because the ability to serve a ball, receive a ball with the forearm pass, and set a ball are basic volleyball skills, test items have content validity.
Reliability. Coefficients of .65 (serve), .73 (forearm pass), and .88 (set test) were found using the intraclass correlation technique.
Serve
Administration and Directions. The court is marked as shown in figure 18.26. Standing in the area indicated, the test performer serves ten times. The serves may be overhand or underhand.
Scoring. The point system was developed with the W-formation of reception in mind. Therefore, test performers are rewarded according to their ability to direct the serve to the areas

of the court with the least coverage. Serves landing on a line score the higher point value; serves contacting the net, antennae, or landing out of bounds receive no score. The test item score is the total points, with a maximum score of 40 points.
Forearm Pass
Administration and Directions. The court is marked as shown in figure 18.27, and a rope is placed on the side of the test performer at a distance of 9'10" (attack line) from the net and 8 feet high. The test performer is given five trials from the right back position (10 feet from right sideline and 5 feet from the baseline) and five trials from the left back position (10 feet from left sideline and 5 feet from the baseline). The test performer receives 10 two-handed overhead tossed balls from the tosser who is positioned across the net at the attack line (14'9" from either sideline). The performer passes the tossed ball over the rope and into the target areas, which have values of 1 to 5 points.
Scoring. The point system rewards the test performer's ability to pass the ball high enough for a setter to easily get under the ball. In most offensive systems, the setter moves to the right center of the court. Therefore, the higher point values are given in the areas of the court where the setter can deliver a good set. Bad tosses may be repeated. Balls landing on a line score the higher point value. Zero points are awarded for (a) illegal contact by the test performer, (b) any ball that contacts or goes under the rope, and (c) any ball that contacts or goes under the net. The item score is the total points for the ten trials, with a maximum score of 50.
Set
Administration and Directions. The court is marked as indicated in figure 18.28, and a rope is placed perpendicular to

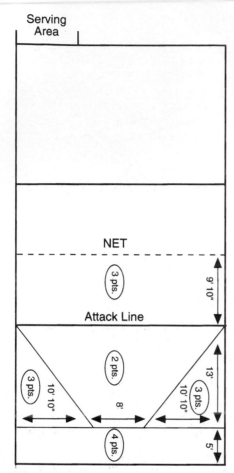

FIGURE 18.26 NCSU volleyball serve test.

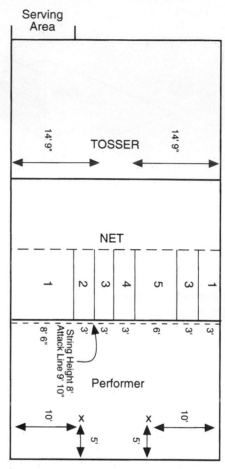

FIGURE 18.27 NCSU volleyball forearm pass test.

the net at a distance of 11 feet from the left sideline and at a height of 10 feet. The rope should extend beyond the attack line. The test performer stands in the marked area (6 feet from right sideline and 5 feet from the net) and receives ten underhand-tossed balls from the tosser who is positioned at midcourt (14'9" from either sideline and 10 feet in front of the baseline). The performer sets the tossed ball over the rope and into the target area, which has values of 1 to 5 points.

Scoring. The point system rewards the test performer's ability to make a high, outside set, which is the most common form of setting for beginners. Therefore, the higher points are given for balls that have the appropriate height and proximity to the sideline and the least points are given to balls closest to the net and/or the center of the court. Bad tosses may be repeated. Balls landing on a line score the higher point value. Zero

points are awarded for (a) illegal or double contacts, (b) any ball that contacts or goes under the rope, and (c) any ball that contacts or goes over the set. The item score is the total points for the ten trials, with a maximum score of 50.

■ Russell-Lange Volleyball Test
(Russell and Lange 1940)

Test Objective. To measure volleyball playing ability.
Age Level. Junior and senior high girls, but the serve item is also appropriate for junior and senior high boys.
Equipment. Volleyballs, floor and wall tape, stopwatch.
Validity. Coefficients of .51 (volley) and .79 (serve) were found when test scores were correlated with ability ratings of seven judges.

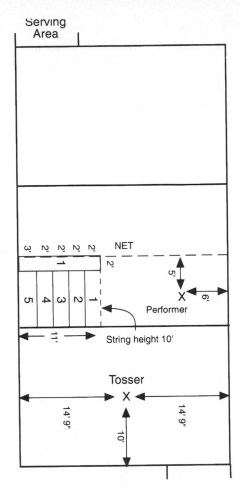

FIGURE 18.28 NCSU volleyball set test.

Reliability. Coefficients of .89 (volley) and .84 (serve) were found.

Volley

Administration and Directions. A line, 2 inches wide and 12 feet long, is placed with the lower edge 7½ feet above the floor. A restraining line is placed 6 feet from and parallel to the wall. Standing behind the restraining line, the test performer uses an underhand movement to toss the ball against the wall, then repeatedly volleys the ball on or above the wall line while remaining behind the restraining line. Three 30-second trials are administered.

Scoring. The legal volleys hit from behind the restraining line that hit on or above the wall line are recorded. The test score is the best score of three trials.

Serve

Administration and Directions. The court is marked as shown in figure 18.29. Standing behind the rear boundary line, the test performer attempts to serve the ball deep into the opponent's court. Two trials of ten legal serves are administered. Serves touching the net but landing in the opponent's court are repeated.

Scoring. Serves landing on a target line are given the highest target value, and serves in which foot faults occur are given a 0 score. The test score is the total points of the best trial.

> ### ► REVIEW PROBLEMS ◄

1. Administer one individual and one team sports skills test to several of your classmates. Ask them to provide constructive criticism of your test administration.

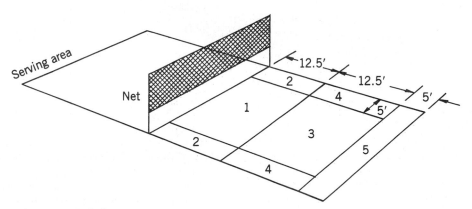

FIGURE 18.29 Russell-Lange volleyball serve test.

2. Additional sports skills tests are presented at the conclusion of this chapter. Review at least one test for each sport, noting the validity and practicability of the test.
3. Ask several physical education instructors of activity classes what sports skills tests they use and why they chose them.

Sources of Additional Sports Skills Tests

Archery

Hyde, E. I. 1937. An achievement scale in archery. *Research Quarterly* 8:109–116.

Shifflett, B., and Schuman, B. 1982. A criterion-referenced test for archery. *Research Quarterly for Exercise and Sport* 53: 330–335.

Zabik, R. M., and Jackson, A. S. 1969. Reliability of archery achievement. *Research Quarterly* 40: 254–255.

Badminton

French, E., and Statler, E. 1949. Study of skill tests in badminton for college women. *Research Quarterly* 20: 257–272.

Lockhart, A., and McPherson, F. A. 1949. The development of a test of badminton playing ability. *Research Quarterly* 20: 402–405.

Miller, F. A. 1951. A badminton wall volley test. *Research Quarterly* 22: 208–213.

Thorpe, J., and West, C. 1969. A test of game sense in badminton. *Perceptual and Motor Skills* 28: 159–169.

Basketball

Boyd, C. A., MacCachren, J. R., and Waglow, L. F. 1955. Predictive ability of a selected basketball test. *Research Quarterly* 26: 364–365.

Broer, M. R. 1958. Reliability of certain skill tests for junior high school girls. *Research Quarterly* 29: 139–145.

Elbel, E. R., and Allen, F. C. 1941. Evaluating team and individual performance in basketball. *Research Quarterly* 5: 538–555.

Knox, R. D. 1947. Basketball ability tests. *Scholastic Coach* 17(3): 45.

Stroup, F. 1955. Game results as a criterion for validating a basketball skill test. *Research Quarterly* 26: 353–357.

Bowling

Martin, J., and Keogh, J. 1964. Bowling norms for college students in elective physical education classes. *Research Quarterly* 35: 325–327.

Olson, J., and Liba, M. R. 1967. A device for evaluating spot bowling ability. *Research Quarterly* 38: 193–201.

Philips, M., and Summers, D. 1950. Bowling norms and learning curves for college women. *Research Quarterly* 21: 377–385.

Field Hockey

Schmithals, M., and French, E. 1940. Achievement tests in field hockey for college women. *Research Quarterly* 11: 84–92.

Football

Borleske, S. E. 1936. Borleske touch football test. In Barrow, H. M., and McGee, R. 1979. *A practical approach to measurement in physical education.* 3d ed. Philadelphia: Lea & Febiger.

Golf

Cotten, D. J., Thomas, J. R., and Plaster, T. 1972. A plastic ball test for golf iron skill. In Johnson, B. L., and Nelson, J. K. 1986. *Practical measurements for evaluation in physical education.* 4th ed. Edina, Minn.: Burgess Publishing.

Rowlands, D. J. 1974. Rowlands golf skills test battery. In Barrow, H. M., and McGee, R. 1989. *A practical approach to measurement in physical education.* 4th ed. Philadelphia: Lea & Febiger.

West, C., and Thorpe, J. 1968. Construction and validation of an eight-iron approach test. *Research Quarterly* 49: 1115–1120.

Handball

Cornish, C. 1949. A study of measurement of ability in handball. *Research Quarterly* 20: 215–222.

Montoye, H. J., and Brotzman, J. 1951. An investigation of the validity of using the results of a doubles tournament as a measurement of handball ability. *Research Quarterly* 22: 214–218.

Pennington, G. G., et al. 1967. A measure of handball ability. *Research Quarterly* 38: 247–253.

Racquetball

Karpman, M., and Isaacs, I. 1979. An improved racquetball skills test. *Research Quarterly* 50: 526–527.

Soccer

Heath, M. L., and Rogers, E. G. 1932. A study in the use of knowledge and skill tests in soccer. *Research Quarterly* 3: 33–53.

Johnson, J. R. 1963. Johnson soccer test. In Johnson, B. L., and Nelson, J. K. 1986. *Practical measurements for evaluation in physical education.* 4th ed. Edina, Minn.: Burgess.

Smith, G. 1947. Smith kick-up test. In Barrow, H. M., and McGee, R. 1979. *A practical approach to measurement in physical education.* 3d ed. Philadelphia: Lea & Febiger.

Vanderhoff, M. 1932. Soccer skills test. *Journal of Health and Physical Education* 3: 42.

Warner, G. F. 1950. Warner soccer test. *Newsletter of the National Soccer Coaches Association of America* 6: 13–22.

Softball

Broer, M. R. 1958. Reliability of certain skill tests for junior high school girls. *Research Quarterly* 29: 139–143.

Fox, M. G., and Young, O. G. 1954. A test of softball batting ability. *Research Quarterly* 25: 26–27.

O'Donnell, D. J. 1950. O'Donnell Softball Skill Test. In Collins, D. R., and Hodges, P. B. 1978. *A comprehensive guide to sports skills tests and measurement.* Springfield, Ill.: Charles C Thomas.

Underkofler, A. 1942. Underkofler softball skills test. In Collins, D. R., and Hodges, P. B. 1978. *A comprehensive guide to sports skills tests and measurement.* Springfield, Ill. Charles C Thomas.

Swimming

Fox, M. G. 1957. Swimming power test. *Research Quarterly* 28: 233–237.

Hewitt, J. E. 1948. Swimming achievement scales for college men. *Research Quarterly* 19: 282–289.

———. 1949. Achievement scale scores for high school swimming. *Research Quarterly* 20: 170–179.

Resentswieg, J. 1968. A revision of the power swimming test. *Research Quarterly* 39: 818–819.

Wilson, C. T. 1934. Coordination tests in swimming. *Research Quarterly* 5: 81–88.

Tennis

Avery, C., Richardson, P., and Jackson, A. 1979. A practical tennis serve test: Measurement of skill under simulated game conditions. *Research Quarterly* 50: 554–564.

Broer, M. R., and Miller, D. M. 1950. Achievement tests for beginning and intermediate tennis. *Research Quarterly* 21: 303–313.

DiGennaro, J. 1969. Construction of forehand drive, backhand drive, and service tennis tests. *Research Quarterly* 40: 496–501.

Dyer, J. T. 1938. Revision of the backboard test of tennis ability. *Research Quarterly* 9: 25–31.

Edwards, J. 1965. Wisconsin wall test for serve. In Barrow, H. M., and McGee, R. 1989. *A practical approach to measurement in physical education.* 4th ed. Philadelphia: Lea & Febiger.

Fox, K. 1953. A study of the validity of the Dyer backboard test and the Miller forehand-backhand test for beginning tennis players. *Research Quarterly* 24: 1–7.

Hewitt, J. E. 1968. Classification tests in tennis. *Research Quarterly* 39: 552–555.

Johnson, J. 1957. Tennis serve of advanced women players. *Research Quarterly* 28: 123–131.

Kemp, J., and Vincent, M. F. 1968. Kemp-Vincent rally test of tennis skill. *Research Quarterly* 39: 1000–1004.

Purcell, K. 1981. A tennis forehand-backhand drive skill test which measures ball control and stroke firmness. *Research Quarterly* 52: 238–245.

Volleyball

Brady, G. F. 1945. Preliminary investigation of volleyball playing ability. *Research Quarterly* 16: 14–17.

Clifton, M. A. 1962. Single hit volley test for women's volleyball. *Research Quarterly* 33: 208–211.

Crogen, C. 1943. A simple volleyball classification test for high school girls. *The Physical Educator* 4: 34–37.

Cunningham, P., and Garrison, J. 1968. High wall volley test for women's volleyball. *Research Quarterly* 39: 486–490.

French, E. L., and Cooper, B. I. 1937. Achievement test in volleyball for high school girls. *Research Quarterly* 8: 150–157.

Kronquist, R. A., and Brumbach, W. B. 1968. A modification of the Brady volleyball test for high school boys. *Research Quarterly* 39: 116–120.

Liba, M. R., and Stauff, M. R. 1963. A test for the volleyball pass. *Research Quarterly* 34: 56–63.

Mohr, D. R., and Haverstick, M. V. 1955. Repeated volleys test for women's volleyball. *Research Quarterly* 26: 179–184.

Russell, N., and Lange, E. 1940. Achievement tests in volleyball for junior high school girls. *Research Quarterly* 11: 33–41.

19 Affective Behavior

Upon completion of this chapter, you should be able to

1. List components of affective behavior;
2. Describe the uses of affective behavior measurement;
3. Describe the Likert scale, semantic differential, rating scale, and questionnaire as they are used in the measurement of social behavior; and
4. Select an instrument to measure social behavior, attitudes, sportsmanship, and leadership.

Affective behavior (also called affective domain) involves the interests, appreciations, attitudes, values, and emotional biases of an individual. It is reflected through an individual's feelings and emotions. Although many teachers are concerned with the affective behavior of students, not all physical educators agree upon how this concern should be expressed. Many physical education teachers list affective objectives for their classes, but because of discomfort in measuring them, they do not attempt to determine if the objectives have been reached. In addition, some physical educators believe that if proper cognitive and psychomotor objectives are attained, the appropriate corresponding affective behavioral objectives will be attained also. Furthermore, for the following reasons, some physical educators feel that the affective domain should not be measured at all:

1. Behaviors change slowly. Knowledge and skills can change in relatively short periods of time, but an individual's attitude, appreciation, and values usually require a longer period of time for change.

2. It is difficult to define and evaluate adjustments, interests, attitudes, appreciations, and values. In addition, affective behavior evaluation procedures are unreliable for everyday use.
3. Feelings are not teachable. How do you teach someone to have a positive attitude toward physical fitness, tennis, golf, and so on?
4. Self-reporting inventories or questionnaires depend on the willingness of the students to state their true beliefs. On occasion, students provide answers that best please the instructors.
5. Physical educators are not adequately trained to evaluate affective behavior.
6. Why should physical education assume responsibility for the development of affective behavior? English and math teachers seldom include the affective objective.
7. There is not adequate time in the physical education class to measure physical skills, knowledge, and affective behavior (Phillips and Hornak 1979; Mood 1982).

In some teaching environments the preceding are valid arguments against measurement of affective behavior, and all physical educators should be aware of these concerns before making any attempt to measure in this domain. There are, however, important uses of affective behavior measurement, and if suitable instruments are properly administered, these measurements can be of value to the physical educator.

Why Measure Affective Behavior?

McGee (1982) provides the following uses of measurement of affective behavior.

Uses for Groups

Measurement of affective behavior can be used to identify the present status of the group. How do students feel about the physical activity that is to be taught? Concerns about sportsmanship and group cohesiveness may also be addressed. This measurement should not be used to evaluate or judge; rather, it should be used to make the teacher aware of the group's attitude toward a particular activity.

Affective behavior measurement can also be used for program evaluation and planning. The strengths and weaknesses of physical education programs may be identified through attitude measurement. If groups repeatedly have no interest in or a bad attitude toward certain activities, it may be wise to make curriculum revisions.

Another important use of affective behavior measurement is to aid in the establishment of teacher-student rapport. If students and teachers work together to plan and implement affective objectives, students usually will know that teachers care about them. When students know the teacher cares about their feelings, they are more likely to cooperate with the teacher.

Finally, affective behavior measurement can be useful for motivation. The planning of affective objectives by both teacher and students can serve to motivate the students to work for attainment of the objectives.

Uses for Individuals

The application of affective behavior measurements to individuals must be done with caution. In fulfilling their counseling responsibilities, all teachers should be aware that some students are more sensitive than others. Receiving a low score in group acceptability may negatively influence many students. When measurement of affective behavior is done for individual use, the teacher must apply the results wisely.

Perhaps the most important individual use of affective behavior measurement is to help students know themselves. Students can become more aware of their attitudes, group acceptance, behavior, values, and self-esteem. Once aware of these measurement results, the students, with the assistance of the teacher, can plan and work for self-improvement. However, programs for self-improvement will not be the same for everyone. Some individuals may not need self-improvement programs.

Furthermore, students who need to be referred to school counselors can be identified, but the physical educator should not attempt to perform this identification and referral alone. There should be consultation with individuals who are better qualified to make these important decisions.

Finally, affective behavior measurement can be used to help select individuals for important roles in class and varsity athletic teams. Attitude, competitiveness, and leadership scores may be used for this purpose.

Categories of Measures

Many instruments are available for measurement of affective behavior in physical education. They can be classified into the following categories:

Attitude inventories. Through responses to the inventory, an individual's feelings about events, people, activities, ideas, policies, or institutions are revealed. One's attitude about an activity will influence future participation in the activity. For example, an individual who has a negative attitude about an activity is unlikely to participate in the activity.

Interest inventories. An individual's likes and dislikes for certain activities and programs are expressed in interest inventories that may be used in selecting activities to be taught and in establishing new programs.

Leadership. Usually members of a group are asked to identify individuals in the group who would make good leaders. These inventories are sometimes used to identify leaders for athletic teams.

Sportsmanship. An individual's responses, or a group's responses, on this survey determine if an individual will abide by the rules, make sacrifices for the good of the group, and be a gracious winner or loser.

Social behavior. Through self-reporting, teacher ratings, or peer ratings, the individual's level of social development is determined. This instrument is often used to determine the student's acceptance by the group or the student's acceptance of the class and school environment.

Personality inventories. Traits such as emotional control, self-confidence, motivation, aggressiveness, determination, poise, and mental toughness may be measured with these inventories. Numerous other personality traits also may be measured.

Behavior ratings. After observing a student over a period of time, the teacher rates the affective behavior of the student. The ratings may include many different aspects of behavior, such as sportsmanship, leadership, attitude, self-control, self-motivation, cooperation, and peer relations.

Types of Items

The types of items most often used in physical education to measure affective behavior are Likert scales, the semantic differential, rating scales, and questionnaires.

Likert Scale

The Likert scale requires individuals to indicate their agreement or disagreement with a series of statements. Typically each statement allows for five degrees of responses. The following are two examples of how the Likert scale may be used for student evaluation of a teacher.

The instructor was enthusiastic about the subject.

1	2	3	4	5
Strongly Disagree	Disagree	Undecided	Agree	Strongly Agree

The instructor was concerned about the student.

1	2	3	4	5
Strongly Disagree	Disagree	Undecided	Agree	Strongly Agree

The responses that best describe the feelings of the respondent are circled. Phrasing the statements so that the high scores reflect the best feeling or attitude provides a basis for statistical analysis of the statements. Thus, a score of 5 is assigned to the most favorable response, 1 to the least favorable, and 2, 3, and 4 to the intervening responses. A group's feelings about a statement are usually reported by averaging the responses.

Fewer or more than five responses can be used. It is not uncommon to find a Likert scale with seven responses, and, for younger children, two categories such as yes-no, like-dislike, or present-absent are sometimes used.

Semantic Differential

The semantic differential scale requires the individual to respond to bipolar adjectives. The bipolar adjectives represent opposite meanings, such as new-old, good-bad, and fair-unfair. The respondent is asked to mark one of seven points that best reflects his or her feelings about a concept. The score for each item ranges from 1 to 7 if the positive adjective of the pair is listed to the right, and from 7 to 1 if the positive adjective is placed to the left.

Three dimensions of a concept can be measured with the semantic differential. *Evaluation,* the most common dimension, involves the "goodness" of the concept. Typical bipolar adjectives used with this concept are good-bad, beautiful-ugly, pleasant-unpleasant, and fair-unfair. A second dimension, *potency,* involves the strength of the rated concept. Examples of bipolar adjectives used to measure this dimension are heavy-light, full-empty, hard-soft, and strong-weak. The third dimension, *activity,* involves action and is measured by such adjectives as happy-sad, fast-slow, tense-relaxed, and active-passive. A semantic differential scale should include at least three items for each dimension.

Bipolar adjectives can measure many different concepts. The following is an example of a semantic differential scale that may be used to evaluate a teacher. With no or only minor adjustments the same scale may be used to rate concepts or a physical activity.

The dimension for each item is identified in the example but should not be included on the form administered to the group. The adjective pairs should be randomly ordered to prevent the clustering of a single factor, and both negative and positive adjectives should appear in each column.

Student's Feelings About the Teacher

Pleasant	—:—:—:—:—:—:—	Unpleasant	(Evaluation)
Lazy	—:—:—:—:—:—:—	Busy	(Activity)
Weak	—:—:—:—:—:—:—	Strong	(Potency)
Fast	—:—:—:—:—:—:—	Slow	(Activity)
Good	—:—:—:—:—:—:—	Bad	(Evaluation)
Relaxed	—:—:—:—:—:—:—	Tense	(Activity)
Unsuccessful	—:—:—:—:—:—:—	Successful	(Evaluation)
Dominant	—:—:—:—:—:—:—	Submissive	(Potency)
Hard	—:—:—:—:—:—:—	Soft	(Potency)
Fair	—:—:—:—:—:—:—	Unfair	(Evaluation)
Excitable	—:—:—:—:—:—:—	Calm	(Activity)
Deep	—:—:—:—:—:—:—	Shallow	(Potency)

Rating Scale

Rating scales are similar in form to Likert scales. Rather than using a standard set of response categories for each statement, however, descriptive terms are presented. The use of descriptive terms ensures that all respondents will rate specific boundaries of behavior. The following examples illustrate how a rating scale may be used to determine the group's feelings toward the teacher.

Concern for Students

1	2	3	4	5
Indifferent	Self-centered	Somewhat concerned	Generally concerned	Deeply and actively concerned

Enthusiasm of Instructor

1	2	3	4	5
Not enthusiastic	Occasionally enthusiastic	Usually enthusiastic	Consistently enthusiastic	Effectively enthusiastic

Questionnaire

A questionnaire consists of a series of questions and is useful for obtaining information from a large number of people. Typically, questionnaires are administered to survey interests, ask opinions, determine values, or gather factual information. Responses are usually in the form of one word, a brief statement, or a selection of a response from a set of options. The responses should be made easily and lend themselves to tabulation.

?ARE YOU ABLE TO DO THE FOLLOWING:

- list the components of affective behavior?
- describe the uses of affective behavior measurement?
- describe the Likert scale, semantic differential, rating scale, and questionnaire as they are used in the measurement of social behavior?

Instruments for Measurement of Affective Behavior

Many instruments have been developed to measure affective behavior. Examples of instruments that measure social behavior, attitudes, sportsmanship, and leadership are presented. All of the described instruments may be used with males and females.

Social Behavior

■ **Cowell Social Adjustment Index**
(Cowell 1958)

Test Objective. To measure the degree of the students' positive and negative social adjustment within their social groups.
Age Level. Twelve through seventeen.
Validity. With the Pupil Who's Who Ratings as a criterion measure, a coefficient of .63 was obtained.
Reliability. .82.

Norms. The original source reports norms for junior high school boys.

Administration and Directions. The student is rated by the teacher on the ten positive items in Form A and the ten negative items in Form B. A mark is placed in the cell that is judged to reflect the degree to which the behavior is displayed. Forms A and B are shown in figure 19.1.

Scoring. The score is the sum of the points for the items in Form A minus the sum of the points for the items in Form B.

■ Blanchard Behavior Rating Scale
(Blanchard 1936)

Test Objective. To measure the character and personality of students.

Age Level. Twelve through seventeen.

Validity. With the criterion of the average of the correlations of each item with the remainder of the items in its category, a coefficient of .93 was found.

Reliability. A coefficient of .71 was found for the correlation between the scores of the teacher and the student raters.

Norms. No norms reported.

Administration and Directions. The scale includes twenty-four items to rate nine character and personality traits of the student. The teacher circles the number (1 through 5) that is judged to reflect the degree to which the behavior is displayed. The scale is shown in figure 19.2.

Scoring. The score is the sum of the numbers that have been circled for the twenty-four items.

■ Cowell's Personal Distance Scale
(Cowell 1958)

Test Objective. To measure a student's degree of acceptance by a social group.

Age Level. Twelve through college-age.

Validity. With Who's Who in My Group ratings as the criterion, a coefficient of .84 was found.

Reliability. .93.

Norms. No norms reported.

Administration and Directions. Using the scale shown in figure 19.3, each student is asked to rate all other students.

Scoring. The average score (to the nearest whole number) for each student is determined. The lower the student's score, the greater the degree of acceptance by the group.

Attitudes

■ Adams Physical Education Attitude Scale
(Adams 1963)

Test Objective. To measure individual and group attitudes toward physical education.

Age Level. High school through college-age.

Validity. A coefficient of .77 was found when correlating the Set 1 scoring scale against the Likert scoring scale.

Reliability. A coefficient of .71 was reported.

Norms. No norms required.

Administration and Directions. Two alternate sets of scales were developed. Set 1 is shown in figure 19.4. The students indicate whether they agree or disagree with the statement by placing a check mark on the appropriate blank. Each statement has a designated weight. These weights should not be printed on the scales that are completed by the students.

Scoring. The total score is the sum of the weights of the "agree" items divided by the number of "agree" items (i.e., the average of the scores for the "agree" items).

■ Wear Attitude Scale
(Wear 1955)

Test Objective. To measure attitudes toward physical education.

Age Level. College-age.

Validity. Face validity.

Reliability. Coefficients of .94 and .96 were reported for Form A and Form B, respectively.

Norms. No norms required.

Administration and Directions. Two alternate forms of the scale, Form A and Form B, were developed. Form A is shown in figure 19.5. The students are instructed to respond to each statement as if physical education is an activity course taught during a regular class period and to let their personal experiences determine their answers. They should answer anonymously, or they should be advised their responses will not affect their physical education grades. The five possible responses are strongly agree, agree, undecided, disagree, and strongly disagree.

Scoring. Positively worded items are scored 5–4–3–2–1, and negatively worded items are scored 1–2–3–4–5. The total test score is the sum of the scores of the thirty items; a high score indicates a positive attitude toward physical education.

■ Kenyon Attitude Scales
(Kenyon 1968a, 1968b)

Test Objective. To measure six attitudes toward physical activity.

Age Level. High school through college.

Validity. Generally, scale scores differed between athletes and nonathletes, and expert opinion confirmed that the six

Instructions: *Think carefully of the student's behavior in group situations; check each behavior trend according to its degree of descriptiveness.*

Descriptive of the Student

Behavior Trends	Markedly (+3)	Somewhat (+2)	Only Slightly (+1)	Not at All (+0)
1. Enters heartily and with enjoyment into the spirit of social intercourse				
2. Frank; talkative and sociable, does not stand on ceremony				
3. Self-confident and self-reliant, tends to take success for granted, strong initiative, prefers to lead				
4. Quick and decisive in movement, pronounced or excessive energy output				
5. Prefers group activities, work or play; not easily satisfied with individual projects				
6. Adaptable to new situations, makes adjustments readily, welcomes change				
7. Is self-composed, seldom shows signs of embarrassment				
8. Tends to elation of spirits, seldom gloomy or moody				
9. Seeks a broad range of friendships, not selective or exclusive in games and the like				
10. Hearty and cordial, even to strangers, forms acquaintanceships very easily				

FIGURE 19.1A Cowell Social Adjustment Index Form A.

Reprinted with permission from *Research Quarterly for Exercise and Sport,* 29, 7–18, 1958 by the American Alliance for Health, Physical Education, Recreation and Dance, 1900 Association Drive, Reston, Virginia 22091.

Instructions: Think carefully of the student's behavior in group situations; check each behavior trend according to its degree of descriptiveness.

Behavior Trends	Descriptive of the Student			
	Markedly (–3)	Somewhat (–2)	Only Slightly (–1)	Not at All (–0)
1. Somewhat prudish, awkward, easily embarrassed in social contacts				
2. Secretive, seclusive, not inclined to talk unless spoken to				
3. Lacking in self-confidence and initiative, a follower				
4. Slow in movement, deliberative or perhaps indecisive. Energy output moderate or deficient..........				
5. Prefers to work and play alone, tends to avoid group activities				
6. Shrinks from making new adjustments, prefers the habitual to the stress of reorganization required by the new				
7. Is self-conscious, easily embarrassed, timid or "bashful"				
8. Tendency of depression, frequently gloomy or moody				
9. Shows preference for a narrow range of intimate friends and tends to exclude others from his or her association				
10. Reserved and distant except to intimate friends, does not form acquaintanceships readily				

FIGURE 19.1B Cowell Social Adjustment Index Form B.

Reprinted with permission from *Research Quarterly for Exercise and Sport,* 29, 7–18, 1958, by the American Alliance for Health, Physical Education, Recreation, and Dance, 1900 Association Drive, Reston, Virginia 22091.

	Frequency of observation						
Personal information	No opportunity to observe	Never	Seldom	Fairly often	Frequently	Extremely often	Score

Leadership
1. Popular with classmates 1 2 3 4 5
2. Seeks responsibility in the classroom 1 2 3 4 5
3. Shows intellectual leadership in the classroom 1 2 3 4 5

Positive active qualities
4. Quits on tasks requiring perseverence 5 4 3 2 1
5. Exhibits aggressiveness in relationships
   with others 1 2 3 4 5
6. Shows initiative in assuming responsibility in
   unfamiliar situations 1 2 3 4 5
7. Alert to new opportunities 1 2 3 4 5

Positive mental qualities
8. Shows keenness of mind 1 2 3 4 5
9. Volunteers ideas 1 2 3 4 5

Self-control
10. Grumbles over decisions of classmates 5 4 3 2 1
11. Takes a justified criticism by teacher or classmate
    without showing anger or pouting 1 2 3 4 5

Cooperation
12. Is loyal to the group 1 2 3 4 5
13. Discharges group responsibilities well 1 2 3 4 5
14. Is cooperative in attitude toward the teacher 1 2 3 4 5

Social action standards
15. Makes loud-mouthed criticisms and comments 5 4 3 2 1
16. Respects the rights of others 1 2 3 4 5

Ethical social qualities
17. Cheats 5 4 3 2 1
18. Is truthful 1 2 3 4 5

Qualities of efficiency
19. Seems satisfied to "get by" with tasks assigned 5 4 3 2 1
20. Is dependable and trustworthy 1 2 3 4 5
21. Has good study habits 1 2 3 4 5

Sociability
22. Is liked by others 1 2 3 4 5
23. Makes a friendly approach to others in the group 1 2 3 4 5
24. Is friendly 1 2 3 4 5

FIGURE 19.2 Blanchard Behavior Rating Scale.

Reprinted with permission from *Research Quarterly for Exercise and Sport,* 7, 56–66, 1936, by the American Alliance for Health, Physical Education, Recreation, and Dance, 1900 Association Drive, Reston, Virginia 22091.

WHAT TO DO:	I WOULD BE WILLING TO ACCEPT HIM OR HER:						
If you had full power to treat each student on this list as you feel, just how would you consider the student? How near would you like to have the student to your family? Check each student in *one* column as to your feeling toward him or her. Circle your own name.	Into my family as a sibling	As a very close friend	As a member of my "gang" or club	On my street as a "next-door neighbor"	Into my class at school	Into my school	Into my city
	1	2	3	4	5	6	7
1. List should							
2. include							
3. names of all							
4. students in							
5. class							

FIGURE 19.3 Cowell's Personal Distance Scale.

Reprinted with permission from *Research Quarterly for Exercise and Sport,* 29, 7–18, 1958, by the American Alliance for Health, Physical Education, Recreation, and Dance, 1900 Association Drive, Reston, Virginia 22091.

dimensions adequately differentiated between active and passive involvement in physical activity.

Reliability. Coefficients ranged from .72 to .89 for the various scales.

Norms. No norms reported.

Administration and Directions. All six scales are administered.

The six scales are as follows:

1. Social experience: A high score on this scale indicates the student values physical activities that provide an opportunity for social relationships.
2. Health and fitness: A high score on this scale indicates the student values activities that contribute to the improvement of physical health and fitness.
3. Pursuit of vertigo: A high score on this scale indicates the student values physical activities that provide an element of thrill or risk to the participant through speed, acceleration, change of direction, or exposure to dangerous situations.
4. Aesthetic experience: A high score on this scale indicates the student values physical activities that are generally pleasing to the observer.
5. Catharsis: A high score on this scale indicates the student values physical activities that provide a release from frustration through some vicarious means.

6. Ascetic experience: A high score on this scale indicates the student values dedication required for championship performance.

Separate scales were developed for males (59 items) and females (54 items). Each item is scored on a 7-point scale, ranging from very strongly disagree to very strongly agree.

Scoring. Each scale is scored separately, so the student will receive six scores. The six scores should not be summed to obtain a single score.

■ **Children's Attitude Toward Physical Activity Inventory**
(Simon and Smoll 1974)

Test Objective. To measure children's attitudes toward vigorous physical activity.

Age Level. Elementary through junior high school.

Validity. Because the Kenyon Attitude Scales were used as a model for this inventory, validity was assumed for the Children's Attitude Toward Physical Activity Inventory.

Reliability. Within a day, coefficients ranged from .80 to .89, and test-retest coefficients ranged from .44 to .62.

Norms. No norms reported.

Administration and Directions. The authors advise that this inventory be used to assess groups and changes in group

Affective Behavior **273**

Weightings
(Not for inclusion
in questionnaire)

A	D	Set I	
_____	_____	1. Physical education gets very monotonous.	3.50
_____	_____	2. I only feel like doing physical education now and then.	5.95
_____	_____	3. Physical education should be disposed of.	1.58
_____	_____	4. Physical education is particularly limited in its value.	4.50
_____	_____	5. I suppose physical education is all right but I don't much care for it.	5.03
_____	_____	6. Physical education is the most hateful subject of all.	1.02
_____	_____	7. I do not want to give up physical education.	8.64
_____	_____	8. On the whole I think physical education is a good thing.	8.00
_____	_____	9. People who like physical education are nearly always good to know.	7.71
_____	_____	10. Anyone who likes physical education is silly.	2.65
_____	_____	11. Physical education has some usefulness.	6.45
_____	_____	12. Physical education is the ideal subject.	10.66
_____	_____	13. Physical education develops good character.	8.92
_____	_____	14. (School) College would be better without physical education.	2.30
_____	_____	15. Physical education has little to offer.	9.39
_____	_____	16. Physical education is my favorite subject.	3.93
_____	_____	17. Physical education gives lasting satisfaction.	9.60
_____	_____	18. Physical education's good and bad points balance out each other.	5.99
_____	_____	19. Physical education is a pleasant break.	7.11
_____	_____	20. Physical education seems useless to me.	3.08

FIGURE 19.4   Adams Physical Education Attitude Scale.

Reprinted with permission from *Research Quarterly for Exercise and Sport,* 34, 91–94, 1963, by the American Alliance for Health, Physical Education, Recreation, and Dance, 1900 Association Drive, Reston, Virginia 22091.

attitudes, not to evaluate individuals. A semantic differential is used, and the students are asked to respond to six dimensions and statements.

1. Physical activity as a social experience: Physical activities that give you a chance to meet new people and be with your friends.
2. Physical activity for health and fitness: Taking part in physical activities to make your health better and to get your body in better condition.
3. Physical activities as a thrill but involving some risk: Physical activities are dangerous. They also can be exciting because you move very fast and must change directions quickly.
4. Physical activity as the beauty in human movement: Physical activities that have beautiful movements. Examples are ballet dancing, gymnastics tumbling, and figure skating on ice.
5. Physical activity for the release of tension: Taking part in physical activities to get away from problems you might have. You can also get away from problems by watching other people in physical activities.
6. Physical activity as long and hard training: Physical activities that have long and hard practices. To spend time in practice you need to give up other things you like to do.

Form A

1. If for any reason a few subjects have to be dropped from the school program, physical education should be one of the subjects dropped.
2. Physical education activities provide no opportunities for learning to control the emotions.
3. Physical education is one of the more important subjects in helping to establish and maintain desirable social standards.
4. Vigorous physical activity works off harmful emotional tensions.
5. I would take physical education only if it were required.
6. Participation in physical education makes no contribution to the development of poise.
7. Because physical skills loom large in importance in youth, it is essential that a person be helped to acquire and improve such skills.
8. Calisthenics taken regularly are good for one's general health.
9. Skill in active games or sports is not necessary for leading the fullest kind of life.
10. Physical education does more harm physically than it does good.
11. Associating with others in some physical education activity is fun.
12. Physical education classes provide situations for the formulation of attitudes, which make one a better citizen.
13. Physical education situations are among the poorest for making friends.
14. There is not enough value coming from physical education to justify the time consumed.
15. Physical education skills make worthwhile contributions to the enrichment of living.
16. People get all the physical exercise they need in just taking care of their daily work.
17. All who are physically able will profit from an hour of physical education each day.
18. Physical education makes a valuable contribution toward building up an adequate reserve of strength and endurance for everyday living.
19. Physical education tears down sociability by encouraging people to attempt to surpass each other in many of the activities.
20. Participation in physical education activities makes for a more wholesome outlook on life.
21. Physical education adds nothing to the improvement of social behavior.
22. Physical education class activities will help to relieve and relax physical tensions.
23. Participation in physical education activities helps a person to maintain a healthful emotional life.
24. Physical education is one of the more important subjects in the school program.
25. There is little value in physical education as far as physical well-being is concerned.
26. Physical education should be included in the program of every school.
27. Skills learned in physical education class do not benefit a person.
28. Physical education provides situations for developing character qualities.
29. Physical education makes for more enjoyable living.
30. Physical education has no place in modern education.

FIGURE 19.5 Wear Attitude Scale.

Reprinted with permission from *Research Quarterly for Exercise and Sport,* 26, 113–119, 1955, by the American Alliance for Health, Physical Education, Recreation, and Dance, 1900 Association Drive, Reston, Virginia 22091.

Each dimension is rated on the basis of eight pairs of bipolar adjectives, which are separated by a 7-point continuum. Figure 19.6 illustrates one dimension with the bipolar adjectives.

Scoring. Each of the six scales is scored separately. The maximum score for each dimension is 56.

Sportsmanship

■ Lakie Attitude Toward Athletic Competition Scale
(Lakie 1964)

Test Objective. To measure the student's attitude toward competition.
Age Level. College-age.
Validity. Face validity.
Reliability. .81.
Norms. No norms reported.
Administration and Directions. Lakie's scale is shown in figure 19.7. The students are advised to circle the number of

the response that best reflects their feelings about each described action.

Scoring. The score is the sum of the item scores. Negative items are scored in a reverse order (5–4–3–2–1). The higher the score, the greater the competitive attitude of the student.

■ Johnson Sportsmanship Attitude Scales
(Johnson 1969)

Test Objective. To measure the student's attitude toward competition.
Age Level. Twelve through fourteen.
Validity. Empirical validity coefficients ranging from −.01 to .43 were found by correlating test scores and behavior ratings.
Reliability. A coefficient of .86 was found between scores of Form A and Form B.
Norms. No norms reported.
Administration and Directions. Johnson developed alternate forms of the scales. Form A is provided in figure 19.8. The

How do you feel about the idea in the box?

| Physical Activity for Health and Fitness |
| Taking part in physical activities to make your health better and to get your body in better condition |

Always think about the idea in the box.

		1	2	3	4	5	6	7	
1.	Good								: Bad
2.	Of no use								: Useful
3.	Not pleasant								: Pleasant
4.	Bitter								: Sweet
5.	Nice								: Awful
6.	Happy								: Sad
7.	Dirty								: Clean
8.	Steady								: Nervous

FIGURE 19.6 Format for the Children's Attitude Toward Physical Activity Inventory.

Reprinted with permission from *Research Quarterly for Exercise and Sport,* 45, 407–415, 1974, by the American Alliance for Health, Physical Education, Recreation, and Dance, 1900 Association Drive, Reston, Virginia 22091.

The following situations describe behavior demonstrated in sports. Circle the category that indicates your feeling toward the behavior described in each of the situations.

1. Strongly approve 2. Approve 3. Undecided 4. Disapprove
5. Strongly disapprove

1 2 3 4 5   1. During a football game team A has the ball on its own 34-yard line, fourth down and 1 yard to go for a first down. The coach of team A signals to the quarterback the play that he wants the team to run.

1 2 3 4 5   2. Team A is the visiting basketball team; and each time a member of the team is given a free shot, the home crowd sets up a continual din of noise until the shot has been taken.

1 2 3 4 5   3. Tennis player A frequently calls out, throws up his or her arms, or otherwise tries to indicate that the opponent's serve is out of bounds when it is questionable.

1 2 3 4 5   4. In a track meet, team A enters a person in the mile run who is to set a fast pace for the first half of the race and then drop out.

1 2 3 4 5   5. In a football game, team B's quarterback was tackled repeatedly after handing off and after he was out of the play.

1 2 3 4 5   6. Sam, playing golf with his friends, hit a drive into the rough. He accidentally moved the ball with his foot; although not improving his position, he added a penalty stroke to his score.

1 2 3 4 5   7. A basketball player was caught out of position on defense; and rather than allow the opponent to attempt a field goal, she fouled her.

1 2 3 4 5   8. Player A during a golf match made quick noises and movements when player B was getting ready to make a shot.

1 2 3 4 5   9. School A has a powerful but quite slow football team. The night before playing a smaller but faster team, they allowed the field sprinkling system to remain on, causing the field to be heavy and slow.

1 2 3 4 5   10. A basketball team used player A to draw the opponent's high scorer into fouling situations.

1 2 3 4 5   11. The alumni of College A pressured the Board of Trustees to lower the admission and eligibility requirements for athletes.

1 2 3 4 5   12. Team A, by use of fake injuries, was able to stop the clock long enough to get off the play that resulted in the winning touchdown.

1 2 3 4 5   13. A tennis player was given the advantage of a bad call in a close match. She then "evened up" the call by intentionally hitting the ball out of bounds.

1 2 3 4 5   14. The coach of basketball team A removed his team from the floor in protest of an official's decision.

1 2 3 4 5   15. Between seasons a coach moved from College A to College B and then persuaded three of College A's athletes to transfer to College B.

1 2 3 4 5   16. After losing a close football game, the coach of the losing team publicly accused the game officials of favoritism when the game movies showed the winning touchdown had been scored by using an illegal maneuver.

FIGURE 19.7   Lakie Attitude Toward Athletic Competition Scale (Continued on Page 278).

Reprinted with permission from *Research Quarterly for Exercise and Sport,* 35, 497–503, 1964, by the American Alliance for Health, Physical Education, Recreation, and Dance, 1900 Association Drive, Reston, Virginia 22091.

1 2 3 4 5   17. College C lowered the admission requirements for athletes awarded athletic scholarships.

1 2 3 4 5   18. Team A's safety man returned a punt for a touchdown. Unseen by the officials, he had stepped out of bounds in front of his team's bench. His coach notified the officials of this fact.

1 2 3 4 5   19. A college with very few athletic scholarships to offer gives athletes preference on all types of campus jobs.

1 2 3 4 5   20. Several wealthy alumni of College C make a monthly gift to several athletes who are in need of financial assistance.

1 2 3 4 5   21. College K has a policy of not allowing any member of a varsity squad to associate with the visiting team until the contest or meet is completed.

1 2 3 4 5   22. The Board of Trustees of College C fired the football coach and gave as the reason for his dismissal his failure to win a conference championship during the past five years.

FIGURE 19.7 *Continued.*

Directions: Read each statement carefully and decide whether you approve or disapprove of the action taken by the person. Circle the ONE response category that tells the way you feel. PLEASE COMPLETE EVERY ITEM.

Example: A pitcher in a baseball game threw a fast ball at the batter to scare him.

⟨Strongly approve⟩   Approve   Disapprove   Strongly Disapprove

(If you strongly approve of this action by the pitcher, you circle the first response category as shown.)

The responses can appear after each item or on an answer sheet.

1. After a basketball player was called by the official for traveling, she slammed the basketball onto the floor.

2. A baseball player was called out as he slid into home plate. He jumped up and down on the plate and screamed at the official.

3. After a personal foul was called against a basketball player, he shook his fist in the official's face.

4. A basketball coach talked very loudly in order to annoy an opponent who was attempting to make a very important free throw shot.

5. After a baseball game, the coach of the losing team went up to the umpire and demanded to know how much money had been paid to "throw" the game.

6. A basketball coach led the spectators in jeering at the official who made calls against her team.

7. After two players were put out on a double-play attempt, a softball coach told the players in her dugout to boo the umpire's decision.

8. As the basketball coach left the gymnasium after the game, he shouted at the officials, "You lost me the game; I never saw such lousy officiating in my life."

FIGURE 19.8 Johnson Sportsmanship Attitude Scale, Form A.

Reprinted with permission from *Research Quarterly for Exercise and Sport,* 40, 312–316, 1969, by the American Alliance for Health, Physical Education, Recreation, and Dance, 1900 Association Drive, Reston, Virginia 22091.

9. A basketball coach put sand on the gym floor to force the opponents into traveling penalties.

10. A football coach left the bench to change the position of a marker dropped by an official to indicate where the ball went out of bounds.

11. During the first half of a football game a touchdown was called back. At halftime the football coach went into the officials' dressing room and cursed the officials.

12. A football player was taken out of the game for unsportsmanlike conduct. The player changed jerseys and the coach sent him back into the game.

13. Following a closely played basketball game, the coach of the losing team cursed her players for not winning.

14. After a basketball game the losing team's coach yelled at spectators to "Go get the Ump."

15. A baseball coach permitted players to use profanity loud enough for the entire park to hear when the players did not like a decision.

16. The basketball coach drank alcoholic beverages while supervising her basketball team on a trip.

17. A college football player was disqualified for misconduct. While on the way to the sideline, the player attacked the official.

18. During a time-out in a basketball game, the clock was accidently left running. The coach whose team was behind ran over to the scoring table and struck the timekeeper.

19. After a basketball player was knocked into a wall, his coach rushed onto the court and hit the player who had fouled.

20. After a baseball player had been removed from the game, the coach met him at the sidelines and hit him.

21. After a runner was called out at first base, the baseball coach went onto the field and wrestled the umpire down to the ground.

FIGURE 19.8 *Continued.*

students are advised to read each statement carefully and to decide if they approve or disapprove of the action taken by the person. They then circle the one response that tells the way they feel.
Scoring. No total test score is recorded. The scale is used to detect attitudes, to detect changes in attitudes, and as material for class discussion.

Leadership

■ Nelson Sports Leadership Questionnaire
(Nelson 1966)

Test Objective. To measure athletic leadership.
Age Level. Junior high through college-age.
Validity. Face validity.
Reliability. Coefficients of .96 with ninth-grade football players, and .78 with varsity college basketball players were reported by Johnson and Nelson (1986).

Norms. No norms reported.
Administration and Directions. Two questionnaires are designed, one for the coaches and one for the students. The students are advised to list a first and a second choice in all cases, excluding their own name. An athlete's name can be used any number of times. Students do not sign their name. The questionnaire for the students is provided in figure 19.9.
Scoring. Five points are awarded for a name appearing in response number 1, and 3 points are awarded for a name appearing in response number 2.

Competition Anxiety

■ Sport Competition Anxiety Test (SCAT)
(Martens 1977)

Test Objective. To measure how anxious individuals generally feel before competition; to describe individual

Do not sign your name to the questionnaire. Fill in the name or names of the squad member that, in your opinion, best fits the question. Give your first and second choice in all cases. *Do not use your own name* on any of the answers. The names of the same players can be used any number of times, and your answers will be kept confidential.

1. If you were on a trip and had a choice of the players you would share the hotel room with, who would they be?
   1. _____ 2. _____
2. Who are the most popular athletes on the squad?
   1. _____ 2. _____
3. Who are the best scholars on the squad?
   1. _____ 2. _____
4. Which players on the team know the most basketball, in terms of strategy, team play, etc.?
   1. _____ 2. _____
5. If the coach were not present for a workout, which players would be the most likely to take charge of the practice?
   1. _____ 2. _____
6. Which players would you listen to first if the team appeared to be disorganized during a crucial game?
   1. _____ 2. _____
7. Your team is behind 1 point with 10 seconds remaining in the game and you could pass to anyone on the squad. Who would it be?
   1. _____ 2. _____
8. Of all the players on your team, who exhibits the most poise on the floor during the crucial parts of the game?
   1. _____ 2. _____
9. Who are the "take charge" athletes on your team?
   1. _____ 2. _____
10. Who are the most consistent ball handlers on your squad?
    1. _____ 2. _____
11. Who are the most consistent shooters on your squad?
    1. _____ 2. _____
12. Who are the most valuable players on your squad?
    1. _____ 2. _____
13. Who are the most unselfish players who are interested most in the team as a whole and who play most "for the team"?
    1. _____ 2. _____
14. Which players have the most overall ability of the squad?
    1. _____ 2. _____
15. Who are the most likable players on the squad?
    1. _____ 2. _____
16. Which players on your team have influenced you the most?
    1. _____ 2. _____
17. Which players have actually helped you the most?
    1. _____ 2. _____
18. Which players do you think would make the best coaches?
    1. _____ 2. _____
19. Which players do you most often look to for leadership?
    1. _____ 2. _____
20. Who are the hardest workers on the squad?
    1. _____ 2. _____

FIGURE 19.9 Nelson Sport Leadership Questionnaire.

Reprinted with permission from *Research Quarterly for Exercise and Sport*, 37, 268–275, 1966, by the American Alliance for Health, Physical Education, Recreation, and Dance, 1900 Association Drive, Reston, Virginia 22091.

TABLE 19.1 SCAT-A Norms for Normal College-Age Adults

	Male		Female	
Raw Score	Standard Score	Percentile	Standard Score	Percentile
30	719	99	652	99
29	698	99	631	93
28	677	97	611	88
27	655	93	590	82
26	634	89	570	75
25	612	86	549	65
24	591	82	529	59
23	570	78	508	53
22	548	74	488	47
21	527	69	467	42
20	505	61	447	35
19	484	50	426	28
18	463	40	406	22
17	441	30	385	15
16	420	24	365	10
15	399	18	344	8
14	377	14	323	6
13	356	9	303	4
12	334	7	282	3
11	313	5	262	2
10	292	1	241	1

Reprinted, by permission, from R. Martens, 1982, Sport Competition Anxiety Test (Champaign, Ill.: Human Kinetics Publishers), 93–94, 96–99.

TABLE 19.2 SCAT-A Norms for Normal Young Adults, Grades 10–12

	Male		Female	
Raw Score	Standard Score	Percentile	Standard Score	Percentile
30	753	99	677	99
29	727	99	654	98
28	702	98	631	92
27	677	98	609	85
26	651	93	586	80
25	626	89	563	74
24	601	87	540	66
23	575	78	518	59
22	550	73	495	50
21	525	67	472	42
20	499	61	450	39
19	474	48	427	30
18	448	39	404	23
17	423	24	381	16
16	398	18	359	10
15	372	12	336	5
14	347	7	313	3
13	322	5	291	3
12	296	2	268	2
11			245	1

Reprinted, by permission, from R. Martens, 1982, Sport Competition Anxiety Test (Champaign, Ill.: Human Kinetics Publishers), 93–94, 96–99.

differences in the perception of competitive situations as threatening and in the response to these situations with feelings of apprehension and tension.

Age Level. Children through adults.

Validity. Six judges assessed the content validity and grammatical clarity. Construct validity was obtained by demonstrating significant relationships between SCAT and other personality constructs; experimental studies also demonstrated construct validity.

Reliability. For grades 5 to 6 and 8 to 9, test-retest coefficients for four time intervals ranged from .57 to .93 with a mean of .77 for all samples combined. The Kuder-Richardson Formula (KR_{20}) produced coefficients of internal consistency ranging from .95 to .97 for both the children and adults versions.

Norms. Tables 19.1 through 19.4 include norms for college-age adults, young adults (grades 10–12), grades 7 to 9, and grades 4 to 6, respectively. Norms also are available for the sports of baseball, basketball, football, soccer, swimming, tennis, volleyball, and wrestling.

Administration and Directions. Tests are available for adults (SCAT-A, see figure 19.10) and children (SCAT-C, see figure 19.11). During the tests, the subjects should be asked to respond to each item according to how they generally feel in competitive sport situations. Directions are included in the tests found in figures 19.10 and 19.11.

TABLE 19.3 SCAT-C Norms for Normal Children, Grades 7–9

Raw Score	Male Standard Score	Percentile	Female Standard Score	Percentile
30	730	99	688	99
29	709	99	669	97
28	687	99	649	96
27	665	97	630	91
26	644	93	610	88
25	622	90	591	84
24	601	85	571	76
23	579	79	552	70
22	558	73	532	63
21	536	66	513	53
20	515	59	493	49
19	493	51	473	42
18	472	43	454	35
17	450	37	434	30
16	429	30	415	26
15	407	24	395	19
14	386	18	376	17
13	364	12	356	12
12	342	8	337	9
11	321	4	317	5
10	299	2	298	2

Reprinted, by permission, from R. Martens, 1982, Sport Competition Anxiety Test (Champaign, Ill.: Human Kinetics Publishers), 93–94, 96–99.

TABLE 19.4 SCAT-C Norms for Normal Children, Grades 4–6

Raw Score	Male Standard Score	Percentile	Female Standard Score	Percentile
30	744	99	734	99
29	722	99	711	99
28	700	99	688	98
27	678	97	666	97
26	656	95	643	92
25	634	90	620	88
24	612	87	597	85
23	590	84	575	80
22	568	77	552	74
21	546	71	529	67
20	524	63	507	56
19	502	56	484	48
18	480	46	461	39
17	458	41	438	31
16	436	33	416	24
15	415	28	393	16
14	393	21	370	14
13	371	13	347	10
12	349	9	325	6
11	327	2	302	2
10	305	1	279	1

Reprinted, by permission, from R. Martens, 1982, Sport Competition Anxiety Test (Champaign, Ill.: Human Kinetics), 93–94, 96–99.

Scoring. The scoring procedure is the same for both forms. Items 2, 3, 5, 8, 9, 12, 14, and 15 are scored as follows: 1 = hardly ever; 2 = sometimes; and 3 = often. Items 6 and 11 are scored as follows: 1 = often; 2 = sometimes; and 3 = hardly ever. Items 1, 4, 7, 10, and 13 are spurious items and are not scored.

Comments. Martens, Vealey, and Burton (1990) have developed the Competitive State Anxiety Inventory-2 (CSAI-2), which measures the anxiety of an athlete right before competition. Included in CSAI-2 are measures of cognitive anxiety (worry), somatic anxiety (physiological), and confidence. The inventory was developed primarily as a research tool, however. Its usefulness as a diagnostic instrument for clinical purposes has not been established.

Other Measures

■ Self-Motivation Inventory (SMI)
(Dishman and Ickes 1981)

Test Objective. To measure self-motivation to persist (originally developed to predict adherence to physical exercise).
Age Level. College-age through older adult.
Validity. Construct validity coefficient of .63.
Reliability. Internal reliability of .91 and test-retest reliability of .92.
Norms. No norms reported.
Administration and Directions. The SMI consists of 40 items in a Likert format. The person is asked to describe how

Directions: Below are some statements about how persons feel when they compete in sports and games. Read each statement and decide if you HARDLY EVER, or SOMETIMES, or OFTEN feel this way when you compete in sports and games. If your choice is HARDLY EVER, blacken the square labeled A, if your choice is SOMETIMES, blacken the square labeled B, and if your choice is OFTEN, blacken the square labeled C. There are no right or wrong answers. Do not spend too much time on any one statement. *Remember* to choose the word that describes how you *usually* feel when competing in *sports and games*.

FIGURE 19.10 Sport competition anxiety test questionnaire: SCAT-A.

Reprinted, by permission, from R. Martens, 1982, Sport Competition Anxiety Test (Champaign, IL: Human Kinetics Publishers), 93–94, 96–99.

	Hardly Ever	Sometimes	Often
1. Competing against others is socially enjoyable.	A ☐	B ☐	C ☐
2. Before I compete I feel uneasy.	A ☐	B ☐	C ☐
3. Before I compete I worry about not performing well.	A ☐	B ☐	C ☐
4. I am a good sport when I compete.	A ☐	B ☐	C ☐
5. When I compete I worry about making mistakes.	A ☐	B ☐	C ☐
6. Before I compete I am calm.	A ☐	B ☐	C ☐
7. Setting a goal is important when competing.	A ☐	B ☐	C ☐
8. Before I compete I get a queasy feeling in my stomach.	A ☐	B ☐	C ☐
9. Just before competing I notice my heart beats faster than usual.	A ☐	B ☐	C ☐
10. I like to compete in games that demand considerable physical energy.	A ☐	B ☐	C ☐
11. Before I compete I feel relaxed.	A ☐	B ☐	C ☐
12. Before I compete I am nervous.	A ☐	B ☐	C ☐
13. Team sports are more exciting than individual sports.	A ☐	B ☐	C ☐
14. I get nervous wanting to start the game.	A ☐	B ☐	C ☐
15. Before I compete I usually get uptight.	A ☐	B ☐	C ☐

characteristic the statement is of herself or himself. Directions for answering each statement are included in figure 19.12.

Scoring. Included in the inventory are 21 positively keyed items and 19 negatively keyed items, with a response scoring range of 40 to 200.

Comments. The authors found that self-motivation, percent body fat, and body weight were the only variables that significantly predicted adherence behavior.

■ Rating of Perceived Exertion
(Borg 1973, 1982)

Test Objective. To rate one's perception of his or her exertion level during exercise.

Age Level. High school age through adult.

Validity. Coefficients between .80 and .90 were reported for the original scale when correlated with heart rate, VO$_2$, and lactic acid.

Administration and Directions. In addition to heart rate as an indicator of exercise intensity, Borg's Rating of Perceived Exertion (RPE) can be used. During exercise stress tests or exercise sessions, individuals are asked to rate on a numerical scale how they feel in relation to their level of exertion. Perceived exertion is defined as the total amount of exertion and physical fatigue. Factors such as breathing difficulties, aches, and pain should not be considered. With proper instruction, it is possible for individuals to exercise at a particular RPE based on their feeling of exertion that relates to objective measures (e.g., heart rate and oxygen consumption). In other words, individuals learn to listen to their body.

Table 19.5 includes the original and revised scales for ratings of perceived exertion. The original scale used the rankings 6 to 20 to approximate the heart values from rest to maximum (60–200). The revised scale represents an attempt to provide a ratio scale of the RPE values. Borg believes that the old scale is the best one for most simple applied studies of perceived exertion, for exercise

Directions: We want to know how you feel about *competition*. You know what competition is. We all compete. We try to do better than our brother or sister or friend at something. We try to score more points in a game. We try to get the best grade in class or win a prize that we want. We all compete in sports and games. Below are some sentences about how boys and girls feel when they compete in sports and games. Read each statement below and decide if *you* HARDLY EVER, or SOMETIMES, or OFTEN feel this way when you compete in sports and games. Mark A if your choice is HARDLY EVER, mark B if you choose SOMETIMES, and mark C if you choose OFTEN. There are no right or wrong answers. Do not spend too much time on any one statement. *Remember* to choose the word which describes how you *usually* feel when competing in *sports and games*.

FIGURE 19.11   Sport competition anxiety test questionnaire: SCAT-C.

Reprinted by permission, from R. Martens, 1982, Sport Competition Anxiety Test (Champaign, IL: Human Kinetics Publishers), 93–94, 96–99.

	Hardly Ever	Sometimes	Often
1. Competing against others is fun.	A ☐	B ☐	C ☐
2. Before I compete I feel uneasy.	A ☐	B ☐	C ☐
3. Before I compete I worry about not performing well.	A ☐	B ☐	C ☐
4. I am a good sport when I compete.	A ☐	B ☐	C ☐
5. When I compete I worry about making mistakes.	A ☐	B ☐	C ☐
6. Before I compete I am calm.	A ☐	B ☐	C ☐
7. Setting a goal is important when competing.	A ☐	B ☐	C ☐
8. Before I compete I get a funny feeling in my stomach.	A ☐	B ☐	C ☐
9. Just before competing I notice my heart beats faster than usual.	A ☐	B ☐	C ☐
10. I like rough games.	A ☐	B ☐	C ☐
11. Before I compete I feel relaxed.	A ☐	B ☐	C ☐
12. Before I compete I am nervous.	A ☐	B ☐	C ☐
13. Team sports are more exciting than individual sports.	A ☐	B ☐	C ☐
14. I get nervous wanting to start the game.	A ☐	B ☐	C ☐
15. Before I compete I usually get uptight.	A ☐	B ☐	C ☐

NAME _____   DATE _____

DIRECTIONS: Read each of the following statements and then blacken the appropriate number to the right of the statement to indicate how it best describes you. Please be sure to answer every item and try to be as honest and accurate as possible in your responses. There are no right or wrong answers. Your answers will be kept in the strictest confidence.

	Very unlike me	Somewhat unlike me	Neither like me nor unlike me	Somewhat like me	Very much like me
1. I'm not very good at committing myself to do things.	1	2	3	4	5
2. Whenever I get bored with projects I start, I drop them to do something else.	1	2	3	4	5
3. I can persevere at stressful tasks, even when they are physically tiring or painful.	1	2	3	4	5

FIGURE 19.12   Self-Motivation Inventory

Source: R. K. Dishman and W. Ickes, Self-motivation and adherence to therapeutic exercise, *Journal of Behavioral Medicine* 4:421–438, 1981. Copyright © Rod K. Dishman, 1978.

	Very unlike me	Somewhat unlike me	Neither like me nor unlike me	Somewhat like me	Very much like me
4. If something gets to be too much of an effort to do, I'm likely to just forget it.	1	2	3	4	5
5. I'm really concerned about developing and maintaining self-discipline.	1	2	3	4	5
6. I'm good at keeping promises, especially the ones I make to myself.	1	2	3	4	5
7. I don't work any harder than I have to.	1	2	3	4	5
8. I seldom work to my full capacity.	1	2	3	4	5
9. I'm just not the goal-setting type.	1	2	3	4	5
10. When I take on a difficult job, I make a point of sticking with it until it's completed.	1	2	3	4	5
11. I'm willing to work for things I want as long as it's not a big hassle for me.	1	2	3	4	5
12. I have a lot of self-motivation.	1	2	3	4	5
13. I'm good at making decisions and standing by them.	1	2	3	4	5
14. I generally take the path of least resistance.	1	2	3	4	5
15. I get discouraged easily.	1	2	3	4	5
16. If I tell somebody I'll do something, you can depend on it being done.	1	2	3	4	5
17. I don't like to overextend myself.	1	2	3	4	5
18. I'm basically lazy.	1	2	3	4	5
19. I have a very hard-driving, aggressive personality.	1	2	3	4	5
20. I work harder than most of my friends.	1	2	3	4	5
21. I can persist in spite of pain or discomfort.	1	2	3	4	5
22. I like to set goals and work toward them.	1	2	3	4	5
23. Sometimes I push myself harder than I should.	1	2	3	4	5
24. I tend to be overly apathetic.	1	2	3	4	5
25. I seldom if ever let myself down.	1	2	3	4	5
26. I'm not very reliable.	1	2	3	4	5
27. I like to take on jobs that challenge me.	1	2	3	4	5
28. I change my mind about things quite easily.	1	2	3	4	5
29. I have a lot of will power.	1	2	3	4	5
30. I'm not likely to put myself out if I don't have to.	1	2	3	4	5
31. Things just don't matter much to me.	1	2	3	4	5
32. I avoid stressful situations.	1	2	3	4	5
33. I often work to the point of exhaustion.	1	2	3	4	5
34. I don't impose much structure on my activities.	1	2	3	4	5
35. I never force myself to do things I don't feel like doing.	1	2	3	4	5
36. It takes a lot to get me going.	1	2	3	4	5
37. Whenever I reach a goal, I set a higher one.	1	2	3	4	5
38. I can persist in spite of failure.	1	2	3	4	5
39. I have a strong desire to achieve.	1	2	3	4	5
40. I don't have much self-discipline.	1	2	3	4	5

FIGURE 19.12 *Continued.*

Affective Behavior   **285**

TABLE 19.5 Rating of Perceived Exertion Scales

Original Rating Scale		New Rating Scale	
6		0	Nothing at all
7	Very, very light	0.5	Very, very weak (just noticeable)
8		1	Very weak
9	Very light	2	Weak (light)
10		3	Moderate
11	Fairly light	4	Somewhat strong
12		5	Strong (heavy)
13	Somewhat hard	6	
14		7	Very strong
15	Hard	8	
16		9	
17	Very hard	10	Very, very strong (almost max)
18			
19	Very, very hard		
20			

Source: G. A. V. Borg, Psychophysical bases of perceived exertion, *Medicine and Science in Sports and Exercise* 14(5): 377–381, 1982.

testing, and for predictions and prescriptions of exercise intensities in sports and medical rehabilitation. The new category scale may be especially suitable for determining other subjective symptoms, such as breathing difficulties, aches, and pains.

▶ REVIEW PROBLEMS ◀

1. Select one of the tests described in this chapter and administer it to a group of students. Score the scale and interpret the results for the group.
2. Review at least one test from each of the areas listed at the conclusion of this chapter.

Sources of Additional Instruments for Measurement of Affective Behavior

Attitudes

McCue, B. F. 1953. Constructing an instrument for evaluating attitudes toward intensive competition in team games. *Research Quarterly* 24: 205–210.

McPherson, B. D., and Yuhasz, M. S. 1968. An inventory for assessing men's attitudes toward exercise and physical activity. *Research Quarterly* 39: 218–219.

Richardson, C. E. 1960. Thurston scale for measuring attitudes of college students toward physical fitness and exercise. *Research Quarterly* 31: 638–643.

Scott, P. M. 1953. Attitudes toward athletic competition in elementary school. *Research Quarterly* 24: 352–361.

Seaman, J. A. 1970. Attitudes of physically handicapped children toward physical education. *Research Quarterly* 41: 439–445.

Body Image

Secord, P. F., and Jourard, S. M. 1953. The appraisal of body cathexis: Body cathexis and the self. *Journal of Consulting Psychology* 17: 343–347.

Self-Esteem

Sonstroem, R. J. 1978. Physical estimation and attraction scales: Rationale and research. *Medicine and Science in Sports* 10: 97–102.

Sportsmanship

Boyer, G. 1963. Children's concepts of sportsmanship in the fourth, fifth, and sixth grades. *Research Quarterly* 34: 282–287.

McAfee, R. A. 1955. Sportsmanship attitudes of sixth, seventh, and eighth grade boys. *Research Quarterly* 26: 120.

Square Root Example

Find the square root of 595.8

$\sqrt{595.\underline{80}}$

1. Begin at the decimal point and mark off two places at a time to the right and to the left. If there is an odd number to the left, mark the one digit. If there is an odd number to the right, add a zero.

$$\begin{array}{r} 2 \\ \sqrt{595.80} \\ 4 \\ \hline 195 \end{array}$$

2. Estimate the square root of the first number (or first two numbers). Square the number (2) and place it under the 5. Subtract 4 from 5 and bring down the next pair of numbers (95).

$$\begin{array}{r} 2 \\ \sqrt{595.80} \\ 4 \\ \hline 40{\overline{)}}195 \end{array}$$

3. Multiply the first root by 2 and add a zero ($2 \times 2 = 4$, add a zero = 40). This number is the new divisor.

$$\begin{array}{r} 24 \\ \sqrt{595.80} \\ 4 \\ \hline 44{\overline{)}}195 \end{array}$$

4. Divide 40 into 195 ($195 \div 40 = 4$). Place 4 as the next digit of the square root. Replace the zero of 40 with 4.

$$\begin{array}{r} 24 \\ \sqrt{595.80} \\ 4 \\ \hline 44{\overline{)}}195 \\ 176 \\ \hline 1980 \end{array}$$

5. Multiply 44 by 4 ($4 \times 44 = 176$) and place the answer under 195. Subtract 176 from 195 ($195 - 176 = 19$). Bring down the next two digits (80).

$$\begin{array}{r} 24.4 \\ \sqrt{595.80} \\ 4 \\ \hline 44{\overline{)}}195 \\ 176 \\ \hline 484{\overline{)}}1980 \\ 1936 \\ \hline 44 \end{array}$$

6. Multiply 24 by 2 ($2 \times 24 = 48$) and add a zero. Divide 480 into 1980 ($1980 \div 480 = 4$). Place 4 as the next digit of the square root. Replace the zero of 480 with 4. Multiply 484 by 4 ($484 \times 4 - 1936$) and place the answer under 1980.

7. If you want to determine another decimal place in the answer, add two zeros and repeat the procedure.

B Values of the Correlation Coefficient *(r)*

df	.05	.01	df	.05	.01
1	.9969	.9999	17	.456	.575
2	.950	.990	18	.444	.561
3	.878	.959	19	.433	.549
4	.811	.917	20	.423	.537
5	.754	.875	25	.381	.487
6	.707	.834	30	.349	.449
7	.666	.798	35	.325	.418
8	.632	.765	40	.304	.393
9	.602	.735	45	.288	.372
10	.576	.708	50	.273	.354
11	.553	.684	60	.250	.325
12	.532	.661	70	.232	.302
13	.514	.641	80	.217	.283
14	.497	.623	90	.205	.267
15	.482	.606	100	.195	.254
16	.468	.590			

Adapted from Table 13 of E. S. Pearson and H. O. Hartley (eds.), *Biometrika Tables for Statisticians,* vol. 1 (3rd ed.), Cambridge University Press for the Biometrika Trustees, 1966. Used with the permission of the Biometrika Trustees.

C Critical Values of t (Two-Tailed Test)

df	.05	.01	df	.05	.01
1	12.706	63.657	18	2.101	2.878
2	4.303	9.925	19	2.093	2.861
3	3.182	5.841	20	2.086	2.845
4	2.776	4.604	21	2.080	2.831
5	2.571	4.032	22	2.074	2.819
6	2.447	3.707	23	2.069	2.807
7	2.365	3.499	24	2.064	2.797
8	2.306	3.355	25	2.060	2.787
9	2.262	3.250	26	2.056	2.779
10	2.228	3.169	27	2.052	2.771
11	2.201	3.106	28	2.048	2.763
12	2.179	3.055	29	2.045	2.756
13	2.160	3.012	30	2.042	2.750
14	2.145	2.977	40	2.021	2.704
15	2.131	2.947	60	2.000	2.660
16	2.120	2.921	120	1.980	2.617
17	2.110	2.898	∞	1.960	2.576

Adapted from Table 12 of E. S. Pearson and H. O. Hartley, eds., *Biometrika Tables for Statisticians,* vol. 1 (3d ed.), Cambridge University Press for the Biometrika Trustees, 1966. Used with the permission of Biometrika Trustees.

D

F-Distribution

p = .05
Values

F-Distribution

Degrees of Freedom for the Denominator, v_2	Degrees of Freedom for the Numerator, v_1								
	1	2	3	4	5	6	7	8	9
1	161.4	199.5	215.7	224.6	230.2	234.0	236.8	238.9	240.5
2	18.51	19.00	19.16	19.25	19.30	19.33	19.35	19.37	19.38
3	10.13	9.55	9.28	9.12	9.01	8.94	8.89	8.85	8.81
4	7.71	6.94	6.59	6.39	6.26	6.16	6.09	6.04	6.00
5	6.61	5.79	5.41	5.19	5.05	4.95	4.88	4.82	4.77
6	5.99	5.14	4.76	4.53	4.39	4.28	4.21	4.15	4.10
7	5.59	4.74	4.35	4.12	3.97	3.87	3.79	3.73	3.68
8	5.32	4.46	4.07	3.84	3.69	3.58	3.50	3.44	3.39
9	5.12	4.26	3.86	3.63	3.48	3.37	3.29	3.23	3.18
10	4.96	4.10	3.71	3.48	3.33	3.22	3.14	3.07	3.02
11	4.84	3.98	3.59	3.36	3.20	3.09	3.01	2.95	2.90
12	4.75	3.89	3.49	3.26	3.11	3.00	2.91	2.85	2.80
13	4.67	3.81	3.41	3.18	3.03	2.92	2.83	2.77	2.71
14	4.60	3.74	3.34	3.11	2.96	2.85	2.76	2.70	2.65
15	4.54	3.68	3.29	3.06	2.90	2.79	2.71	2.64	2.59
16	4.49	3.63	3.24	3.01	2.85	2.74	2.66	2.59	2.54
17	4.45	3.59	3.20	2.96	2.81	2.70	2.61	2.55	2.49
18	4.41	3.55	3.16	2.93	2.77	2.66	2.58	2.51	2.46
19	4.38	3.52	3.13	2.90	2.74	2.63	2.54	2.48	2.42
20	4.35	3.49	3.10	2.87	2.71	2.60	2.51	2.45	2.39
21	4.32	3.47	3.07	2.84	2.68	2.57	2.49	2.42	2.37
22	4.30	3.44	3.05	2.82	2.66	2.55	2.46	2.40	2.34
23	4.28	3.42	3.03	2.80	2.64	2.53	2.44	2.37	2.32
24	4.26	3.40	3.01	2.78	2.62	2.51	2.42	2.36	2.30
30	4.17	3.32	2.92	2.69	2.53	2.42	2.33	2.27	2.21
40	4.08	3.23	2.84	2.61	2.45	2.34	2.25	2.18	2.12
60	4.00	3.15	2.76	2.53	2.37	2.25	2.17	2.10	2.04
120	3.92	3.07	2.68	2.45	2.29	2.17	2.09	2.02	1.96
∞	3.84	3.00	2.60	2.37	2.21	2.10	2.01	1.94	1.88

Adapted from Table 18 of E. S. Pearson and H. O. Hartley, eds., *Biometrika Tables for Statisticians,* vol. 1 (3d ed.), Cambridge University Press for the Biometrika Trustees, 1966. Used with the permission of Biometrika Trustees.

p = .05 Values	F-Distribution								
Degrees of Freedom for the Denominator, v_2	**Degrees of Freedom for the Numerator, v_1**								
	10	12	15	20	30	40	60	120	∞
1	241.9	243.9	245.9	248.0	250.1	251.1	252.2	253.3	254.3
2	19.40	19.41	19.43	19.45	19.46	19.47	19.48	19.49	19.50
3	8.79	8.74	8.70	8.66	8.62	8.59	8.57	8.55	8.53
4	5.96	5.91	5.86	5.80	5.75	5.72	5.69	5.66	5.63
5	4.74	4.68	4.62	4.56	4.50	4.46	4.43	4.40	4.36
6	4.06	4.00	3.94	3.87	3.81	3.77	3.74	3.70	3.67
7	3.64	3.57	3.51	3.44	3.38	3.34	3.30	3.27	3.23
8	3.35	3.28	3.22	3.15	3.08	3.04	3.01	2.97	2.93
9	3.14	3.07	3.01	2.94	2.86	2.83	2.79	2.75	2.71
10	2.98	2.91	2.85	2.77	2.70	2.66	2.62	2.58	2.54
11	2.85	2.79	2.72	2.65	2.57	2.53	2.49	2.45	2.40
12	2.75	2.69	2.62	2.54	2.47	2.43	2.38	2.34	2.30
13	2.67	2.60	2.53	2.46	2.38	2.34	2.30	2.25	2.21
14	2.60	2.53	2.46	2.39	2.31	2.27	2.22	2.18	2.13
15	2.54	2.48	2.40	2.33	2.25	2.20	2.16	2.11	2.07
16	2.49	2.42	2.35	2.28	2.19	2.15	2.11	2.06	2.01
17	2.45	2.38	2.31	2.23	2.15	2.10	2.06	2.01	1.96
18	2.41	2.34	2.27	2.19	2.11	2.06	2.02	1.97	1.92
19	2.38	2.31	2.23	2.16	2.07	2.03	1.98	1.93	1.88
20	2.35	2.28	2.20	2.12	2.04	1.99	1.95	1.90	1.84
21	2.32	2.25	2.18	2.10	2.01	1.96	1.92	1.87	1.81
22	2.30	2.23	2.15	2.07	1.98	1.94	1.89	1.84	1.78
23	2.27	2.20	2.13	2.05	1.96	1.91	1.86	1.81	1.76
24	2.25	2.18	2.11	2.03	1.94	1.89	1.84	1.79	1.73
30	2.16	2.09	2.01	1.93	1.84	1.79	1.74	1.68	1.62
40	2.08	2.00	1.92	1.84	1.74	1.69	1.64	1.58	1.51
60	1.99	1.92	1.84	1.75	1.65	1.59	1.53	1.47	1.39
120	1.91	1.83	1.75	1.66	1.55	1.50	1.43	1.35	1.25
∞	1.83	1.75	1.67	1.57	1.46	1.39	1.32	1.22	1.00

F-Distribution

Degrees of
Freedom for the
Denominator,
v_2

Degrees of Freedom for the Numerator, v_1

	1	2	3	4	5	6	7	8	9
1	4052	4999.5	5403	5625	5764	5859	5928	5981	6022
2	98.50	99.00	99.17	99.25	99.30	99.33	99.36	99.37	99.39
3	34.12	30.82	29.46	28.71	28.24	27.91	27.67	27.49	27.35
4	21.20	18.00	16.69	15.98	15.52	15.21	14.98	14.80	14.66
5	16.26	13.27	12.06	11.39	10.97	10.67	10.46	10.29	10.16
6	13.75	10.92	9.78	9.15	8.75	8.47	8.26	8.10	7.98
7	12.25	9.55	8.45	7.85	7.46	7.19	6.99	6.84	6.72
8	11.26	8.65	7.59	7.01	6.63	6.37	6.18	6.03	5.91
9	10.56	8.02	6.99	6.42	6.06	5.80	5.61	5.47	5.35
10	10.04	7.56	6.55	5.99	5.64	5.39	5.20	5.06	4.94
11	9.65	7.21	6.22	5.67	5.32	5.07	4.89	4.74	4.63
12	9.33	6.93	5.95	5.41	5.06	4.82	4.64	4.50	4.39
13	9.07	6.70	5.74	5.21	4.86	4.62	4.44	4.30	4.19
14	8.86	6.51	5.56	5.04	4.69	4.46	4.28	4.14	4.03
15	8.68	6.36	5.42	4.89	4.56	4.32	4.14	4.00	3.89
16	8.53	6.23	5.29	4.77	4.44	4.20	4.03	3.89	3.78
17	8.40	6.11	5.18	4.67	4.34	4.10	3.93	3.79	3.68
18	8.29	6.01	5.09	4.58	4.25	4.01	3.84	3.71	3.60
19	8.18	5.93	5.01	4.50	4.17	3.94	3.77	3.63	3.52
20	8.10	5.85	4.94	4.43	4.10	3.87	3.70	3.56	3.46
21	8.02	5.78	4.87	4.37	4.04	3.81	3.64	3.51	3.40
22	7.95	5.72	4.82	4.31	3.99	3.76	3.59	3.45	3.35
23	7.88	5.66	4.76	4.26	3.94	3.71	3.54	3.41	3.30
24	7.82	5.61	4.72	4.22	3.90	3.67	3.50	3.36	3.26
30	7.56	5.39	4.51	4.02	3.70	3.47	3.30	3.17	3.07
40	7.31	5.18	4.31	3.83	3.51	3.29	3.12	2.99	2.89
60	7.08	4.98	4.13	3.65	3.34	3.12	2.95	2.82	2.72
120	6.85	4.79	3.95	3.48	3.17	2.96	2.79	2.66	2.56
∞	6.63	4.61	3.78	3.32	3.02	2.80	2.64	2.51	2.41

Degrees of Freedom for the Denominator, v_2	Degrees of Freedom for the Numerator, v_1								
	10	12	15	20	30	40	60	120	∞
1	6056	6106	6157	6209	6261	6287	6313	6339	6366
2	99.40	99.42	99.43	99.45	99.47	99.47	99.48	99.49	99.50
3	27.23	27.05	26.87	26.69	26.50	26.41	26.32	26.22	26.13
4	14.55	14.37	14.20	14.02	13.84	13.75	13.65	13.56	13.46
5	10.05	9.89	9.72	9.55	9.38	9.29	9.20	9.11	9.02
6	7.87	7.72	7.56	7.40	7.23	7.14	7.06	6.97	6.88
7	6.62	6.47	6.31	6.16	5.99	5.91	5.82	5.74	5.65
8	5.81	5.67	5.52	5.36	5.20	5.12	5.03	4.95	4.86
9	5.26	5.11	4.96	4.81	4.65	4.57	4.48	4.40	4.31
10	4.85	4.71	4.56	4.41	4.25	4.17	4.08	4.00	3.91
11	4.54	4.40	4.25	4.10	3.94	3.86	3.78	3.69	3.60
12	4.30	4.16	4.01	3.86	3.70	3.62	3.54	3.45	3.36
13	4.10	3.96	3.82	3.66	3.51	3.43	3.34	3.25	3.17
14	3.94	3.80	3.66	3.51	3.35	3.27	3.18	3.09	3.00
15	3.80	3.67	3.52	3.37	3.21	3.13	3.05	2.96	2.87
16	3.69	3.55	3.41	3.26	3.10	3.02	2.93	2.84	2.75
17	3.59	3.46	3.31	3.16	3.00	2.92	2.83	2.75	2.65
18	3.51	3.37	3.23	3.08	2.92	2.84	2.75	2.66	2.57
19	3.43	3.30	3.15	3.00	2.84	2.76	2.67	2.58	2.49
20	3.37	3.23	3.09	2.94	2.78	2.69	2.61	2.52	2.42
21	3.31	3.17	3.03	2.88	2.72	2.64	2.55	2.46	2.36
22	3.26	3.12	2.98	2.83	2.67	2.58	2.50	2.40	2.31
23	3.21	3.07	2.93	2.78	2.62	2.54	2.45	2.35	2.26
24	3.17	3.03	2.89	2.74	2.58	2.49	2.40	2.31	2.21
30	2.98	2.84	2.70	2.55	2.39	2.30	2.21	2.11	2.01
40	2.80	2.66	2.52	2.37	2.20	2.11	2.02	1.92	1.80
60	2.63	2.50	2.35	2.20	2.03	1.94	1.84	1.73	1.60
120	2.47	2.34	2.19	2.03	1.86	1.76	1.66	1.53	1.38
∞	2.32	2.18	2.04	1.88	1.70	1.59	1.47	1.32	1.00

Values of the Studentized Range *(q)*

(p = .05) df for Denominator	Number of Groups (k)								
	2	3	4	5	6	7	8	9	10
1	18.0	27.0	32.8	37.1	40.4	43.1	45.4	47.4	49.1
2	6.09	8.3	9.8	10.9	11.7	12.4	13.0	13.5	14.0
3	4.50	5.91	6.82	7.50	8.04	8.48	8.85	9.18	9.46
4	3.93	5.04	5.76	6.29	6.71	7.05	7.35	7.60	7.83
5	3.64	4.60	5.22	5.67	6.03	6.33	6.58	6.80	6.99
6	3.46	4.34	4.90	5.31	5.63	5.89	6.12	6.32	6.49
7	3.34	4.16	4.68	5.06	5.36	5.61	5.82	6.00	6.16
8	3.26	4.04	4.53	4.89	5.17	5.40	5.60	5.77	5.92
9	3.20	3.95	4.42	4.76	5.02	5.24	5.43	5.60	5.74
10	3.15	3.88	4.33	4.65	4.91	5.12	5.30	5.46	5.60
11	3.11	3.82	4.26	4.57	4.82	5.03	5.20	5.35	5.49
12	3.08	3.77	4.20	4.51	4.75	4.95	5.12	5.27	5.40
13	3.06	3.73	4.15	4.45	4.69	4.88	5.05	5.19	5.32
14	3.03	3.70	4.11	4.41	4.64	4.83	4.99	5.13	5.25
15	3.01	3.67	4.08	4.37	4.60	4.78	4.94	5.08	5.20
16	3.00	3.65	4.05	4.33	4.56	4.74	4.90	5.03	5.15
17	2.98	3.63	4.02	4.30	4.52	4.71	4.86	4.99	5.11
18	2.97	3.61	4.00	4.29	4.49	4.67	4.82	4.96	5.07
19	2.96	3.59	3.98	4.25	4.47	4.65	4.79	4.92	5.04
20	2.95	3.58	3.96	4.23	4.45	4.62	4.77	4.90	5.01
24	2.92	3.53	3.90	4.17	4.37	4.54	4.68	4.81	4.92
30	2.89	3.49	3.84	4.10	4.30	4.46	4.60	4.72	4.83
40	2.86	3.44	3.79	4.04	4.23	4.39	4.54	4.63	4.74
60	2.83	3.40	3.74	3.98	4.16	4.31	4.44	4.55	4.65
120	2.80	3.36	3.69	3.92	4.10	4.24	4.36	4.48	4.56
∞	2.77	3.31	3.63	3.86	4.03	4.17	4.29	4.39	4.47

Adapted from Table 29 of E. S. Pearson and H. O. Hartley, eds., *Biometrika Tables for Statisticians,* vol. 1 (3d ed.), Cambridge University Press for the Biometrika Trustees, 1966. Used with the permission of Biometrika Trustees.

(p = .01) df for Denominator	Number of Groups (k)								
	2	3	4	5	6	7	8	9	10
1	90.0	135	164	186	202	216	227	237	246
2	14.0	19.0	22.3	24.7	26.6	28.2	29.5	30.7	31.7
3	8.26	10.6	12.2	13.3	14.2	15.0	15.6	16.2	16.7
4	6.51	8.12	9.17	9.96	10.6	11.1	11.5	11.9	12.3
5	5.70	6.97	7.80	8.42	8.91	9.32	9.67	9.97	10.2
6	5.24	6.33	7.03	7.56	7.97	8.32	8.61	8.87	9.10
7	4.95	5.92	6.54	7.01	7.37	7.68	7.94	8.17	8.37
8	4.74	5.63	6.20	6.63	6.96	7.24	7.47	7.68	7.87
9	4.60	5.43	5.96	6.35	6.66	6.91	7.13	7.32	7.49
10	4.48	5.27	5.77	6.14	6.43	6.67	6.87	7.05	7.21
11	4.39	5.14	5.62	5.97	6.25	6.48	6.67	6.84	6.99
12	4.32	5.04	5.50	5.84	6.10	6.32	6.51	6.67	6.81
13	4.26	4.96	5.40	5.73	5.98	6.19	6.37	6.53	6.67
14	4.21	4.89	5.32	5.63	5.88	6.08	6.26	6.41	6.54
15	4.17	4.83	5.25	5.56	5.80	5.99	6.16	6.31	6.44
16	4.13	4.78	5.19	5.49	5.72	5.92	6.08	6.22	6.35
17	4.10	4.74	5.14	5.43	5.66	5.85	6.01	6.15	6.27
18	4.07	4.70	5.09	5.38	5.60	5.79	5.94	6.08	6.20
19	4.05	4.67	5.05	5.33	5.55	5.73	5.89	6.02	6.14
20	4.02	4.64	5.02	5.29	5.51	5.69	5.84	5.97	6.09
24	3.96	4.54	4.91	5.17	5.37	5.54	5.69	5.81	5.92
30	3.89	4.45	4.80	5.05	5.24	5.40	5.54	5.65	5.76
40	3.82	4.37	4.70	4.93	5.11	5.27	5.39	5.50	5.60
60	3.76	4.28	4.60	4.82	4.99	5.13	5.25	5.36	5.45
120	3.70	4.20	4.50	4.71	4.87	5.01	5.12	5.21	5.30
∞	3.64	4.12	4.40	4.60	4.76	4.88	4.99	5.08	5.16

References and Additional Reading

AAHPER. 1965. *Football: Skills test manual.* Washington, D.C.: American Association for Health, Physical Education and Recreation.

———. 1967. *Archery for boys and girls: Skills test manual.* Washington, D.C.: American Association for Health, Physical Education and Recreation.

AAHPERD. 1976a. *AAHPERD youth fitness test manual.* Reston, Va.: American Alliance for Health, Physical Education, Recreation and Dance.

———. 1976b. *Special fitness test manual for mildly mentally retarded persons.* Reston, Va.: American Alliance for Health, Physical Education, Recreation and Dance.

———. 1980a. *AAHPERD health related physical fitness test manual.* Reston, Va.: American Alliance for Health, Physical Education, Recreation and Dance.

———. 1980b. *Testing for impaired, disabled and handicapped individuals.* Reston, Va.: American Alliance for Health, Physical Education, Recreation and Dance.

———. 1984. *Technical manual for health related physical fitness.* Reston, Va.: American Alliance for Health, Physical Education, Recreation and Dance.

———. 1988. *Physical best.* Reston, Va.: American Alliance for Health, Physical Education, Recreation and Dance.

———. 1989. *Tennis skills test manual.* Reston, Va.: American Alliance for Health, Physical Education, Recreation and Dance.

———. 1991. *Softball skills test manual.* Reston, Va.: American Alliance for Health, Physical Education, Recreation and Dance.

Adams, R. S. 1963. Two scales for measuring attitude toward physical education. *Research Quarterly* 34: 91–94.

Ahmann, J. S., and Glock, M. D. 1958. *Evaluating pupil growth.* Boston: Allyn & Bacon.

Althoff, S. A., Heyden, S. M., and Robertson, L. D. 1988a. Back to the basics—Whatever happened to posture? *Journal of Physical Education, Recreation and Dance* 59(7): 20–24.

———. 1988b. Posture screening—A program that works. *Journal of Physical Education, Recreation and Dance* 58(8): 26–32.

Amateur Athletic Union. 1994. *AAU physical fitness program.* Bloomington, Ind.: Amateur Athletic Union.

American College of Sports Medicine. 1998. *ACSM fitness book.* 2d ed. Champaign, Ill.: Human Kinetics 7.

American College of Sports Medicine. 1998. Position stand: Exercise and physical activity for older adults. *Medicine and Science in Sports and Exercise* 30: 992–1008.

American Health and Fitness Foundation. 1986. *FTY program manual.* Austin, Tex.: American Health and Fitness Foundation.

Arnheim, D. D., and Sinclair, W. A. 1979. *The clumsy child: A program of motor therapy.* 2d ed. St. Louis: C. V. Mosby.

———. 1985. *Physical education for special populations: A developmental, adapted, and remedial approach.* Englewood Cliffs, N.J.: Prentice-Hall.

Barrow, H. M. 1954. Tests of motor ability for college men. *Research Quarterly* 25: 253–260.

Barrow, H. M., and McGee, R. 1979. *A practical approach to measurement in physical education.* 3d ed. Philadelphia: Lea & Fabiger.

Bartlett, J., et al. 1991. Development of a valid volleyball skills test battery. *Journal of Physical Education, Recreation and Dance* 62(2): 19–21.

Bass, R. I. 1939. An analysis of the components of tests of semi-circular canal function and of static and dynamic balance. *Research Quarterly* 10: 33–52.

Baumgartner, T. A., and Jackson, A. S. 1982. *Measurement for evaluation in physical education.* 2d ed. Dubuque, Iowa: Wm. C. Brown.

Baumgartner, T. A., and Wood, S. S. 1984. Development of shoulder-girdle strength endurance in elementary children. *Research Quarterly for Exercise and Sport* 55: 169–171.

Baumgartner, T. A., et al. 1984. Equipment improvements and additional norms for the modified pull-ups test. *Research Quarterly for Exercise and Sport* 55: 64–68.

Bennett, C. L. 1956. Relative contributions of modern dance, folk dance, basketball, and swimming to motor abilities of college women. *Research Quarterly* 27: 253–257.

Blanchard, B. E. 1936. A behavior frequency rating scale for the measurement of character and personality traits in a physical education classroom situation. *Research Quarterly* 7: 56–66.

Bloom, S. B., Madaus, G. F., and Hastings, J. T. 1981. *Evaluation to improve learning.* New York: McGraw-Hill.

Body composition (a roundtable). 1986. *The Physician and Sportsmedicine* 14(3): 144–152, 157, 161, 162.

Bonci, C. M., Hensel, F. J., and Torg, J. S. 1986. A preliminary study on the measurements of static and dynamic motion at the glenohumeral joint. *The American Journal of Sports Medicine* 14: 12–17.

Borg, G. A. V. 1973. Perceived exertion: A note on "history" and methods. *Medicine and Science in Sports* 5: 90–93.

———. 1982. Psychophysical bases of perceived exertion. *Medicine and Science in Sports* 14: 377–381.

Bosco, J. S., and Gustafson, W. F. 1983. *Measurement and evaluation in physical education, fitness, and sports.* Englewood Cliffs, N.J.: Prentice-Hall.

Bowerman, W. J., and Harris, W. D. 1967. *Jogging.* New York: Grosset & Dunlap.

Brady, G. F. 1945. Preliminary investigations of volleyball playing ability. *Research Quarterly* 16: 14–17.

Broer, M. R. 1973. *Efficiency of human movement.* 3d ed. Philadelphia: W. B. Saunders.

Brouha, L. 1943. The step test: A simple method of measuring physical fitness for muscular work in young men. *Research Quarterly* 14: 31–36.

Brouha, L., and Ball, M. V. 1952. *Canadian Red Cross Society's meal study.* Toronto: University of Toronto Press.

Brown, F. G. 1983. *Principles of educational and psychological testing.* 3d ed. New York: Holt, Rinehart & Winston.

Brumbach, W. B. 1967. *Beginning volleyball, a syllabus for teachers.* Revised ed. Eugene, Oreg.: W. B. Brumbach. In Collins, D. R., and Hodges, P. B. 1978. *A comprehensive guide to sports skills tests and measurement.* Springfield, Ill.: Charles C Thomas.

Bucher, C. A., and Prentice, W. E. 1985. *Fitness for college and life.* St. Louis: Times Mirror/Mosby.

Buell, C. E. 1982. *Physical education and recreation for the visually handicapped.* Reston, Va.: American Alliance for Health, Physical Education, Recreation and Dance.

Bunn, J. W. 1955. *Scientific principles of coaching.* Englewood Cliffs, N.J.: Prentice-Hall.

Burton, B. T., and Foster, M. D. 1985. Health implications of obesity: An NIH consensus development conference. *Journal of the American Dietetic Association* 85: 1117–1121.

Canadian Society for Exercise Physiology. 1998. *The Canadian physical activity, fitness & lifestyle appraisal (CPAFLA): CSEP's plan for healthy active living.* 2d ed. Ottawa, Canada: Canadian Society for Exercise Physiology.

Chapman, N. L. 1982. Chapman ball control test—Field hockey. *Research Quarterly for Exercise and Sport* 53: 239–242.

Chase, C. I. 1978. *Measurement for educational evaluation.* 2d ed. Reading, Mass.: Addison-Wesley.

Cirn, J. T. 1986. True/false versus short answer questions. *College Teaching* 34(4): 34–37.

Clark, H. H., ed. 1975. Exercise and fat reduction. *Physical fitness research digest.* Washington, D.C.: President's Council on Physical Fitness, Series 5, April.

———. 1979. Posture. *Physical fitness research digest.* Washington, D.C.: President's Council on Physical Fitness and Sports, Series 9, January.

Clark, H. H., and Clark, D. H. 1987. *Application of measurement to physical education.* 6th ed. Englewood Cliffs, N.J.: Prentice-Hall.

Claxton, D., and Faribault, J. 1988. *Tennis.* Scottsdale, Ariz.: Gorsuch, Scarisbrick.

Clevett, M. A. 1931. An experiment in teaching methods of golf. *Research Quarterly* 2: 104–112.

Coleman, R., et al. 1987. Validation of 1-mile walk test for estimating VO_2 max in 20–29 year olds. *Medicine and Science in Sports and Exercise* 19 (Suppl. 2): S29.

Collins, D. R., and Hodges, P. B. 1978. *A comprehensive guide to sports skills tests and measurement.* Springfield, Ill.: Charles C Thomas.

Cooper, K. H. 1982. *The aerobics program for total well-being.* New York: M. Evans & Company.

Cooper Institute for Aerobics Research. 1999. *FITNESSGRAM Test Administration Manual.* 2d ed. Champaign, Ill.: Human Kinetics.

Corbin, C. B. 1987. Physical fitness in the K–12 curriculum: Some defensible solutions to perennial problems. *Journal of Physical Education, Recreation and Dance* 58(7): 49–54.

Corbin, C. B., and Lindsey, R. 1985. *Concepts of physical fitness.* 5th ed. Dubuque, Iowa: Wm. C. Brown.

Corbin, C. B., and Noble, L. 1980. Flexibility: A major component of physical fitness. *Journal of Physical Education and Recreation* 51(6): 23–24, 57–60.

Cornelius, W. L., and Hinon, M. M. 1980. The relationship between isometric contractions of hip extensors and subsequent flexibility in males. *The Journal of Sports Medicine and Physical Fitness* 20: 75–80.

Cowell, C. C. 1958. Validating an index of social adjustment for high school use. *Research Quarterly* 29: 7–10.

Cratty, B. J. 1975. *Remedial motor activity for children.* Philadelphia: Lea & Febiger.

Cureton, K. J., and Warren, G. L. 1990. Criterion-referenced standards for youth health-related fitness tests: A tutorial. *Research Quarterly for Exercise and Sport* 61: 7–19.

Custer, S. J., and Chaloupka, V. A. 1977. Relationship between predicted maximal oxygen consumption and running performance of college females. *Research Quarterly* 48: 47–50.

Darling-Hammond, L. 1994. Setting standards for students: The case for authentic assessment. *The Educational Forum* 59 (Fall): 14–20.

DiPietro, L. 1996. The epidemiology of physical activity and physical function in older people. *Medicine and Science in Sports and Exercise* 28: 596–600.

Dishman, R. K., and Ickes, W. 1981. Self-motivation and adherence to therapeutic exercise. *Journal of Behavioral Medicine* 4: 421–438.

Doolittle, T. L., and Bigbee, R. 1968. The twelve-minute run-walk: A test of cardiorespiratory fitness of adolescent boys. *Research Quarterly* 39: 491–495.

Dotson, C. 1988. Health fitness standards: Aerobic endurance. *Journal of Physical Education, Recreation and Dance* 59(7): 26–31.

Dotson, C. O., and Kirkendall, D. R. 1974. *Statistics for physical education, health, and recreation.* New York: Harper & Row.

Downie, N. M., and Heath, R. W. 1974. *Basic statistical methods.* 4th ed. New York: Harper & Row.

Dunn, J. M., Morehouse, J. W., and Fredericks, H. D. 1986. *Physical education for the severely handicapped: A systematic approach to a data based gymnasium.* Austin, Tex.: Pro-Ed.

Ebel, R. L. 1979. *Essentials of educational measurement.* 3d ed. Englewood Cliffs, N.J.: Prentice Hall.

Edgren, H. 1932. An experiment in the testing of ability and progress in basketball. *Research Quarterly* 3: 159–171.

Fait, H. F., and Dunn, J. M. 1984. *Special physical education: Adapted, individualized, and developmental.* 5th ed. Philadelphia: Saunders College Publishing.

Franks, B. D., and Deutsch, H. 1973. *Evaluating performance in physical education.* New York: Academic.

Franks, B. D., Morrow, J. R., and Plowman, S. A. 1988. Youth fitness testing: Validation, planning, and politics. *Quest* 40: 197–199.

French, R. W., and Jansma, P. 1982. *Special physical education.* Columbus: Charles E. Merrill.

Fringer, M. N. 1961. A battery of softball skill tests for senior high school girls. Master's thesis, University of Oregon, Eugene, Oregon. In Collins, D. R., and Hodges, P. B.

1978. *A comprehensive guide to sports skills tests and measurement.* Springfield, Ill.: Charles C Thomas.

Fry, P. F. 1983. Measurement of psychosocial aspects of physical education. *Journal of Physical Education, Recreation and Dance* 54(8): 26–27.

Gabbard, C., et al. 1983. Effects of grip and forearm position on flexed-arm hang performance. *Research Quarterly for Exercise and Sport* 54: 198–199.

Gallagher, J. R., and Brouha, L. 1943. A simple method for testing the physical fitness of boys. *Research Quarterly* 14(1): 24–30.

Gates, D. P., and Sheffield, R. P. 1940. Tests of change of direction as measurement of different kinds of motor ability in boys of 7th, 8th, and 9th grades. *Research Quarterly* 11: 136–147.

Going, S., and Williams, D. 1989. Understanding fitness standards. *Journal of Physical Education, Recreation and Dance* 60(6): 34–38.

Golding, L. A., Myers, C. R., and Sinning, W. E., eds. 1989. *The Y's way to physical fitness.* 3d ed. Chicago, Ill.: Human Kinetics.

Gould, D. 1985. *Tennis, anyone?* 4th ed. Palo Alto, Calif.: Mayfield.

Grady, J. B. 1994. Authentic assessment and tasks: Helping students demonstrate their abilities. *NASSP Bulletin* 78(566): 92–98.

Green, J. A. 1975. *Teacher-made tests.* 2d ed. New York: Harper & Row.

Griffin, P. S. 1982. Second thoughts on affective evaluation. In Wiese, C. E. (ed.). Doing well and feeling good. *Journal of Physical Education, Recreation and Dance* 53(2): 15–25, 86.

Guralnik, J. M., et al. 1989. Physical performance measures in aging research. *Journal of Gerontology* 44: M141–146.

Harris, M. L. 1969. A factor analysis study of flexibility. *Research Quarterly* 40: 62–70.

Hensley, L. D., East, W. B., and Stillwell, J. L. 1979. A racquetball skills test. *Research Quarterly* 50: 114–118.

Hensley, L. D., Morrow, J. R., and East, W. B. 1990. Practical measurement to solve practical problems. *Journal of Physical Education, Recreation and Dance* 6(3): 42–44.

Hewitt, J. E. 1965. Revision of the Dyer backboard tennis test. *Research Quarterly* 36: 153–157.

———. 1966. Hewitt's tennis achievement test. *Research Quarterly* 37: 231–237.

Hodgkins, J., and Skubic, V. 1963. Cardiovascular efficiency test scores for college women in the United States. *Research Quarterly* 34: 454–461.

Holt, L. E., Travis, T. M., and Okita, T. 1970. A comparative study of three stretching techniques. *Perceptual and Motor Skills* 31: 611–616.

Hopkins, D. R., Shick, J., and Plack, J. J. 1984. *Basketball for boys and girls: Skills test manual.* Reston, Va.: American Alliance for Health, Physical Education, Recreation and Dance.

Humphrey, L. D. 1981. Flexibility. *Journal of Physical Education, Recreation and Dance* 52(7): 41–43.

Jackson, A., et al. 1982. Baumgartner's modified pull-up test for male and female elementary school aged children. *Research Quarterly for Exercise and Sport* 53: 163–164.

Jackson, A. S., and Coleman, E. 1976. Validation of distance run tests for elementary school children. *Research Quarterly* 47: 86–94.

Jackson, A. S., and Pollock, M. L. 1985. Practical assessment of body composition. *The Physician and Sportsmedicine* 13(5): 76–90.

Jackson, A. S., et al. 1995. Changes in aerobic power of men, ages 25–70 years. *Medicine and Science in Sports and Exercise* 27: 113–120.

Jansma, P., ed. 1988. *The psychomotor domain and the seriously handicapped.* 3d ed. Lanham, Md.: University Press of America.

Jensen, C. R., and Hirst, C. C. 1980. *Measurement in physical education and athletics.* New York: Macmillan.

Jensen, C. R., Schultz, G. W., and Bangerter, B. L. 1983. *Applied kinesiology and biomechanics.* 3d ed. New York: McGraw-Hill.

Jequier, E. 1987. Energy, obesity, and body weight standards. *American Journal of Clinical Nutrition* 45: 1035–1047.

Johnson, B. L., and Nelson, J. K. 1986. *Practical measurements for evaluation in physical education.* 4th ed. Edina, Minn.: Burgess.

Johnson, L., and Londeree, B. 1976. *Motor fitness testing manual for the moderately mentally retarded.* Reston, Va.: American Alliance for Health, Physical Education, Recreation and Dance.

Johnson, M. L. 1969. Construction of sportsmanship attitude scales. *Research Quarterly* 40: 312–316.

Johnson, P. B., et al. 1975. *Sport, exercise and you.* New York: Holt, Rinehart & Winston.

Johnson, R., and Christian, V. 1982. *Laboratory experiences in measurement and evaluation: Theory to application.* Boone, N.C.: Appalachian State University.

Johnson, R. E., and Lavay, B. 1988. *Kansas adapted/special physical education test manual.* Topeka, Kans.: Kansas State Department of Education.

Kalakian, L. H., and Eichstaedt, C. B. 1982. *Developmental/adapted physical education: Making ability count.* Minn.: Burgess.

Katch, F. I., and McArdle, W. D. 1977. *Nutrition, weight control, and exercise.* Boston: Houghton Mifflin.

Kenyon, G. S. 1968a. A conceptual model for characterizing physical activity. *Research Quarterly* 39: 96–105.

———. 1968b. Six scales for assessing attitude toward physical activity. *Research Quarterly* 39: 566–574.

Kirby, R. F. 1971. A simple test of agility. *Coach and Athlete* (June): 30–31.

Kirkendall, D. R., Gruber, J. J., and Johnson, R. E. 1980. *Measurement and evaluation for physical educators.* Dubuque, Iowa: Wm. C. Brown.

Kline, G., et al. 1987. Estimation of VO_2 max from a one-mile track walk, gender, age, and body weight. *Medicine and Science in Sports and Exercise* 19: 253–259.

Kryspin, W. J., and Feldusen, J. F. 1974. *Developing classroom tests: A guide for writing and evaluating test items.* Edina, Minn.: Burgess.

Lafuze, M. 1951. A study of the learning of fundamental skills by college freshman women of low motor ability. *Research Quarterly* 22: 149–157.

Lakie, W. L. 1964. Expressed attitudes of various groups of athletes toward athletic competition. *Research Quarterly* 35: 497–503.

Logan, G. A., and McKinney, W. C. 1982. *Anatomic kinesiology.* 3d ed. Dubuque, Iowa: Wm. C. Brown.

Lohman, G. A. 1982. Measurement of body composition in children. *Journal of Physical Education, Recreation and Dance* 53(8): 67–70.

Lohman, G. A., and Pollock, M. L. 1981. Which caliper? How much training? *Journal of Physical Education, Recreation and Dance* 52(1): 27–29.

Lohman, T. G. 1982. Body composition methodology in sports medicine. *The Physician and Sports Medicine* 10(12): 46–58.

Lund, J. 1992. Assessment and accountability in secondary physical education. *Quest* 44: 352–360.

Luttgens, K., and Wells, K. F. 1982. *Kinesiology: Scientific basis of human motion.* 7th ed. Philadelphia: Saunders College Publishing.

Lyman, H. B. 1963. *Test scores and what they mean.* Englewood Cliffs, N.J.: Prentice-Hall.

Magid, L. J. 1996. *The little PC book.* 2d ed. Berkeley, Calif.: Peachpit.

Manitoba Education and Training. 1989. *Manitoba schools fitness.* Winnipeg, Manitoba: Manitoba Education and Training.

Marsh, J. J. 1984. Measuring affective objectives in physical education. *Physical Educator* 41(2): 77–81.

Martens, R. 1977. *Sport competition anxiety test.* Champaign, Ill.: Human Kinetics.

Martens, R., Vealey, R. S., and Burton, D. 1990. *Competitive anxiety in sport.* Champaign, Ill.: Human Kinetics.

Masley, J. W., Hairabedian, A., and Donaldson, D. N. 1953. Weight training in relation to strength, speed, and coordination. *Research Quarterly* 24: 308–315.

Masters, L. F., Mori, A. A., and Lange, E. K. 1983. *Adapted physical education: A practitioner's guide.* Rockville, Md.: Aspen Publication.

Mattson, D. E. 1981. *Statistics: Difficult concepts, understandable explanations.* St. Louis: C. V. Mosby.

McArdle, W. D., et al. 1972. Reliability and interrelationships between maximal oxygen intake, physical work capacity, and step test scores in college women. *Medicine and Science in Sports* 4: 182–186.

McClenaghan, B. A., and Gallahue, D. L. 1978. *Fundamental movement: A developmental and remedial approach.* Philadelphia: W. B. Saunders.

McCloy, C. H., and Young, N. D. 1954. *Tests and measurements in health and physical education.* 3d ed. New York: Appleton-Century-Crofts.

McDonald, L. G. 1951. The construction of a kicking test as an index of general soccer ability. Master's thesis, Springfield College, Springfield, Mass. In Collins, D. R., and Hodges, P. B. 1978. *A comprehensive guide to sports skills tests and measurement.* Springfield, Ill.: Charles C Thomas.

McGee, R. 1982. Uses and abuses of affective measurement. In Wiese, C. E. (ed.). Doing well and feeling good. *Journal of Physical Education, Recreation and Dance* 53(2): 15–25, 86.

McKeachie, W. J. 1969. *Teaching tips: A guidebook for the beginning college teacher.* Lexington, Mass.: D. C. Heath.

Melograno, V. J. 1994. Portfolio assessment: Documenting authentic student learning. *Journal of Physical Education, Recreation and Dance* 65(8): 50–55, 58–61.

Metheny, E. 1982. *Body mechanics.* New York: McGraw-Hill.

Metropolitan Life Insurance Company. 1983. *1983 height and weight tables announced.* New York: Metropolitan Life Insurance Company.

Miller, A. G., and Sullivan, J. V. 1982. *Teaching physical activities to impaired youth: An approach to mainstreaming.* New York: John Wiley & Sons.

Miller, D. K. 1970. A comparison of the effects of individual and team sports programs on the motor ability of male college freshmen. Unpublished doctoral dissertation, Florida State University.

———. 1983. *The well being–good health handbook.* New York: Leisure.

Miller, D. K., and Allen, T. E. 1990. *Fitness: A lifetime commitment.* 4th ed. New York: Macmillan.

Mitchell, J. R. 1963. The modification of the McDonald skill test for upper elementary school boys. Master's thesis, University of Oregon, Eugene, Oregon. In Collins, D. R., and Hodges, P. B. 1978. *A comprehensive guide to sports skills tests and measurement.* Springfield, Ill.: Charles C Thomas.

Mood, D. P. 1980. *Numbers in motion: A balanced approach to measurement and evaluation in physical education.* Palo Alto, Calif.: Mayfield.

———. 1982. Evaluation in the affective domain? No! In Wiese, C. E. (ed.). Doing well and feeling good. *Journal of Physical Education, Recreation and Dance* 53(2): 15–25, 86.

Moore, M. 1983. New height-weight tables gain pounds, lose status. *The Physician and Sportsmedicine* 11(5): 25.

Morehouse, C. A., and Stull, G. A. 1975. *Statistical principles and procedures with applications for physical education.* Philadelphia: Lea & Febiger.

Nelson, D. O. 1966. Leadership in sports. *Research Quarterly* 37: 268–275.

Nichols, D. B., Arsenault, D. R., and Giuffre, D. L. 1980. *Motor activities for the underachiever.* Springfield, Ill.: Charles C Thomas.

North Carolina Department of Public Instruction. 1977. *North Carolina motor fitness battery.* Raleigh, N.C.: North Carolina Department of Public Instruction.

Osness, W. H., et al. 1996. *Functional Fitness Assessment for Adults Over 60 Years.* 2d ed. Dubuque, Iowa: Kendall/Hunt Publishing.

Pate, R. R., ed. 1983. *South Carolina physical fitness test manual.* 2d ed. Columbia, S.C.: South Carolina Association for Health, Physical Education, Recreation and Dance.

Pate, R. R. 1985. *Norms for college students: Health related physical fitness test.* Reston, Va.: American Alliance for Health, Physical Education, Recreation, and Dance.

———. 1995. Physical activity and public health. *Journal of the American Medical Association* 273: 402–407.

Pate, R. R., et al. 1987. The modified pull-up. *Journal of Physical Education, Recreation, and Dance* 58(10): 71–73.

Petray, C., et al. 1989. Designing the fitness testing environment. *Journal of Physical Education, Recreation and Dance* 60(1): 35–38.

Phillips, D. A., and Hornak, J. E. 1979. *Measurement and evaluation in physical education.* New York: John Wiley & Sons.

Physical fitness–motor ability test. 1973. Austin, Tex.: Texas Governor's Commission on Physical Fitness.

Piscopo, J., and Baley, J. A. 1981. *Kinesiology: The science of movement.* New York: John Wiley & Sons.

Pollock, M. L., Wilmore, J. H., and Fox, S. M. 1978. *Health and fitness through physical activity.* New York: John Wiley & Sons.

Poole, J., and Nelson, J. K. 1970. Construction of a badminton skills test battery. Unpublished study. In Johnson, B. L., and Nelson, J. K. 1986. *Practical measurements for evaluation in physical education.* 4th ed. Edina, Minn.: Burgess.

President's Council on Physical Fitness and Sports. 1986. *Presidential physical fitness award program.* Washington, D.C.: President's Council on Physical Fitness and Sports.

———. 1998. Physical activity and aging: Implications for health and quality of life in older persons. *Research Digest,* Series 3, no. 4 (December).

———. 1999. Physical activity and fitness for persons with disabilities. *Research Digest,* Series 3, no. 5 (March).

———. 1999. Physical activity promotion and school physical education. *Research Digest,* Series 3, no. 7 (September)..

———. 1999. *The president's challenge physical fitness program.* Washington, D.C.: President's Council on Physical Fitness and Sports.

Radford, K. W., Schincariol, L., and Hughes, A. S. 1995. Enhance performance through assessment. *Strategies* 8(6): 5–9.

Rarick, G. L., Widdop, J. H., and Broadhead, G. D. 1970. The physical fitness and motor performance of educable mentally retarded children. *Exceptional Children* 36: 509–519.

Rikli, R. E., and Jones, C. J. 1997. Assessing physical performance in independent older adults: Issues and guidelines. *Journal of Aging and Physical Activity* 5: 244–261.

———. 1999a. Development and validation of a functional fitness test for community-residing older adults. *Journal of Aging and Physical Activity* 7: 129–161.

———. 1999b. Functional fitness normative scores for community-residing older adults, ages 60–94. *Journal of Aging and Physical Activity* 7: 162–182.

Rippe, J. M. 1991. *One mile walk test.* Marlboro, Mass.: Rockport.

Roach, E. G., and Kephart, N. C. 1966. *The Purdue perceptual-motor survey.* Columbus, Ohio: Charles E. Merrill.

Robbins, G., Powers, D., and Burgess, S. 1991. *A wellness way of life.* Dubuque, Iowa: Wm. C. Brown.

———. 1994. *A wellness way of life.* 2d ed. Dubuque, Iowa: Brown & Benchmark.

Ross, R. M., and Jackson, A. S. 1990. *Understanding exercise: Concepts, calculations, and computers.* Houston: MacJr/CSI Publishing.

Rothstein, A. L. 1985. *Research design and statistics for physical education.* Englewood Cliffs, N.J.: Prentice-Hall.

Russell, N., and Lange, E. 1940. Achievement tests in volleyball for junior high school girls. *Research Quarterly* 11: 33–41.

Safrit, M. J. 1981. *Evaluation in physical education.* 2d ed. Englewood Cliffs, N.J.: Prentice-Hall.

———. 1986. *Introduction to measurement in physical education and exercise science.* St. Louis: Times Mirror/Mosby College.

Safrit, M. J., and Wood, T. M. 1989. *Measurement concepts in physical education and exercise science.* Champaign, Ill.: Human Kinetics.

Sargent, D. A. 1921. The physical test of a man. *American Physical Education Review* 26(4): 188–194.

Scott, M. G., and French, E. 1959. *Measurement and evaluation in physical education.* Dubuque, Iowa: Wm. C. Brown.

Scott, M. G., et al. 1941. Achievement examination in badminton. *Research Quarterly* 12: 242–253.

Seashore, H. G. 1947. The development of a beam-walking test and its use in measuring development of balance in children. *Research Quarterly* 18: 246–258.

Seils, L. G. 1951. The relationship between measures of physical growth and gross motor performance of primary-grade school children. *Research Quarterly* 22: 244–260.

Sheehan, T. J. 1971. *An introduction to the evaluation of measurement data in physical education.* Reading, Mass.: Addison-Wesley.

Sheldon, W., Stevens, S. S., and Tucker, W. B. 1970. *The varieties of human physique.* Darien, Conn.: Hafner.

Shephard, R. J. 1993. Exercise and aging: Extending independence in older adults. *Geriatrics* 48: 61–64.

Sherrill, C. 1976. *Adapted physical education and recreation.* Dubuque, Iowa: Wm. C. Brown.

Shick, J. 1970. Battery of defensive softball skills tests for college women. *Research Quarterly* 41: 82–87.

Shick, J., and Berg, N. G. 1983. Indoor golf skill test for junior high school boys. *Research Quarterly for Exercise and Sport* 54: 75–78.

Simon, J. A., and Smoll, F. L. 1974. An instrument for assessing children's attitude toward physical activity. *Research Quarterly* 45: 407–415.

Skubic, V., and Hodgkins, J. 1963. Cardiovascular efficiency test scores for girls and women. *Research Quarterly* 34: 191–198.

———. 1964. Cardiovascular efficiency test scores for junior and senior high school girls in the United States. *Research Quarterly* 35: 184–192.

Smith, J. A. 1956. Relation of certain physical traits and abilities to motor learning in elementary school children. *Research Quarterly* 27: 220–228.

Society of Actuaries. 1959. *Build and blood pressure study.* New York: Metropolitan Life Insurance Company.

Society of Actuaries and Association of Life Insurance Medical Directors of America. 1980. *1979 build study.* New York: Metropolitan Life Insurance Company.

Spence, J. T., et al. 1968. *Elementary statistics.* 2d ed. New York: Appleton-Century-Crofts.

Stamford, B. 1986. Somatotypes and sports selection. *The Physician and Sportsmedicine* 14(7): 176.

Sterner, T. G., and Burke, E. J. 1986. Body fat assessment: A comparison of visual estimation and skinfold techniques. *The Physician and Sportsmedicine* 14(4): 101–107.

Stodola, Q., and Stordahl, K. 1967. *Basic educational tests and measurements.* Chicago: Science Research Associates.

Stoner, L. J. 1982. Evaluation in the affective domain? Yes! In Wiese, C. E. (ed.). Doing well and feeling good. *Journal of Physical Education, Recreation and Dance* 53(2): 15–25, 86.

Thomas, J. R., Pierce, C., and Ridsale, S. 1977. Age differences in children's ability to model motor behavior. *Research Quarterly* 48: 592–597.

Torshen, K. P. 1977. *The mastery approach to competency-based education.* New York: Academic.

Tyson, K. W. 1970. A handball skill test for college men. Master's thesis, University of Texas, Austin, Texas. In Collins, D. R., and Hodges, P. B. 1978. *A comprehensive guide to sports skills tests and measurement.* Springfield, Ill.: Charles C Thomas.

Ulrich, D. A. 1986. *Test of gross motor development.* Austin, TX: PRO-ED.

The University of the State of New York. 1966. *New York State physical fitness test.* Albany, N.Y.: The State Education Department.

U.S. Bureau of the Census. 1996. *Sixty-five plus in the United States: Current population reports* (P23-P190). Washington, D.C.: U.S. Department of Commerce.

U.S. Department of Agriculture and U.S. Department of Health and Human Services. 1990. *Nutrition and your health: Dietary guidelines for Americans.* 3d ed. Home Garden Bulletin No. 232. Washington, D.C.: U.S. Government Printing Office.

Vars, G. F. 1983. Missiles, marks, and the middle level student. *NASS Principal's Bulletin* 67(5): 72–77.

Veal, M. L. 1988a. Pupil assessment issues: A teacher educator's perspective. *Quest* 40: 151–161.

———. 1988b. Pupil assessment perceptions and practices of secondary teachers. J*ournal of Teaching Physical Education* 7: 327–342.

———. 1992. The role of assessment in secondary physical education—A pedagogical view. *Journal of Physical Education, Recreation and Dance* 63(7): 88–92.

———. 1995. Assessment as an instructional tool. *Strategies* 8(6): 10–15.

Veal, M. L., and Taylor, M. 1995. A case for teaching about assessment. *Journal of Physical Education, Recreation and Dance* 66(1): 54–59.

Verducci, F. M. 1980. *Measurement concepts in physical education.* St. Louis: C. V. Mosby.

Vincent, W. J. 1976. *Elementary statistics in physical education.* Springfield, Ill.: Charles C Thomas.

———. 1995. *Statistics in kinesiology.* Champaign, Ill.: Human Kinetics.

Wallin, D., et al. 1985. Improvement in muscle flexibility: A comparison between two techniques. *The American Journal of Sports Medicine* 13: 263–268.

Wear, C. L. 1955. Construction of equivalent forms of an attitude scale. *Research Quarterly* 26: 113–119.

Weber, J. C., and Lamb, D. R. 1970. *Statistics and research in physical education.* St. Louis: C. V. Mosby.

Wessel, J. 1961. *Movement fundamentals.* 2d ed. Englewood Cliffs, N.J.: Prentice-Hall.

Wiese, C. E. 1982. Is affective evaluation possible? In Wiese, C. E. (ed.). Doing well and feeling good. *Journal of Physical Education, Recreation and Dance* 53(2): 15–25, 86.

Wiggins, G. 1993. Assessment: Authenticity, context, and validity. *The Delta Kappa* 75(3): 200–208, 210–214.

Williford, N. H. 1986. Evaluation of warm-up for improvement in flexibility. *The American Journal of Sports Medicine* 14: 316–319.

Williford, N. H., and Smith, J. F. 1985. A comparison of proprioceptive neuromuscular facilitation and static stretching techniques. *American Corrective Therapy Journal* 39: 30–33.

Winnick, J. P. 1995. *Adapted physical education and sport.* 2d ed. Champaign, Ill.: Human Kinetics.

Winnick, J. P., and Short, F. X. 1999. *The Brockport Physical Fitness Test Manual.* Champaign, Ill.: Human Kinetics.

Youjie, H., et al. 1998. Physical fitness, physical activity, and functional limitation in adults aged 40 and older. *Medicine and Science in Sports and Exercise* 30: 1430–1435.

INDEX